Nelson Yuan-sheng Kiang

rcvd. 11/81

PHARMACOLOGY *of* HEARING

PHARMACOLOGY *of* HEARING

Experimental and Clinical Bases

Co-Editors

R. DON BROWN, PH.D.

Professor of Pharmacology
Louisiana State University School
of Medicine in Shreveport

ERNEST A. DAIGNEAULT, PH.D.

Professor and Head
Department of Pharmacology
East Tennessee State University
College of Medicine

A Wiley-Interscience Publication

JOHN WILEY & SONS, New York • Chichester • Brisbane • Toronto

Library of Congress Cataloging in Publication Data
Main entry under title:

Pharmacology of hearing.

"A Wiley-Interscience publication."
Includes index.
1. Ototoxic agents. 2. Auditory pathways—Effect of drugs on. 3. Vestibular apparatus—Effect of drugs on. I. Brown, Richard Don. II. Daigneault, Ernest A.
[DNLM: 1. Ear—Drug effects. 2. Drug therapy—Adverse effects. 3. Hearing—Drug effects. WV 270 P536]
RF285.083P47 615′.78 81-437
ISBN 0-471-05074-1 AACR1
Printed in the United States of America
10 9 8 7 6 5 4 3 2 1

PREFACE

There are pharmacological agents that affect one or more of the basic physiological or biochemical processes involved in the perception of sound. These agents include potential neurotransmitter substances, drugs that alter synaptic physiology, those that affect energy transport, and the ototoxic agents, which produce a frank impairment in hearing. The purpose of this book is to review the emerging field of auditory pharmacology and place it in perspective with the many new developments in the anatomy, physiology, and biochemistry of hearing. A chapter on the pharmacology of audiogenic seizures is also included to (1) show how pharmacologic manipulation of hearing and/or central nervous system monoamines (norepinephrine, 5-hydroxytryptamine, and/or dopamine) results in the production of an animal model for the study of convulsive disorders and (2) give an insight into the interplay between the ascending auditory pathways and those pathways that are not normally considered to be functionally related to hearing. Furthermore, a number of drugs which affect hearing also alter equilibrium. Therefore, a chapter on vestibular pharmacology is included so that the similarities, as well as the differences, can be emphasized.

It is hoped that this volume will serve as a useful text for graduate students and researchers in otolaryngology, neurology, and auditory physiology and pharmacology as well as an important reference for the practicing clinician.

R. Don Brown
Ernest A. Daigneault

Shreveport, Louisiana
Johnson City, Tennessee
May 1981

ACKNOWLEDGMENTS

Editing a book requires the assistance of many others. We gratefully acknowledge the extent of cooperation that exists among people who are interested in promoting scientific knowledge. It is reaffirmation that the principles learned about science and the scientific community during our idealistic youths are true and thriving.

The support that every scientist receives from his everyday associates and family is especially important. In particular, the secretarial assistance of Ms. Susie Fessler and Mrs. Helen Higdon and the additional editorial tasks performed by Ms. Fessler made our task much easier and we thank them for their help. Finally, the moral support, understanding and encouragement from our wives, Fronie Brown and Claire Daigneault, were constant forces which made our work both feasible and worthwhile; we love you for being who you are.

R. D. BROWN
ERNEST A. DAIGNEAULT

CONTENTS

CHAPTER 1

Anatomy of the Inner Ear

R. DON BROWN, Ph.D.

Professor of Pharmacology
Louisiana State University School
of Medicine in Shreveport
Department of Pharmacology and Therapeutics
Shreveport, Louisiana

CONTENTS

1.1 INTRODUCTION

This chapter is being written from the perspective of a pharmacologist. Therefore one of its purposes is to furnish a description of the potential sites of action of drugs that affect hearing and/or equilibrium and to describe the accessibility of those sites to drugs.

Its other purpose is to provide the reader with sufficient background to interpret the material presented in subsequent chapters. It is not intended to be an in-depth survey of the anatomy of the inner ear; these details can be found in publications by authorities in this area.[1-13]

1.1.1 Gross Anatomy

The inner ear (labyrinth) lies within the petrous portion of the temporal bone and consists of the cochlea and vestibular apparatus. This entire structure is a series of interconnected bony cavities (osseous labyrinth) within which lie a number of communicating membranous sacs and ducts (membranous labyrinth). The fluid filling the space between the osseous and membranous labyrinths is perilymph (Figure 1.1), which has a composition similar to that of extracellular fluid; it is apparently formed by an influx of cerebrospinal fluid and by ultrafiltration from the vessels lying in the tissue covering the inner walls of the osseous labyrinth.[14] The potassium-rich fluid within the membranous labyrinth is endolymph (Figure 1.1), which is similar to intracellular fluid in ionic composition. This fluid is thought to originate from the stria vascularis of the cochlea and the differentiated, nonsensory epithelia of the vestibular apparatus.[6,15] The fluid surrounding the sensory receptors (hair cells) of the cochlea and vestibular apparatus is isolated from endolymph by tight junctions on the epithelia lining the endolymphatic compartment.[16]

1.1.2 Microscopic Anatomy

The cochlea is a coiled, fluid-filled tube encased in a bony capsule. The two outer fluid compartments, the scala vestibuli and scala tympani, are connected by the helicotrema, an opening at the apex of the cochlea (Figure 1.1). The central compartment, the scala media, is roughly triangular and is bounded by Reissner's membrane, the basilar membrane, and the stria vascularis (Figure 1.2). The organ of Corti rests on the basilar membrane and includes one row of inner hair cells, three rows of outer hair cells, supporting cells (Deiters, Hensen, and Claudius), the rods, pillars, and tunnel of Corti, the pillar cells, the afferent and efferent nerve endings, and the basilar and tectorial membranes. The enclosure formed by Reissner's membrane and the basilar membrane is called the cochlear duct or cochlear partition. (Some investigators exclude the organ of Corti from the cochlear duct by defining the tectorial membrane rather than the basilar membrane as one of the

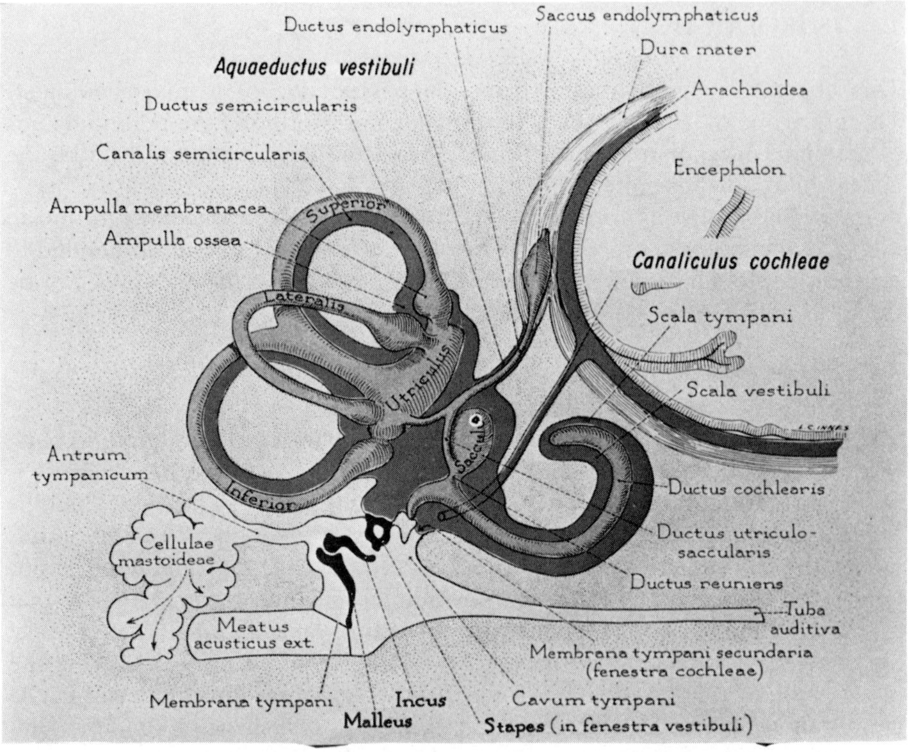

Figure 1.1 Schematic representation of the vestibular and cochlear aqueducts in relation to the labyrinthine systems for endolymph and perilymph (perilymphatic compartment darkest shade). Reproduced by permission from Anson et al.[1]

boundaries of the cochlear duct.) The superior surface of the hair cells, the framework of supporting cell processes that holds them in place, and the superior aspects of the rods of Corti constitute the reticular lamina of the cochlea. Running up through the center of the coiled tube of the cochlea is the modiolus, which contains the spiral ganglia (nerve cell bodies of the primary auditory afferents) and the intraganglionic spiral bundles (axons of the cochlear efferents). Cochlear afferent and efferent nerve fibers penetrate the temporal bone through the habenula perforata and take one of several courses to the sensory epithelia. (These courses are described later in detail.)

The vestibular apparatus contains several specialized areas of epithelia: the ampullar cristae and the saccular and utricular maculae. The lining of the endolymphatic compartment is a one-layered epithelium, below which is a layer of connective tissue. Most of the epithelial lining is undifferentiated and squamous. In the areas of specialization, however, the epithelium is differentiated into a secretory epithelium and a sensory epithelium.[6] The epithelium and connective tissue stroma which line the endolymphatic com-

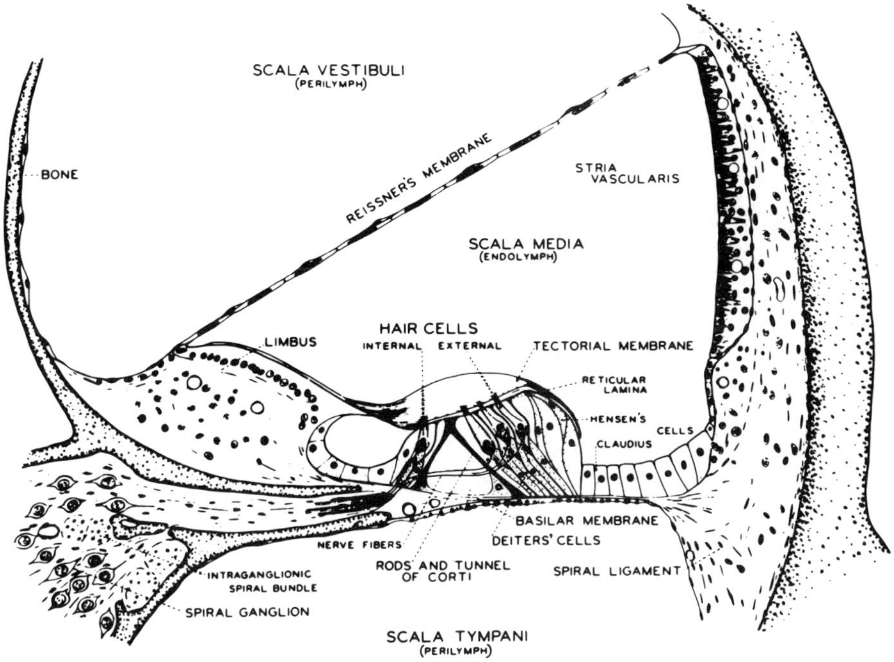

Figure 1.2 Cross section of the second turn of the guinea pig cochlea. Reproduced by permission from Davis et al.[13]

partment are secured to the outer boundary of the perilymphatic compartment by loose connective tissue (Figure 1.3); there are no vestibular structures analogous to Reissner's and the basilar membranes of the cochlea. The nerve cell bodies of the vestibular afferents constitute Scarpa's ganglion and are located in the bony capsule that surrounds the labyrinth. Vestibular afferent and efferent fibers penetrate the temporal bone through the cribrose macula and course directly to the sensory epithelia (Figure 1.3).

1.2 DRUGS AND THE INNER EAR

1.2.1 Distribution

Several factors govern the distribution of drugs within the fluid compartments of the inner ear and, as a result, their accessibility to the sensory receptors and associated nerve endings. Figure 1.1 shows that gross anatomical connections exist between the cochlea and vestibular apparatus for the endolymphatic and perilymphatic fluid compartments. On closer examination, however, the endolymphatic compartment is found to be discontinuous. The endolymphatic connection between the saccule and utricle is

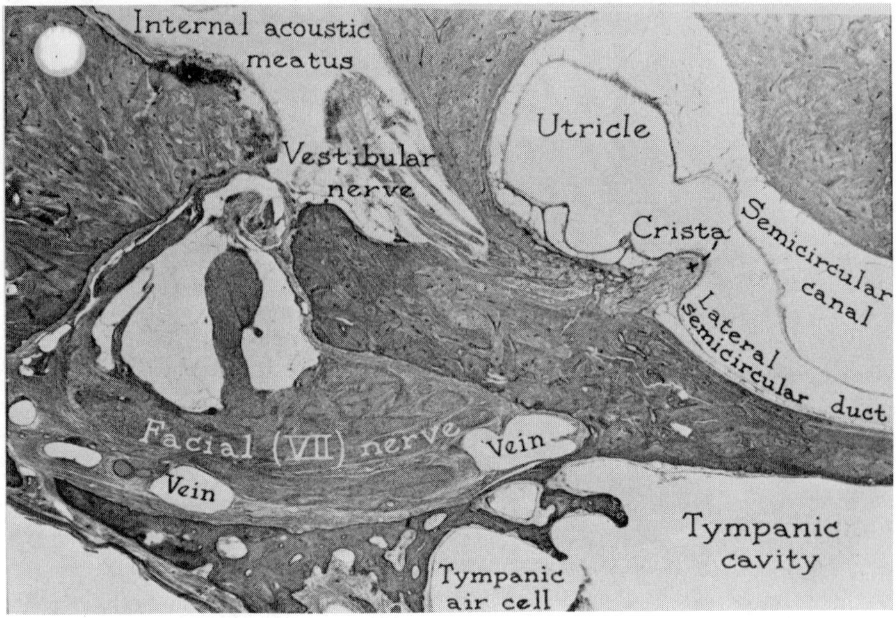

Figure 1.3 Utricle and portion of lateral semicircular canal with its crista. Reproduced by permission from Anson and Donaldson.[7]

very small in most animal species and in some cases is closed by a valve on the utricular side of the endolymphatic duct; furthermore, endolymph circulation in the vestibular apparatus is separate from that in the cochlea.[17] Thus it does not appear likely that drugs that enter the endolymph of the cochlea or vestibular apparatus would be distributed by it to the other system. (It should be recognized, however, that hydrostatic pressure changes in disease states can be reflected through both systems, as it is in Meniere's disease.[18-19])

In contrast, the perilymphatic fluid compartment of the cochlea does appear to be continuous with that of the vestibular apparatus.* Furthermore, it has been proposed that cortilymph, the interstitial fluid within the organ of Corti proper (Figure 1.2), is similar to perilymph in ionic composition and is continuous with the perilymph of the scala tympani.[14] In the vestibular apparatus there is no structure analogous to the basilar membrane that might limit access of perilymph to the vestibular sensory epithelia. Therefore drugs that gain access to the perilymphatic fluid could be distributed throughout

*In some animals, notably the guinea pig, a connective tissue boundary membrane divides the perilymphatic compartment into vestibular and cochlear divisions.[11] Even in this animal, however, it is unclear whether an anatomical communication exists between the two divisions, and there is no proof that this membrane serves as an effective diffusion barrier to ions, nutrients, or drugs.

that compartment and conceivably to the cochlear and vestibular sensory receptors and their nerve endings.

The stria vascularis of the cochlea appears to form another compartmentalized area of the inner ear (Figure 1.4).[16] Diffusion or active transport of drugs into this compartment may explain the selective cochlear toxicity of the loop diuretics. These drugs exert their initial action on the stria vascularis of the cochlea.[20] On the other hand, the secretory epithelium, the analogous tissue of the vestibular apparatus, is not compartmentalized; this could account for the relative lack of vestibular toxicity of the loop diuretics.

Another way for drugs to gain access to the area of the receptors is by passive or active transport from the capillary beds of the vascular system that supplies those specific areas; that is, the arterioles of the basilar membrane of the cochlea and the arterioles that serve the ampullae and the utricle and saccule. A blood-cochlea barrier is present, however (Figure 1.4). This barrier seems to be similar to the "blood-brain barrier"[21–22] and most certainly plays an important role in determining which drugs find their way into

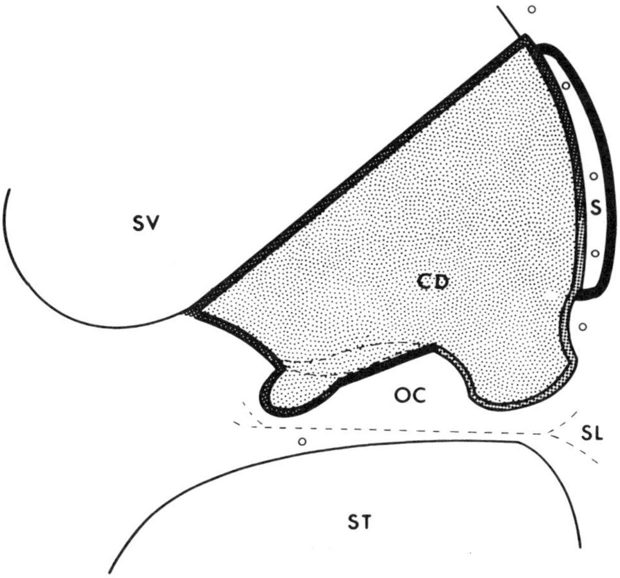

Figure 1.4 The perilymph-endolymph barrier of the cochlea and the stria vascularis. This diagram summarizes the results of observations on tight junctions that seal the cochlear duct and the intercellular spaces of the stria vascularis. SV = scala vestibuli, ST = scala tympani, CD = cochlear duct, OC = organ of Corti, S = stria vascularis, SL = spiral ligament. All nonsensory epithelia, which line the cochlear duct, have zonulae occludentes of the intermediate to tight type (dotted line). In contrast, the zonulae occludentes of the cochlear sensory epithelium and junctions of basal cells of the stria vascularis are very tight (thick black line). The circles represent blood vessels, all of which have tight junctions such that their nonfenestrated endothelia also form barriers. Reproduced by permission from Jahnke.[16]

the cochlea. (It is not known whether a similar barrier exists in the vestibular portion of the inner ear.)

1.2.2 Possible Sites of Action

Logical sites of action of drugs within the inner ear include (1) the sensory receptors (mechanoreceptors; i.e., hair cells), (2) their afferent and/or efferent nerve endings, (3) the stria vascularis of the cochlea and/or the analogous structure of the vestibular apparatus, and (4) the vasculature of the cochlea or the vestibular apparatus. (In addition, the brainstem is the presumed site of action of antimotion sickness drugs; this, however, is discussed in Chapter 11).

Hair Cells

Two types of mechanoreceptor are found in the cochlea and the vestibular apparatus, each with a different basic shape and pattern of innervation (Figures 1.5 and 1.6). Both types of hair cell possess stereocilia and it is thought that their mechanical distortion initiates the transduction processes of the inner ear. The Type I hair cell is flaskshaped and synapses directly with afferent fibers. In contrast, the efferent fibers synapse with the afferent dendrites rather than with the hair cell itself. The inner hair cell of the

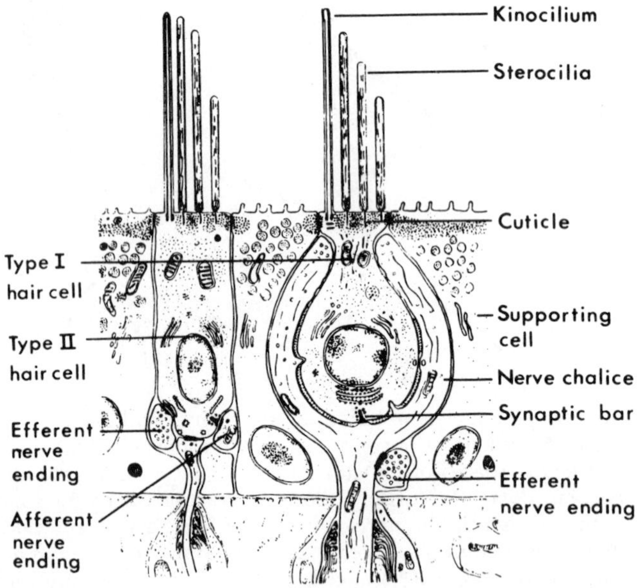

Figure 1.5 Schematic drawing of the two types of sensory apparatus which show the fine structure organization of Type I and Type II sensory cells of the vestibular apparatus and their innervation. Reproduced by permission from Wersall and Bagger-Sjoback.[6]

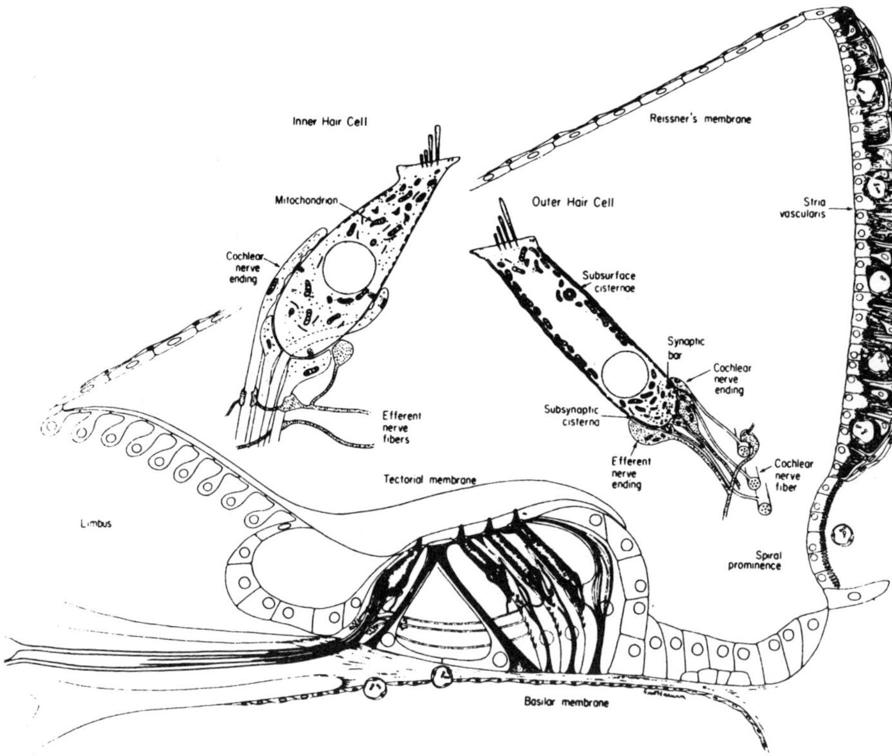

Figure 1.6 Drawing of the cochlear duct, second turn, guinea pig cochlea. Only recent findings are shown in detail. Reproduced by permission from Smith.[5]

cochlea and the vestibular hair cell with the afferent nerve chalice are Type I hair cells. The Type II hair cell is cylindrical and has direct synaptic contact with the afferent and efferent nerve terminals. The outer hair cells of the cochlea and the vestibular hair cells which lack the afferent nerve chalice are Type II hair cells. The aminoglycosides seem to produce their ototoxicity primarily by direct action on the hair cells, selective cochlear and/or vestibular toxicity being dependent on the specific aminoglycoside.

Afferent and Efferent Synapses

The morphology of the afferent and efferent synapses of the inner ear is presented later in this chapter and the physiology and pharmacology of these synapses are subjects of subsequent chapters. It should be pointed out at this juncture, however, that alteration of afferent and/or efferent synaptic physiology, due to direct action on these synapses, has not been demonstrated as an important part of any drug's therapeutic or toxic effect.

Stria Vascularis and Vestibular Secretory Epithelia

As previously stated, the stria vascularis of the cochlea and the analogous tissue of the vestibular apparatus (the differentiated, nonsensory epithelium) are the apparent sources of endolymph. The stria vascularis is also thought to be responsible for the generation of the positive cochlear endolymphatic dc potential; the analogous tissue of the vestibular system is presumed to be the source of the smaller, positive vestibular endolymphatic dc potential.[10,20,23-24] The loop diuretics appear to exert their ototoxic effect by interfering with the functions of these specialized, secretory tissues.

Vasculature

The labyrinthine or internal auditory branch of the anterior inferior cerebellar artery, a branch of the basilar artery, supplies the entire membranous labyrinth (Figure 1.7). The main cochlear artery spirals up through the modiolus and serves most of the cochlea by breaking up into many arterioles that feed capillary beds for the pertinent cochlear structures. The rest of the cochlea, the basal portion, is supplied in an analogous fashion by the cochlear ramus of the vestibulo-cochlear artery.[11-12]

The blood supply to the vestibular apparatus is not so complex as that of the cochlea. It consists primarily of capillary beds formed beneath each area of specialized epithelia by arterioles and venules which follow the nerves

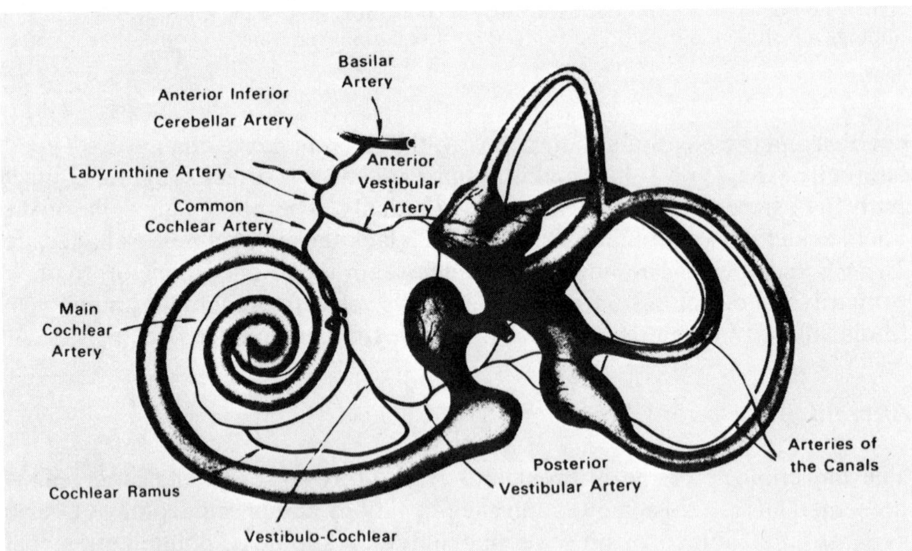

Figure 1.7 Diagrammatic sketch which shows the arterial system of the mammalian membranous labyrinth. Reproduced by permission from Schuknecht.[11]

that supply these structures. A separate, loosely connected set of capillaries is formed by arterioles and venules that extend throughout the connective tissue which forms the outer boundary of the vestibular division of the perilymphatic fluid compartment.[11]

The vasculature of the inner ear has been postulated as the site of action involved in the ototoxicity of nonsteroidal antiinflammatory agents and quinine.[20] In addition, disruption of the blood supply to the inner ear by a clot is thought to be responsible for the sudden hearing loss that has occurred in females who take oral contraceptives; vasodilator therapy has been given in an attempt to restore their cochlear circulation to normal.[25]

1.3 AFFERENT AND EFFERENT SYNAPSES OF THE INNER EAR

The morphology of the synapses in the inner ear is similar to that of other synapses that are chemically mediated.[9,26] Two types of receptoneural synapse occur: the afferent are found on Type I and Type II hair cells (Figures 1.5 and 1.6). The other receptoneural synapse occurs primarily between Type II hair cells (e.g., the outer hair cell of the cochlea) and their efferent nerve terminals (Figures 1.5 and 1.6); only rarely does an efferent terminal make contact with a Type I hair cell.

A third type of synapse occurs in the region immediately beneath the Type I hair cell between vesiculated enlargements of the efferent fibers and the afferent dendrites coursing from the cell (Figures 1.5 and 1.6); only rarely is it found in the region beneath the Type II hair cell.

The most recently discovered synapse is the dendro-dendritic. So far this synapse has been identified only in the cochlea and is apparently confined to synapses between the afferent dendrites that innervate the outer hair cells. Bodian[26] states that these junctions "between pairs of presumptive afferent processes suggest the possibility of dendro-dendritic interaction confined to the outer hair cell system."

Finally, it must be pointed out that an anatomical substrate has not been conclusively identified for the much speculated-about functional interaction between cochlear inner and outer hair cells. (See Chapter 2 for further discussion.) The only candidates for this role at the present time are the atypical, desmosomelike junctions in the spiral ganglion reported by Adamo and Daigneault.[27]

1.4 INNERVATION OF THE COCHLEA

This portion of the chapter is restricted to a general description of the innervation of the cochlea. Details of the innervation of the vestibular apparatus are presented, as needed, in Chapter 11.

1.4.1 Cochlear Afferents

Afferent Innervation Pattern

The pattern of afferent innervation of the cochlea has been clarified by experiments that involve sectioning of cranial nerve VIII.[28–29] Three types of spiral ganglion cell are evident. The preponderance of the spiral ganglion cells (≃95%), or Type I neurons (Figure 1.8), are associated with the inner radial fibers that course directly to the inner hair cell. As many as 20 of these neurons innervate each inner hair cell (Figure 1.9).

Type II spiral ganglion cells (≃5%) give rise to the outer spiral fibers which course below the tunnel of Corti and, turning up the cochlea, innervate the outer hair cells in a diffuse manner. Each Type II neuron innervates 10 or more outer hair cells.

The Type III spiral ganglion cell (<1%) is similar to the Type I cell but is surrounded only by a satellite cell; it lacks a myelin sheath. Each of these neurons connects several inner hair cells.

The physiological implications of the afferent innervation pattern are discussed in Chapter 2, but a seemingly paradoxical effect of cochlear toxicity

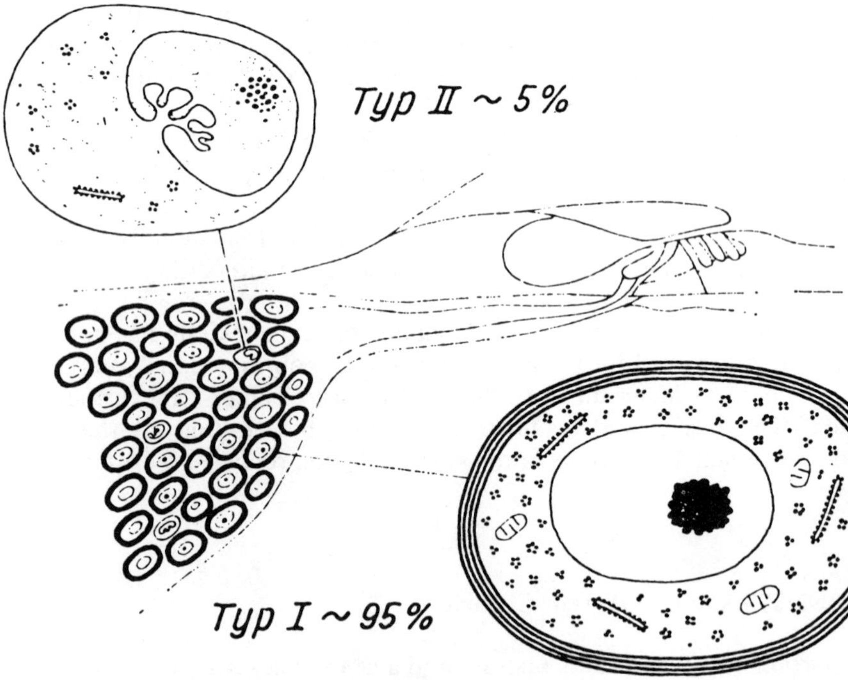

Figure 1.8 Schematic representation of two types of ganglion cell in the spiral ganglion and their relative percentage. Reproduced by permission from Spoendlin.[28]

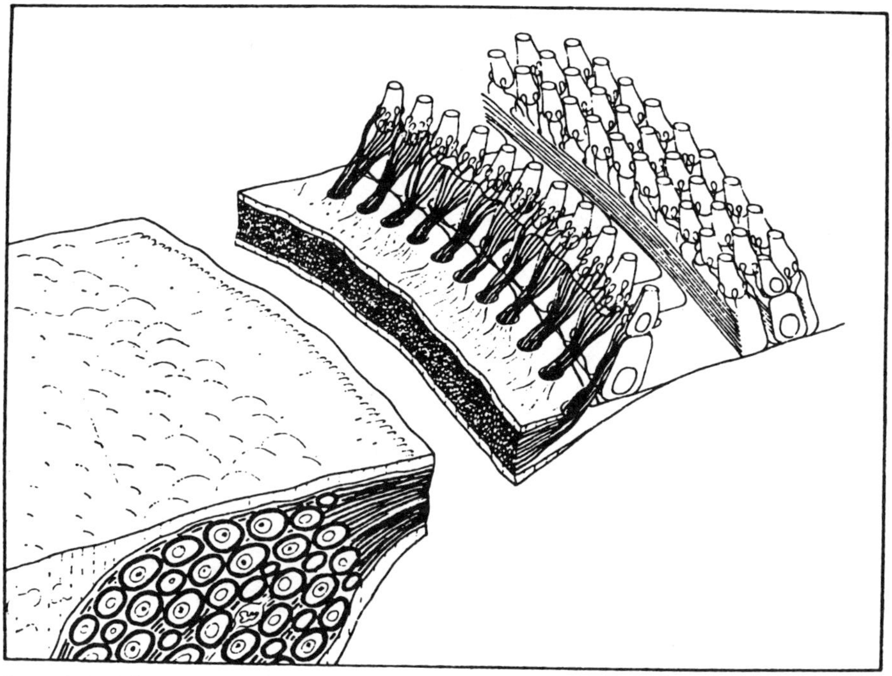

Figure 1.9 Schematic representation which summarizes the afferent innervation pattern of the organ of Corti, where all spiral ganglion cells are present. Reproduced by permission from Spoendlin.[28]

should be pointed out. The outer hair cells are much more sensitive to the toxic effect of drugs than the inner hair cells and their (OHC) selective destruction does cause serious impairment in hearing. This impairment occurs in spite of 95% of the afferent input to the central nervous system (CNS) which arises from fibers that discretely innervate the inner hair cells. These observations can be interpreted in two ways; either loss of the outer hair cells disrupts a functional interaction between inner and outer hair cells or it disrupts the structural and/or ionic integrity of the organ of Corti. The answer to this seeming paradox must await further investigation.

The Ascending Auditory Pathway

The cochlea is tonotopically organized; the highest frequencies cause localized displacement of the basilar membrane at the very base of the cochlea. As the frequencies become progressively lower, they displace larger portions of the basilar membrane, with the peak displacement moving toward the apex.[30] The ascending auditory pathway is also tonotopically organized.[31] The classical ascending (and descending) auditory pathway is schematically represented in Figure 1.10. (A detailed discussion of the as-

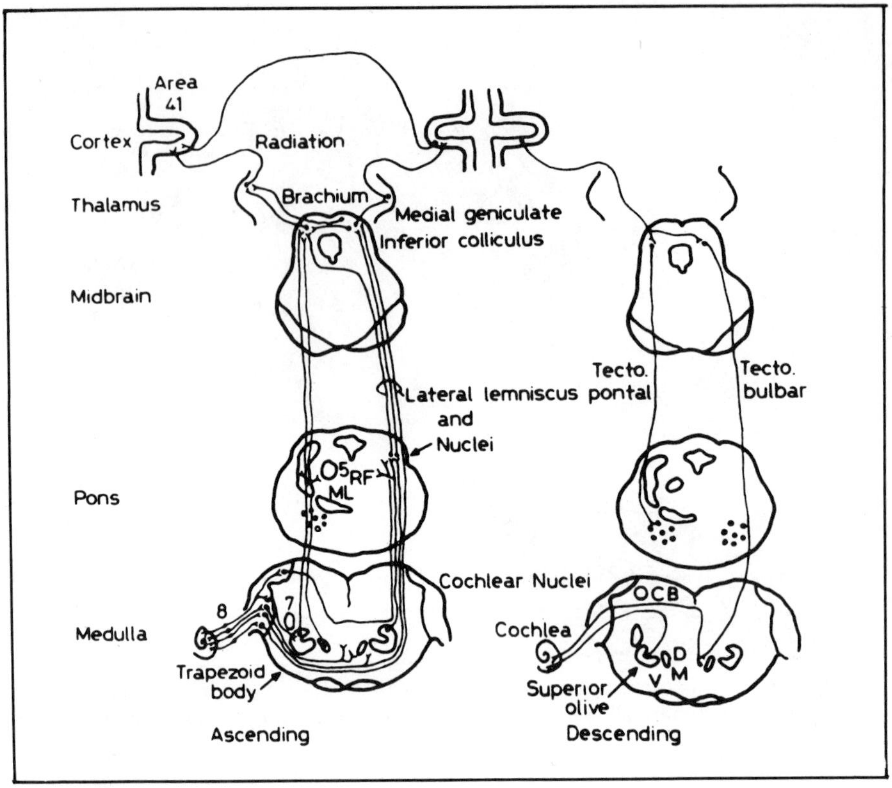

Figure 1.10 The main ascending and decending pathways of the auditory system. D = dorsomedial peri-olivary nucleus; M = medial nucleus of trapezoid body; ML = medial lemniscus; OCB = crossed and uncrossed olivocochlear bundles; RF = reticular formation; V = ventral nucleus of trapezoid body; 5 = trigeminal nucleus; 7 = facial nucleus; 8 = spiral ganglion. Reproduced by permission from Morest.[31]

cending auditory pathway can be found in an excellent review by Harrison and Howe.[32])

1.4.2 Cochlear Efferents

Origin and Course

The origin and course of the contralateral or crossed efferents to the cochlea were first described by Rasmussen in 1942.[33] In 1953 he added to this knowledge a description of the origin and course of the homolateral cochlear efferents.[34] These two bundles of efferent fibers are called the contralateral and homolateral olivocochlear bundles (COCB and HOCB) because their cell bodies lie in the superior olivary complex; those of the COCB are contained in the dorsomedial periolivary nucleus of the opposite side and those of the HOCB lie in the dorsolateral periolivary nucleus of the same side (Figure 1.10).

The COCB fibers leave their nucleus of origin dorsally and cross the floor of the medulla. The HOCB fibers course dorsolaterally and join the COCB immediately dorsal to the descending tract of cranial nerve V. The joined bundles leave the brainstem and course with the vestibular division of cranial nerve VIII, enter the vestibulo-cochlear anastomosis (Oort's bundle) and then follow the course of the cochlear division of cranial nerve VIII into the modiolous, becoming the intraganglionic spiral bundles (Figure 1.2). Three-fourths or more of the fibers in the intraganglionic spiral bundles are COCB fibers.[35]

Efferent Innervation Pattern

Cochlear efferent ramification is extensive (Figure 1.11).[29] About 500 efferent fibers arrive in the intraganglionic spiral bundles, from which originate the inner spiral bundles (50–200 fibers) and the upper tunnel radial bundles ($\simeq$ 8000 fibers). From the upper tunnel radial bundles originate approximately 40,000 efferent terminals which synapse with the outer hair cells. The fibers of the inner spiral bundles terminate on the afferent dendrites to the inner hair cell but no estimates have been reported of the extent of their branching.

In the basal turn of the cochlea each outer hair cell is provided with six to

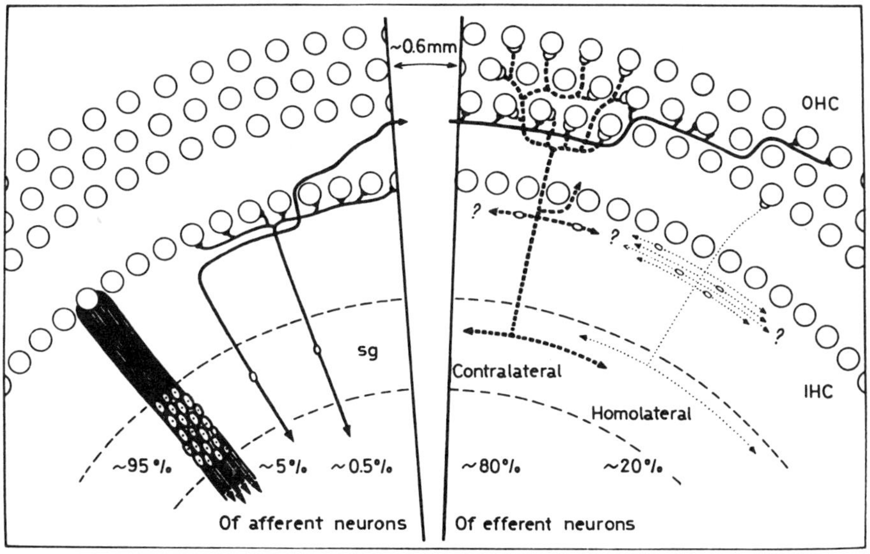

Figure 1.11 Horizontal innervation schema of the organ of Corti with the different types of afferent neuron on the left and efferent neuron on the right with corresponding approximate percentages. Reproduced by permission from Spoendlin.[29]

eight efferent nerve endings. This number is reduced progressively to the point at which efferent nerve endings disappear entirely in the upper turns of the cochlea.

Degeneration studies of the cochlear efferents reveal that the COCB innervates the outer hair cells and, in some species, contributes as well to the inner spiral fibers; almost all the HOCB fibers end up as inner spiral fibers (Figure 1.11).[29] Thus the HOCB seems to be related functionally to the dendrites of the inner hair cell and the COCB, primarily to the outer hair cell. The functional implications of these efferents are discussed in subsequent chapters of this book.

1.4.3 Sympathetic Innervation

The sympathetic innervation of the cochlea has its origin in the cervical sympathetic ganglia.[36–37] It undergoes a dual distribution (Figure 1.12).[9,37–38]

One group of sympathetic fibers is perivascular and is presumed to have vasomotor function. A specific role postulated for these fibers is the adrenergic regulation of fluid balance in the cochlea.[37]

The other group of sympathetic fibers courses independently of blood vessels among nerve fibers of the auditory division of cranial nerve VIII. On arriving at the modiolus this group forms a terminal plexus at the level of the habenula perforata (Figure 1.12), their terminals found where the myelinated fibers lose their myelin sheaths. It has also been postulated that this group of fibers may influence auditory afferent activity at the site of generation of the action potential.[37]

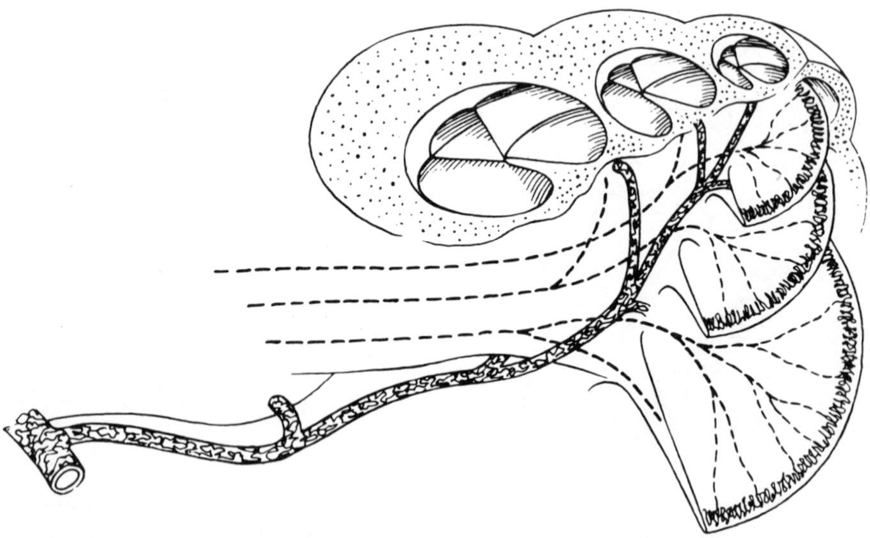

Figure 1.12 Schematic representation of the two types of adrenergic innervation of the cochlea. Reproduced by permission from Spoendlin.[9]

Regardless of the speculations based on anatomical grounds, the fact remains that the function of both groups of sympathetic fibers is unknown. Investigations of the role of the cochlear sympathetics have not yielded definitive information,[9,37] perhaps because of the bimodal distribution of these fibers.

ACKNOWLEDGMENTS

I gratefully acknowledge the assistance of Susan Bairnsfather, Susie Fessler, and David Glenn and the past and present research support of the Southern Medical Association, the LSU Foundation, and NIGMS (RO1 GM22097).

REFERENCES

1. B. J. Anson, R. L. Warpeha, and M. J. Rensink, *Ann. Otol. Rhinol. Laryngol.*, **77**, 583 (1968).
2. H. Engstrom and J. Wersall, *Exp. Cell Res. Suppl.*, **5**, 460 (1958).
3. S. Iurato, in W. D. Keidel and W. D. Neff, Eds., *Handbook of Sensory Physiology*, Vol. V/1, Springer-Verlag, New York, 1974, pp. 261–282.
4. C. A. Smith, *Ann. Otol. Rhinol. Laryngol.*, **70**, 504 (1961).
5. C. A. Smith, in E. L. Eagles, Ed., *The Nervous System*, Vol. 3, Raven, New York, 1975, pp. 1–18.
6. J. Wersall and D. Bagger-Sjobac, in H. H. Kornhuber, Ed., *Handbook of Sensory Physiology*, Vol. VI/1, Springer-Verlag, New York, 1974, pp. 123–170.
7. B. J. Anson and J. A. Donaldson, *Surgical Anatomy of the Temporal Bone and Ear*, 2nd ed. Saunders, Philadelphia, 1973, p. 492.
8. J. Wersall, *Acta Oto Laryngol. Suppl.*, **126**, 1 (1956).
9. H. Spoendlin, in L. Ruedi, Ed., *Advances in Oto-Rhino-Laryngology*, Vol. 13, Karger, Basel, Switzerland, 1966, p. 227.
10. C. A. Smith, in M. M. Paparella, Ed., *Biochemical Mechanisms of Hearing and Deafness*, Thomas, Springfield, 1970, pp. 171–185.
11. H. F. Schuknecht, *Pathology of the Ear*, Harvard University Press, Cambridge, MA, 1974, p. 503.
12. A. Axelsson, in W. D. Keidel and W. D. Neff, Eds., *Handbook of Sensory Physiology*, Vol. V/1, Springer-Verlag, New York, 1974, pp. 213–260.
13. H. Davis and Associates, *J. Acoust. Soc. Am.*, **25**, 1180 (1953).
14. E. A. Schnieder, *Ann. Otol. Rhinol. Laryngol.*, **83**, 76 (1974).
15. R. D. Brown, *Medikon*, **4**, 33 (1975).
16. K. Jahnke, *Acta Oto Laryngol. Suppl.*, **336**, 1 (1975).
17. H. F. Schuknecht and R. A. McNeill, *J. Laryngol. Otol.*, **80**, 1 (1966).
18. S.K. Juhn, *Ann. Otol. Rhinol. Laryngol.*, **86**, 689 (1977).
19. M. E. Glasscock, G. W. Miller, F. D. Drake, and M. M. Kanok, *Laryngoscope*, **87**, 1668 (1977).
20. R. D. Brown and A. M. Feldman, *Ann. Rev. Pharmacol. Toxicol.*, **18**, 233 (1978).
21. E. A. Daigneault and R. D. Brown, *Arch. Int. Pharmacodyn. Ther.*, **162**, 20 (1966).

22. R. Klinke and N. Galley, *Physiol. Rev.*, **54,** 316 (1974).
23. R. S. Kimura, *Ann. Otol. Rhinol. Laryngol.*, **78,** 542 (1969).
24. Y. Nakai and D. A. Hilding, *Acta Oto Laryngol.*, **66,** 120 (1968).
25. J. Sudaka, *Nouv. Presse Med.*, **5,** 2807, 1976.
26. D. Bodian, *Proc. Nat. Acad. Sci. USA*, **75,** 4582 (1978).
27. N. J. Adamo and E. A. Daigneault, *J. Neurocytol.*, **2,** 91 (1973).
28. H. Spoendlin, *Acta Oto Laryngol.*, **73,** 234 (1972).
29. H. Spoendlin, *Audiology*, **14,** 383 (1975).
30. G. von Bekesy, *Experiments in Hearing*, McGraw-Hill, New York, 1960, pp. 500–510.
31. D. K. Morest, in E. L. Eagles, Ed., *The Nervous System*, Vol. 3, Raven, New York, 1975, pp. 19–29.
32. J. M. Harrison and M. E. Howe, in W. D. Keidel and W. D. Neff, Eds., *Handbook of Sensory Physiology*, Vol. V/1, Springer-Verlag, New York, 1974, pp. 284–336.
33. G. L. Rasmussen, *Anat. Rec.*, **82,** 441 Abstr. (1942).
34. G. L. Rasmussen, *J. Comp. Neurol.*, **99,** 61 (1953).
35. J. M. Harrison and M. E. Howe, in W. D. Keidel and W. D. Neff, Eds., *Handbook of Sensory Physiology*, Vol. V/1, Springer-Verlag, New York, 1974, pp. 364–388.
36. Y. Terayama, E. Holz, and C. Beck, *Ann. Otol. Rhinol. Laryngol.*, **75,** 69 (1966).
37. M. D. Ross, *Acta Oto Laryngol. Suppl.*, **286,** 1 (1972).
38. O. Densert and A. Flock, *Acta Oto Laryngol.*, **77,** 185 (1974).

CHAPTER 2

Physiology of Hearing

RICHARD P. BOBBIN, Ph.D.

Associate Professor of Otorhinolaryngology and Pharmacology
Kresge Hearing Research Laboratory of the South
Louisiana State University Medical Center
Department of Otorhinolaryngology
New Orleans, Louisiana

DENNIS L. KISIEL, Ph.D.

Director
Cleveland Hearing and Speech Center
Cleveland, Ohio

CONTENTS

2.1 INTRODUCTION

The physiology of audition encompasses such a wealth of knowledge that it cannot be reviewed to any completeness in one chapter. Therefore our goal is to outline several mechanisms that operate in the sensory process of audition, to formulate a conceptualization of the system for interpreting the action of drugs.

This chapter is outlined in the order of peripheral-to-central function. Emphasis is placed on the peripheral systems, even though "hearing" is a psychological function, the expression of which is determined by verbal or manual modes. This is illustrated in Figure 2.1 by an audiogram of an individual before and during dosing with excessive amounts of aspirin. The audiogram measures hearing by requiring subjects to carry out a manual task—to raise an arm when a tone presented to one ear at a particular frequency and intensity is heard. The lowest intensity at which the sound must be presented to be "heard" is then plotted in relation to a normalized curve. In this particular case the aspirin dosage seems to have decreased the ability of the individual to "hear" sound at a given intensity; in reality, however, aspirin only decreased the ability of the individual to respond. Where and how the drug acted on the global psychomotor system is undetermined. In the following discussion a small part of this psychomotor system is reviewed, and hopefully the reader will be able to suggest sites at which aspirin may act to influence the psychomotor system used in the process of hearing.

2.2 PHYSICS OF SOUND

Sound is a longitudinal compression-rarefaction wave phenomenon which may be conceptualized as a sine wave with the two dimensional coordinates of degree of compression and time. A period is the interval necessary for a cyclic phenomenon to complete one cycle. Frequency (f) is then defined as

$$f = \frac{1}{\text{period (sec)}}$$

Wavelength (λ) is the distance between two cycles or the speed of sound (c; 1090 ft/sec, 2.2×10^4 cm/sec) divided by f:

$$\lambda = \frac{c}{f}$$

The intensity of sound is measured perpendicular to the direction of the sound, both in terms of power (energy/time, watts) per unit area and pressure (force/area, pascals). [Review of units of measure: (1) *force,* a unit of weight: 1 gm = 980 dynes or 10^5 dynes = 1 newton; (2) *pressure,* force per unit area: 1 bar = 1 dyne/cm^2 or 1 newton/cm^2 = 10^5 dynes/cm^2 = 10^4

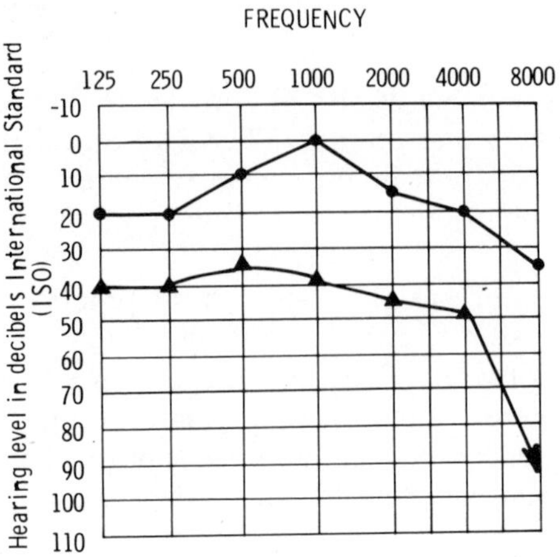

Figure 2.1 Hearing level obtained from one ear of a subject during (-▲-▲-) dosing with aspirin (16 × 400 mg/day for more than two days and 10 × 400 mg/day for several days before that) compared with the hearing level obtained one month later after the subject had discontinued the aspirin (-●-●-). Note losses are indicated as positive rather than negative dB values.

pascals; (3) *energy*, force over distance: 1 newton/m = 1 joule = 10^7 ergs; (4) *power*, energy/time: 1 W = 1 joule/sec = 10^7 ergs/sec.] Sound intensity is described by decibel (dB) notation. Two sounds are compared in terms of dB by multiplying the logarithm of their power (P) ratios by 10 or their pressure (p) ratios by 20:

$$\text{dB} = 10 \log \frac{P_1}{P_2} = 20 \log \frac{p_1}{p_2}$$

(For an in-depth discussion of the use of dB see Berlin.[1]) Standard convention defines the reference pressure (p_2) as 20 micropascals (20 μPa) and reference power (P_2) as 10^{-16} W/cm^2. Sound intensity measured in relation to this sound-pressure, standard-reference pressure, or power is called the dB sound pressure level or dB SPL. Thus the term 10 dB SPL implies, without saying, that the reference used was that standard. Human hearing for optimal frequencies ranges from 0 dB (20 μPa) to 120 dB (sensation of pain), a 10^6 range in the pressure ratio and 10^{12} range in the power ratio. Clinically, hearing loss is expressed not in terms of dB SPL but of a relative measure, labeled dB international standard (ISO); the mean threshold level of the general population is set at 0 dB and losses or gains are compared with this dB ISO. This measure is illustrated in Figure 2.1. With certain sounds, such as clicks and bursts, it is difficult to measure the intensity accurately. To overcome this problem authors have different methods, one of which is to use as a reference the unattenuated voltage to the earphone. Another method sets a continuous tone to the same peak-to-peak voltage at the transducer or speaker as the sound to be measured and then measures the sound pressure of the continuous tone and states it as an equivalent intensity.

In contrast to the physical measurement of intensity, loudness is a psychophysical correlate of intensity that varies according to frequency and intensity, as demonstrated in Figure 2.2. Note that the threshold of hearing

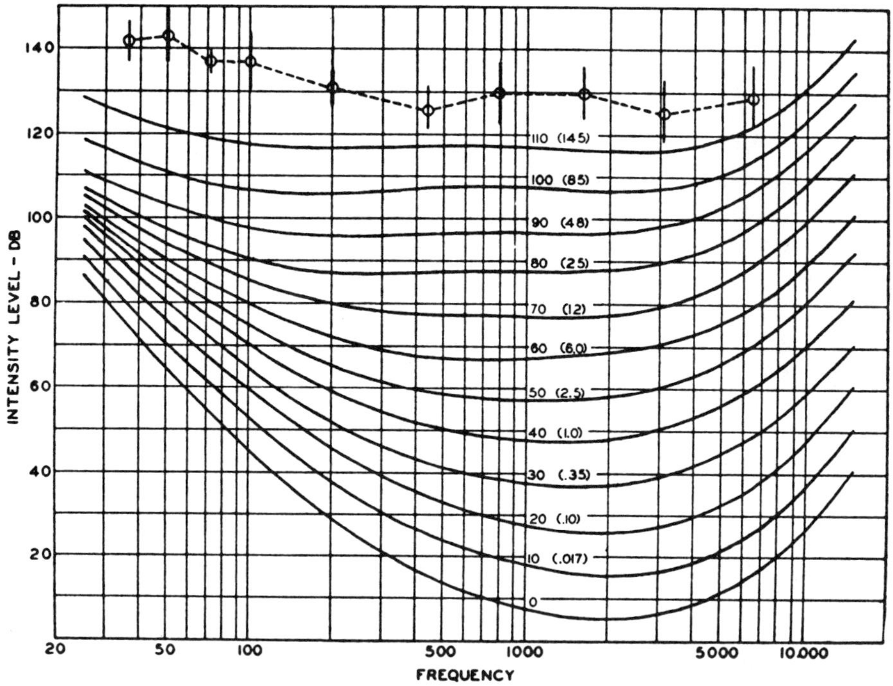

Figure 2.2 Equal-loudness contours plotted against intensity (dB above the reference pressure of 0.0002 dyne/cm²). The zero contour is the curve for minimum audible pressure. The dotted curve represents the threshold of feeling. The numbers in the center of the figure are the loudness levels in dB of the 1000-Hz tone above threshold (first number) and loudness, in sones (one sone = the loudness of a 1000-Hz tone 40 dB above threshold), of the tones represented by each contour (number in parentheses). (From Stevens and Davis.[2])

for humans occurs in the 1 to 4 kHz region (lowest minimum audible pressure). At high intensities the sensation of loudness becomes equal at all frequencies.

Sound is usually a complex signal that contains multiple frequencies at varying intensities. A click is an example of a complex signal that is generated in response to a pulse with infinite rise/fall characteristics. Physical systems cannot react with infinite on-and-off times; instead they respond by generating frequencies limited by the characteristics of a particular physical system. Because these systems vary between laboratories, displays of frequency versus intensity content of the sounds used are necessary if experimental results are to be duplicated.

2.3 EXTERNAL EAR

Sound energy is conducted through the external and middle ear into the inner ear, where the transduction process takes place. On the way all structures between the sound source and point of transduction modify or transform the physical dimensions of the sound energy.

From the formula for wavelength (λ) = c/f it is apparent that low-frequency sounds have long wavelengths (109 Hz = 10 ft) compared with high frequencies (10900 Hz = 0.1 ft). Large objects, such as buildings, interfere with and attenuate all frequencies of sound, but trees and corners mainly obstruct high-frequency (short wavelength) sounds. Likewise, the head attenuates high-frequency sound (short wavelength) more than low-frequency sound.

The concha and external canal act as resonators that modify the free-field sound intensity to amplify the input by as much as 10 dB at certain frequencies (a peak occurs at 3.8 kHz in man) when sound is monitored at the tympanic membrane (for review see Shaw[3]). Any changes in the shape of these structures will affect this frequency-intensity relationship. Most common changes in which foreign objects and cerumen (earwax) block conduction through the canal are hygienic. Microtresia, or complete absence of the canal and pinna, is present in certain birth defects. Complete closure results in a 20 to 30 dB hearing loss.

2.4 MIDDLE EAR

While incoming sound energy is air-borne, the transduction process takes place in the fluid-filled inner ear. At an air-water interface 99.9% of the incident sound energy (I_i) is reflected (I_r) and only 0.1% is transmitted (I_t) into the fluid. This is due to the large difference in the impedance of air (Z_a) compared with the impedance of the cochlear fluids (Z_b). The amount of transmitted energy (I_t) is given by the formula

$$I_t = I_i - I_r$$

or

$$= \frac{4Z_b/Z_a}{(1 + Z_b/Z_a)^2} I_i$$

The middle ear (i.e., the tympanic membrane or TM, malleus, incus, stapes, and oval window) evolved as an impedance-matching transformer to enable air-conducted sound to be conducted efficiently across the air-water interface (for reviews, see Wever and Lawrence,[4] Dallos,[5] and Moller[6]). A force (F) [i.e., pressure (p) $\times$ area (A)] and a pressure (p) [i.e., force (F) per area (A)] amplification method is used by these structures to match the air-water interface. The larger area of the TM (A_{TM}) compared with the area (A) of the stapes footplate (A_{S}) amplifies the pressure (p) at the TM (p_{TM}) by a factor of $A_{\text{TM}}/A_{\text{S}}$ for delivery as pressure at the stapes (p_s):

$$F = p \times A \qquad (1)$$

$$p_{TM} \times A_{TM} = p_S \times A_S \tag{2}$$

$$p_S = p_{TM} \times \frac{A_{TM}}{A_S} \tag{3}$$

The force (F) of the TM (F_{TM}) is amplified by the lever action of the fulcrum formed by the larger length of the malleus (L_M) and shorter incus (L_I) to give the force at the stapes (F_S). Thus

$$F_{TM} \times L_M = F_S \times L_I \tag{4}$$

or by substituting equation 1 into 4

$$p_{TM} \times A_{TM} \times L_M = p_S \times A_S \times L_I \tag{5}$$

yields

$$\frac{p_{TM}}{p_S} = \frac{A_S \times L_I}{A_{TM} \times L_M} \tag{6}$$

To arrive at a formulation for impedance transformation $Z = p/v$ is substituted for p in equation 6, where p is pressure and v is velocity:

$$\frac{Zv_{TM}}{Zv_S} = \frac{A_S \times L_I}{A_{TM} \times L_M} \tag{7}$$

The mechanical transformation includes a velocity transfer; then, because

$$\frac{v_{TM}}{v_S} = \frac{L_M}{L_I} \tag{8}$$

and by substituting into equation 7

$$\frac{Z_{TM}}{Z_S} \times \frac{L_M}{L_I} = \frac{A_S \times L_I}{A_{TM} \times L_M} \tag{9}$$

and

$$\frac{Z_{TM}}{Z_S} = \frac{A_S}{A_{TM}} \times \frac{L_I}{L_M} \times \frac{L_I}{L_M} \quad \text{or} \quad \frac{Z_{TM}}{Z_S} = \frac{A_S}{A_{TM}} \times \left(\frac{L_I}{L_M}\right)^2 \tag{10}$$

By substituting for Z_S the specific impedance of seawater (144,000 dynes sec/cm^3) and for the anatomical parameters the measures from von Bekesy and Rosenblith[7] ($A_{TM} = 0.55$ cm^2, $A_S = 0.032$ cm^2, $L_I/L_M = 0.77$) yields the calculated value for Z_{TM} as 4968 dynes sec/cm^3. For a perfect impedance match Z_{TM} should be equal to 41.5 dynes sec/cm^3 compared with the calculated 4968 dynes sec/cm^3 value. This impedance disparity or mismatch, together with other mechanical losses such as friction, has been calculated as an estimated 40% loss or a transmission of 60% of the energy delivered to the drum.[5]

Mass and stiffness properties of the middle ear affect its transfer function in the intensity and frequency domains; for example, Dallos[5] has shown that the middle-ear transfer function contributes to the determination of an animal's behaviorally monitored hearing sensitivity and cochlear microphonic (CM) sensitivity recorded from the round window. Likewise, pathologies such as otosclerosis, which increase the stiffness of the ossicular chain, produce losses in the low-frequency transfer capability. On the other hand, the mass of the ossicular chain places limits on the high-frequency transfer function. The middle-ear cavity proper plays a role in the transfer function and in some animals has evolved to enhance their low-frequency hearing for survival.[8,9] Accumulation of fluid in this cavity produces a hearing loss by interfering with the transfer function of the middle ear.

Two muscles, the tensor tympani and the stapedius, are attached to the malleus and stapes, respectively. Their action is reviewed by Wever and Lawrence[4] and Moller.[10] Contraction of the tensor tympani pulls the malleus inward and forward and contraction of the stapedius pulls the stapes in a posterior direction. The action that results is an increased tension at right angles to the course of the ossicular chain, which causes a change in the transmission characteristics of sound through the middle ear. Bilateral contraction of the middle-ear muscles, which is triggered by sound, voluntary contraction, vocalization, or noxious stimuli to the face, occurs by way of a reflex arc mediated through the brain stem olivary region.

2.5 BASILAR MEMBRANE MOTION

As discussed in the anatomy chapter, the enclosure formed by Reissner's membrane and the basilar membrane is called the cochlear duct or cochlear partition. The cochlear duct extends the length of the cochlea (35 mm in the adult human[4]) to end blindly at the helicotrema. The cochlear partition contains the hair cells and other anatomical structures for the transduction of sound into nerve impulses. It has been known for some time that sound conducted to the cochlear fluids by the ossicles was translated into cochlear-partition movement, which triggered action-potential generation in the auditory nerve in an unknown manner. Because there were no numerical assessments of the mechanical properties of the cochlear partition available, a plethora of cochlear-partition movement hypotheses were proposed. It occurred to one man, Georg von Bekesy, to open a cochlea to determine the mechanical properties of the cochlear partition. He not only discovered these properties but also demonstrated how the partition moved in response to ossicular motion. In recognition of his pioneering efforts von Bekesy was awarded the Nobel Prize (for physiology or medicine) in 1961.

Von Bekesy[11] directly observed the basilar membrane pattern-of-motion in response to sound stimulation. He measured the phase and amplitude of the sinusoidal motion of the cochlear partition at several points and arrived at the fact that the partition was moving from base to apex in traveling-wave fashion (see Figure 2.3). If attention were focused on one point along the cochlear partition during a traveling wave, it would be noted that the fre-

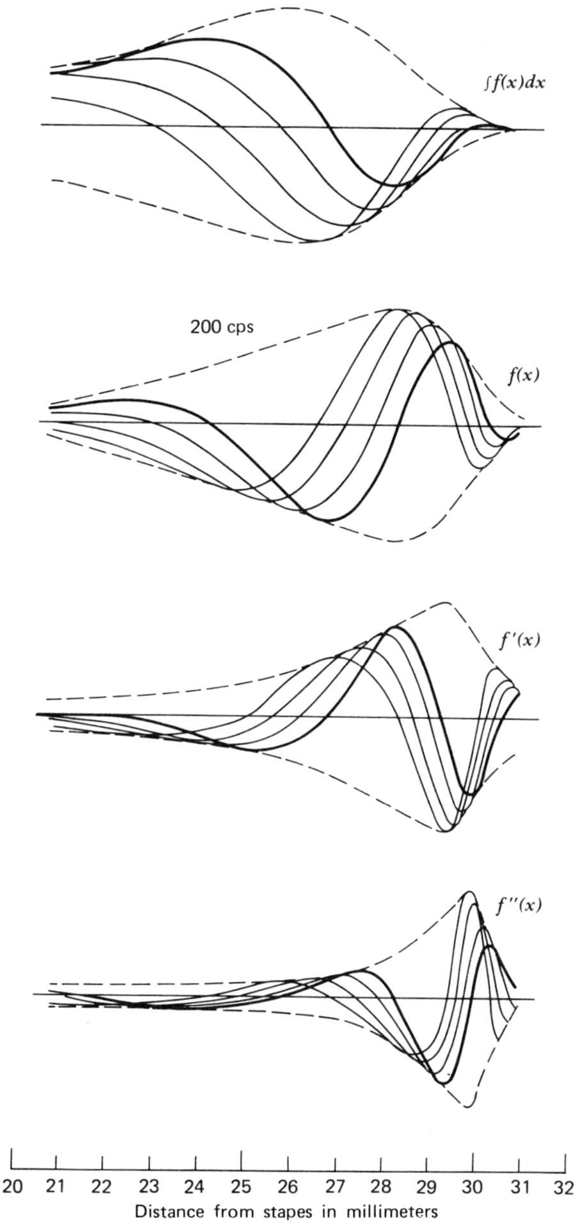

Figure 2.3 Traveling waves along the basilar membrane of a human cochlea for a tone of 200 Hz. Shown are the displacement wave [$f(x)$], its integral [$f(x)\,dx$], which shows the area under the curves, and its first two differentials [$f'(x)$] and [$f''(x)$], which demonstrate velocity and acceleration, respectively. Within each envelope constructed with dashed lines the different waves represent different time periods; the darker line represents most recent times. (From von Bekesy.[12])

quency of vibration of that point was the same as the frequency of the sound used to generate the motion.

The dotted lines in Figure 2.3 enclose the maximal excursions of the cochlear partition during passage of a traveling wave and outline the "envelope" of the traveling wave. Figure 2.4 shows one-half of the envelope of vibration for a sequence of increasing frequencies. The point of maximal vibration (the point of maximum on the envelope) is displaced toward the basal end with an increase in frequency of vibration, which indicates that high frequencies have their points of maximal stimulation at the basal end, whereas low frequencies have their maximal excursions toward the apex. Another point to note about the traveling-wave envelope is that for any frequency the pattern of vibration is attenuated more sharply toward the apex than toward the base.

The pressure wave (sound stimulus) applied to the fluid travels throughout the cochlear fluids nearly instantaneously [25 microseconds (μsec)]; yet the traveling wave takes 3000 μsec (3 msec) to move from base to apex. The traveling wave is the response of the cochlear partition to the pressure wave.

What are the mechanical properties of the cochlear partition that underlie this traveling-wave phenomenon? Von Bekesy pointed out that among the structures in the cochlear partition the basilar membrane's mechanical characteristics account for the traveling-wave phenomenon. Among the several mechanical properties of the basilar membrane described by von Bekesy the most important are the longitudinal coupling without tension and the change in elastic properties along the membrane's length.

To measure the elastic properties of the basilar membrane glass threads or human hairs were pressed at right angles on the surface of the basilar membrane; this process resulted in circular patterns that showed the same elastic properties in longitudinal and transverse directions. Fine cuts made in the basilar membrane did not draw apart, thus indicating that the basilar membrane was not under tension. The hairs bent when they exerted a certain maximum pressure and therefore were used to measure the compliance of the cochlear partition. Only the basilar membrane exhibited changes in the elastic properties along the length of the cochlea.

Another method used to measure the compliance of the basilar membrane involved the attachment of a fluid-filled tube to the pierced round window and blocking the helicotrema with a mixture of agar and gelatin. With this procedure von Bekesy produced a static differential pressure between the scala tympani and scala vestibuli. The displacement of the cochlear partition was then observed and measured because it is proportional to the compliance of the cochlear partition. The compliance from the oval window to the helicotrema changed by a factor of 100 and appeared to be the basis for the characteristic pattern of vibration of the cochlear partition.

The transduction of the traveling wave into neural impulses of the cochlear nerve delivers sound into the nervous system but how it occurs is

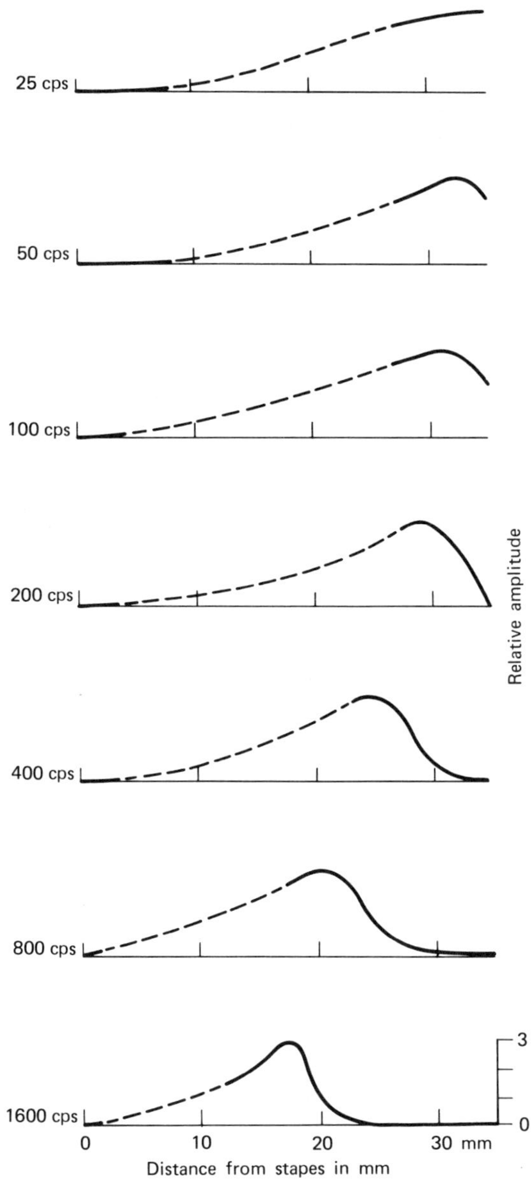

Figure 2.4 One-half of the envelope's force sequence of traveling waves in response to an increasing frequency of vibration. (From von Bekesy.[13])

unknown. Von Bekesy believed that it probably involved deformation or stress applied to the hair cells and observed that at the position of maximum vibration of the cochlear partition the hair cells showed an "up-and-down" movement. Because the tectorial membrane is attached at a different rotational point from the basilar membrane, the up-and-down motion could cause bending or shearing of the stereocilia on the hair cells.

2.6 TRANSDUCTION

There is little argument over von Bekesy's traveling-wave theory. This is in contrast to the controversy surrounding the manner in which this motion is translated into excitation of nerve elements in the auditory nerve. As pointed out in the chapter on anatomy, the hair cells possess stereocilia. Davis[14] suggested that the up-and-down motion of the cochlear partition produced a shearing action in the stereocilia embedded in the tectorial membrane, which somehow produced a depolarization of the hair cells and resulted in the release of transmitter (see Section 2.7 for further discussion). The cochlea has two types of hair cell (discussed in Chapter 1) called inner and outer. The inner hair cells constitute a single row, receive 95% of the afferents with little branching, have no efferent nerve endings (they occur on the nerve fibers under the hair cells), their cilia do not touch the tectorial membrane, and their afferents degenerate under traumatic insult. In contrast, the outer hair cells constitute three rows, receive 5% of the afferents with a lot of branching, have efferent nerve endings, appear to have cilia imbedded in the tectorial membrane, and have afferents that apparently remain after the hair cells have been lost. The relationship between these microanatomical differences and the micromotion of the cell groups is currently speculative.

Because only the tallest cilia of the outer hair cells appear to be embedded in the tectorial membrane,[15,16] shearing can apply only to these cells. This would also imply fluid-flow-induced bending rather than shearing.[17] It has been suggested[18,19] that the outer hair cells respond to displacement (shearing) and that the inner hair cells respond to velocity, the first derivative of displacement induced by fluid flow. On the other hand, several studies[20,21] suggest that the outer hair cells interact with the inner hair cells to enhance the sensitivity of 95% of the afferents. This interaction was thought to be neural until it was demonstrated[22,23] that the inner hair cells generate a potential that appears to mirror the sensitivity of the afferent nerve fibers.

All of this resulted in an interesting speculation at a recent meeting (Association for Research in Otolaryngology, St. Petersburg Beach, Florida, January 30–February 1, 1978). It was based on the demonstration of actin elements[24] in the stereocilia and the concept that the inner hair cells are the primary receptors that respond to the velocity of fluid flow under the tectorial membrane. This suggested that the flow may be altered by the up-and-down distance of the tectorial membrane, which, in turn, would be controlled by the degree of contraction exerted by the outer hair cell stereocilia on the tectorial membrane. Along these lines of speculation, the function of the small number of afferents and efferents which synapse on the outer hair cells would be to alter the tension on the stereocilia through the hair cell in a central loop. Thus the function of the outer hair cells may be analogous to the gamma motor neurons that change the tension on the spindle system of muscle.

The differences between inner and outer hair cells, together with the differences in vesicular-membrane structures at the point at which transmitter may be released,[25,26] have led to the suggestion that the afferent transmitter substance and/or the afferent postsynaptic transmitter action may differ between inner and outer hair cells. Whether the process is chemical or electrical is not completely resolved (see Chapter 5), but there is no lack of electrical events for the pharmacologist to monitor or interpret.

2.7 COCHLEAR POTENTIALS

Historically (see Stevens and Davis[2]) it was determined early that recording electrodes on tissue near the cochlear registered an alternating current (ac) voltage change when sound was led into the cochlea and that this voltage change, when amplified and used to drive an audio monitor, produced what "sounded like" the initial air-borne stimulus to the cochlea. This voltage was called the microphonic action of the cochlea or the cochlear microphonic (CM) or cochlear ac potential. Later the use of the terminology of alternating or ac cochlear potential was urged.[27] Experimental manipulation and calculations by von Bekesy[28] indicated that the energy so generated in this voltage was greater than that which entered the cochlea and concluded that an active element (endogenous energy) was involved in its generation. Von Bekesy discovered the active elements in the cochlea in the form of two direct current (dc) or resting voltages.

Von Bekesy[29] was the first to describe the potential in the endolymphatic space, now called the endocochlear or endolymphatic dc potential (EP), as a voltage in the scala media of about 80 mV magnitude with a positive polarity in relation to the extracellular fluid. Others[30] have since described the source of the EP as the stria vascularis, the extreme sensitivity of the EP to anoxia and drugs that affect metabolism,[31] and the relationship of the EP to the high K^+, low Na^+ that exists in the scala media.[32,33] The negative resting (dc) potential in the cells of the organ of Corti was also described by von Bekesy.[29]

Since the discovery of the negative organ of Corti potential there has been considerable debate over its origin, with some authors[30,34] claiming that the dc potential is found in the fluid spaces surrounding the hair cells and supporting structures. Sohmer et al.,[35] however, failed to record a stable, negative dc potential in the fluid spaces of the organ of Corti. They argue, together with Dallos,[36] that the dc potential represents the intracellular resting potential of cells in the organ of Corti. Suga and Hattler[37] (p. 99), recording from animals with no organ of Corti, call the negative dc potential they found the ". . . negative resting potential of the basilar membrane. . . ," apparently attributing it to the basilar membrane. It appears, then, that a negative dc "shift" is first obtained when a microelectrode penetrates the basilar membrane and, later, when a microelectrode penetrates a cell of the organ of Corti. Thus Konishi and Kelsey[38] label the first negative dc shift as due to penetration of the basilar membrane and the later negative dc shift as due to penetration of (cells in) the organ of Corti. In addition, a negative dc shift can be identified on penetration of the round-window membrane (see Sohmer et al.,[35] their Figure 12) or on penetration of Reissner's membrane (von Bekesy,[11] p. 652). On the other hand, a negative dc potential is recordable from cells in the organ of Corti.[22,23,39-46]

Many authors[47-50] have proposed models to explain the generation of the CM. Currently the most popular, but challenged,[50a,b] model is one proposed by Davis,[14] a "battery theory" model, which has since been tested[51] and modified with active elements.[52] In this model the EP (+ 80 mV) adds with the dc resting potential in the hair cells (− 60 mV) in a series circuit to produce a 140-mV voltage source that generates current (probably due to K^+)[41a] through the hair cells. The current flow is thought to be modulated by a variable resistor in the form of stereocilia, which change their resistance value with the act of shearing. The CM is envisioned as a voltage monitor of the current flow. It is interesting that the CM, when monitored along the cochlear partition and displayed properly, will demonstrate the form of the traveling wave and confirm that the CM appears to be an electrical analog of the traveling wave.[53]

The CM is made up of components of many frequencies other than the fundamental frequency of the signal source. The quantity and frequency of these components vary with the manner and place of recording and the sound used to generate the CM (see Dallos[5] for a complete discussion). One that has received much attention is a dc component, termed the summating potential (SP) by Davis and his colleages.[54-56] Composed of many components, it includes a positive and negative polarity component that depends on such parameters as place-of-recording and intensity and frequency of sound stimulus.[5] Destruction of the outer hair cells greatly diminishes (30 to 40 dB) the CM and SP.[57]

The peak-to-peak magnitude of the classical CM component is related to the intensity of sound used to evoke the CM (Figure 2.5, Curve A). It is both an indirect and a remote monitor of cochlear function because its magnitude varies with such parameters as the magnitudes of the EP, hair-cell resting potential, the mechanical properties of the cochlear partition, the number of hair cells that contributes to the response, and even the recording site. With this complex dependency it is not surprising to see a variety of changes in the

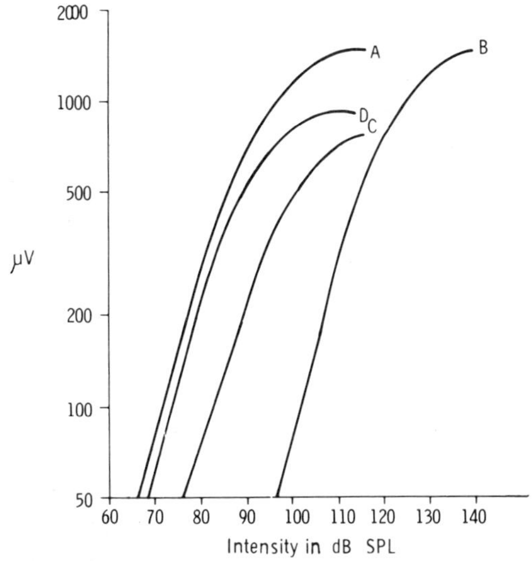

Figure 2.5 Peak-to-peak output curves for the cochlear microphonic response of the first turn of guinea pig cochlea to 6000-Hz tone bursts. (See text for explanation of Curves A–D.)

CM output curve following experimental manipulations. Figure 2.5 shows three of these changes. Curve A represents the normal CM output. The first change is the parallel shift (Curve B), which may be accounted for by a mechanical change in the sound-conduction system of the ear. Curve C shows a parallel shift in CM sensitivity and a decrease in maximum voltage. This type of change occurs in trauma due to intense sound exposure or damage to the hair cells.[58] The third type of curve (Figure 2.5, Curve D) is observed when the EP is reduced and is characterized by a slight change in sensitivity and a much larger drop in maximum voltage.[59]

The SP and other CM components are much more complex in their output functions and their response to noxious stimuli is much more difficult to interpret. This may explain their notable absence in the literature as monitoring parameters during drug testing and in the assessment of pathologies.[60–62] The reader is referred to Dallos[5] for a discussion of their various output curves.

What is the relationship between the CM, SP, and transmitter release at the inner and outer hair cells? This question currently remains unanswered. Recordings from individual hair cells have revealed that the CM,[39,41,41a] the SP,[22,23] or both[43] may be the potential change in the hair cells which results in the release of transmitter substance. In those animals with inner and outer hair cells it is possible that the CM reflects the release of transmitter from the outer hair cells[57] and the SP, the release from the inner hair cells. On the other hand, both may be epiphenomena and may not have a causal role in the transduction process.

2.8 NERVE ACTION POTENTIAL

The fast, all-or-none change in the neuronal membrane potential, the action potential, is believed to occur first at the point at which myelination of the cochlear afferents begins, close to the bony lip of the basilar membrane, called the foramina nervosa (the termination of the habenula perforata). Experimental recording of these potentials has been carried out from the area of the ganglion cells[63,64] and the areas central to these structures.[65–67] To date the only recordings that can be attributed to the unmyelinated nerve fibers are those of excitatory postsynaptic potentials in goldfish[68,69] and lateral line organs in lower animals.[41,42] Part of the CM-distortion products, the SP, may represent activity from the unmyelinated nerve fibers.[70]

Except for a small population of fibers, most first-order cochlear afferent neurons exhibit a level of spontaneous firing.[66,71,72] The cause of this firing is unknown but it may be related to spontaneous release of transmitter. The single nerve-fiber response of the first-order neurons to tonal stimuli is illustrated in Figure 2.6, which shows the typical initial overshoot and a drop to a flat level while the tone is on. When the tone is turned off, the unit becomes silent; it then returns to the pretone spontaneous level. The units respond over a 40-dB sound-intensity range by increasing their firing rate and then leveling off or decreasing their rate. In contrast to the response to a continuous tone a sharp, short-duration sound such as a click produces a poststimulus-time histogram, illustrated in Figure 2.7, which shows multiple firings and earlier firing to rarefaction (stapes moving out) than condensation (stapes moving in) clicks.

All first-order neurons exhibit a best, or characteristic, frequency at which the intensity of sound necessary to change the firing rate is lower than at any other frequency. Plots of frequency versus intensity necessary to evoke a standard unit response (tuning curves) are illustrated in Figure 2.8 for several primary units. Note that the curves tend to be more sharply tuned on the high-frequency side than on the low. At high intensities low-frequency "tails" also appear.

All of these characteristics of tuning curves have been correlated to basilar membrane mechanics and the motion of a traveling wave on the basilar membrane. Thus the shapes of the tuning curves seem to show (1) the point of maximal displacement of the traveling wave by the existence of a best frequency for a given unit; (2) the sharp cutoff on the apical end of the traveling-wave envelope due to the absence of stimulation of the unit by frequencies much higher than the best frequency; and (3) the gradual slope of the basal end of the traveling-wave envelope by the low-frequency tails obtained by making frequencies lower than the best sufficiently intense to stimulate afferent fibers synapsing basalward of the point of maximum displacement.

The tuning curves do not reflect the same slopes as the plots of basilar membrane motion.[73] Figure 2.9 illustrates mechanical tuning curves (see

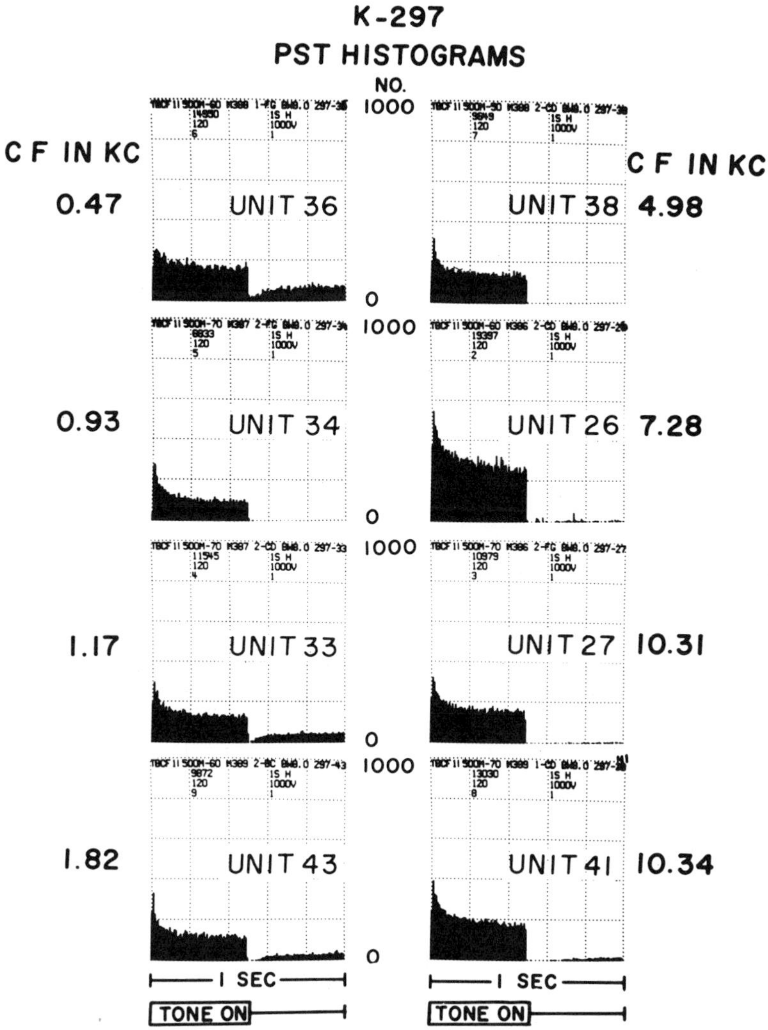

Figure 2.6 Poststimulus time (PST) histogram response patterns of primary auditory neurons to tone bursts. (From Kiang et al.[66]) CF = characteristic frequency; KC = kilocycles per second.

Bekesy, Johnstone, and Rhode curves) and compares them with the neural tuning curves (see Kiang-Wilson and Moller curves) obtained by various investigators as improvements were made in the techniques of measuring basilar membrane motion.

As illustrated, the high-frequency slopes (mechanical = 100 dB/octave; neural = 200 dB/octave) and low-frequency slopes (mechanical = 24 dB/octave; neural = 200 dB/octave) differ. To explain this discrepancy a second filter that would sharpen or in some way transform the mechanical motion to

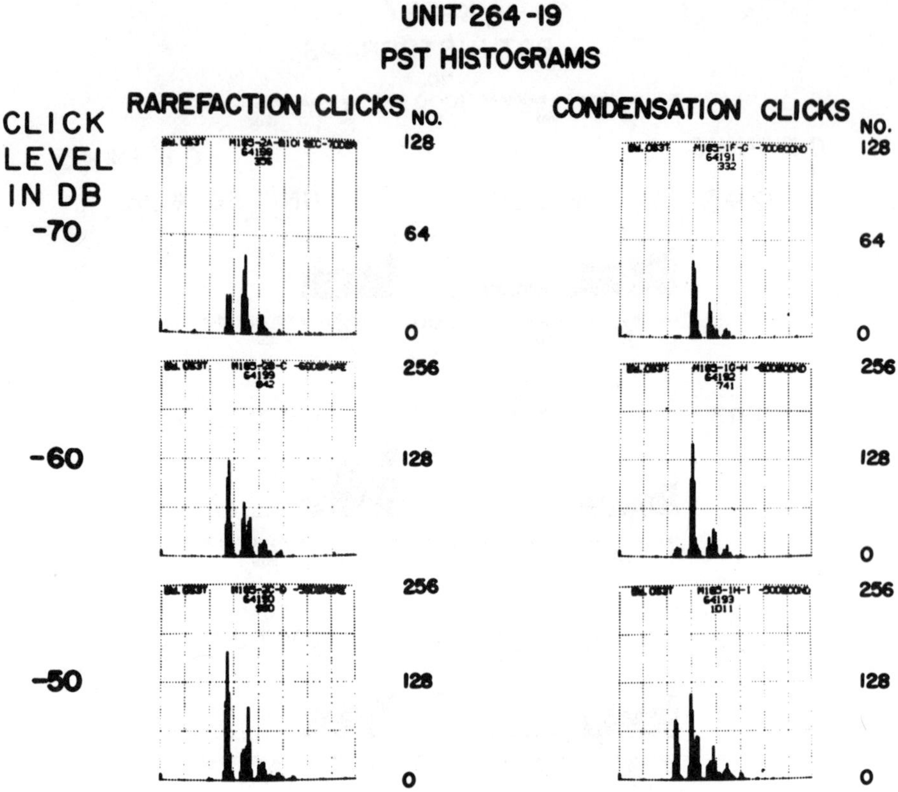

Figure 2.7 Poststimulus time (PST) histogram response patterns to rarefaction and condensation clicks as functions of click level. Stimulus levels are given in terms of dB attenuation of the input voltage (4 V) to the earphone (i.e., −20 dB is at a 40 dB greater intensity level than −60 dB). (From Kiang et al.[66])

yield the neural tuning curves[67] has been proposed. This filter has taken the form of nerve-nerve interaction,[20,75] hair cell-hair cell interaction,[76] and a fluid-flow system.[17,77] It is surprising that the apparent tuning curve of the claimed receptor potential generated by the inner hair cells is as sharp as that of the nerve fibers.[22,23] This has led to the suggestion that the sharpening effects of the second filter must occur before the generation of this potential, thus seemingly eliminating a posthair cell, nerve-nerve interaction.

Only recently have the effects of drugs been studied on single-unit activity. The removal of perilymph, drugs, toxic substances, destruction of hair cells, and stimulation of the crossed olivocochlear bundle (COCB) all appear to have the same effect on the tuning curves and all produce an elevation of the sharply tuned, low-threshold tips of the tuning curves in relation to the broadly tuned, high-threshold tails.[71,78–83] To some this implies that the sharp-

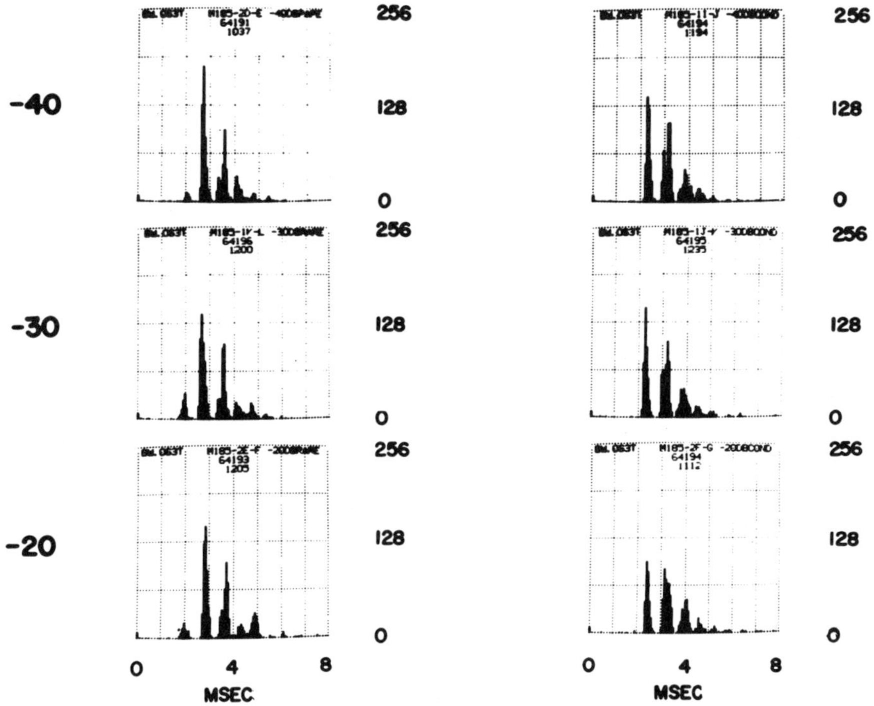

Figure 2.7 (Continued)

ening filter is dependent on the presence of intact outer hair cells;[84] it is also metabolism-dependent, oxygen-, temperature-, and cyanide-sensitive,[85–87] and/or depends on the EP (i.e., furosemide-sensitive[86]). On the other hand, insult to the inner hair cells may have caused a loss of sharp tuning.[88] Overall, the effect of drugs and other toxic substances seems to progress from an initial effect on the sharp portion of the tuning curve to an effect on the remaining portion.

2.9 COMPOUND ACTION POTENTIAL OF THE AUDITORY NERVE (CAP)

Figure 2.10A illustrates a complex waveform recorded from an anesthetized and paralyzed guinea pig in response to a high-intensity (≃100 dB SPL), short-duration (20 msec), 10-kHz tone burst with a rise/fall time of 0.5 msec. The recording was made single-ended by a silver wire (200 μ) inserted through a hole in the scala tympani of the basal turn, referenced to neck muscle. The signal was amplified 1000 times [Tektronix, Model 122 preamplifier, band-pass (3 dB/octave) 0.2 Hz–40 kHz] and routed through a filter (Krohn-Hite, 24 dB/octave) to an oscilloscope. The complex waveform

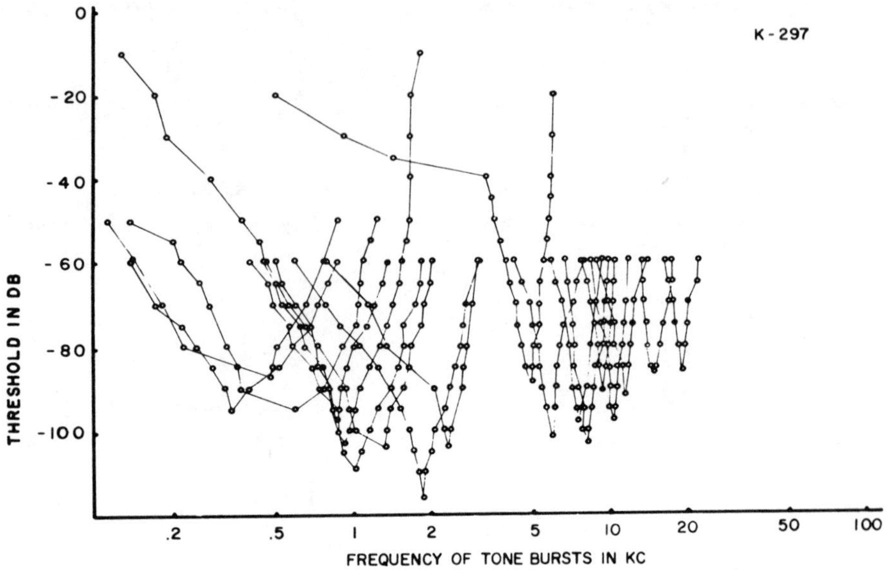

Figure 2.8 A sampling of tuning curves obtained for several primary units in a single cat. Stimulus levels are given in terms of dB attenuation of the input voltage (200 volts) to the earphone as in Figure 7. (From Kiang et al.[66])

shown in Figure 2.10A can be separated into three parts by band-pass filtering at certain points. The following are illustrated in Figure 2.10:

1 Figure 2.10B, a band-pass of 0.2 Hz to 2 kHz [high pass (HP) = 0.2 Hz, 3 dB/octave; low pass (LP) = 2 kHz, 48 dB/octave] yields a compound action potential of the auditory nerve (CAP) and SP combination.
2 Figure 2.10C, a band-pass of 6 to 40 kHz [HP = 6 kHz, 48 dB/octave; LP = 40 kHz, 3 dB/octave] yields the CM alone.
3 Figure 2.10D, a band-pass of 200 Hz to 2 kHz [HP = 200 Hz, 24 dB/octave; LP = 2 kHz, 24 dB/octave] yields the CAP alone.
4 Figure 2.10E, a band-pass of 0.2 to 200 Hz [HP = 0.2 Hz, 3 dB/octave; LP = 200 Hz, 48 dB/octave] yields the (positive) SP alone.

Similar recordings can be obtained by using a short-duration sound such as a click. The potentials with dominant frequency components in the 1-kHz range are called the cochlear action potential (CAP) and, as illustrated in Figure 2.10D, various bumps have been labeled in order and according to polarity, N_1 representing the first, N_2 the second, and N_3 the third negative wave and P_0 representing the first, P_1 the second, and P_2 the third position wave. The N_1 portion of the CAP appears to represent the synchronous discharge of many primary fibers in the auditory nerve.[53,89] The source of the

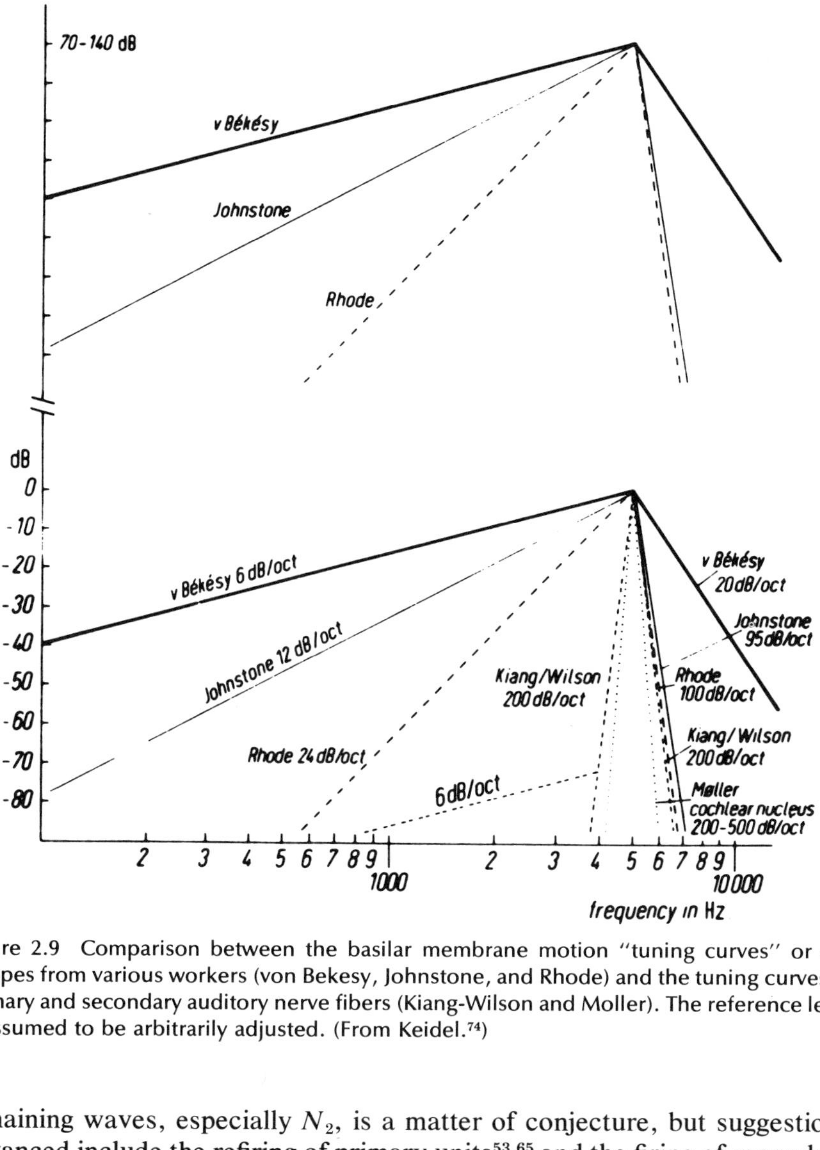

Figure 2.9 Comparison between the basilar membrane motion "tuning curves" or envelopes from various workers (von Bekesy, Johnstone, and Rhode) and the tuning curves of primary and secondary auditory nerve fibers (Kiang-Wilson and Moller). The reference level is assumed to be arbitrarily adjusted. (From Keidel.[74])

remaining waves, especially N_2, is a matter of conjecture, but suggestions advanced include the refiring of primary units[53,65] and the firing of secondary auditory units in the cochlear nucleus.[5,67]

The CAP may be recorded from several locations in and around the cochlea with slight changes in the waveform.[90,91] The potential may be recorded at a greater distance from the source, depending on the amplification and signal-detection equipment available; for instance, the CAP has been recorded from a site as remote as the external canal[92,93] and the scalp (see Section 2.10).

The magnitude and latency of the CAP varies with the rate of onset and

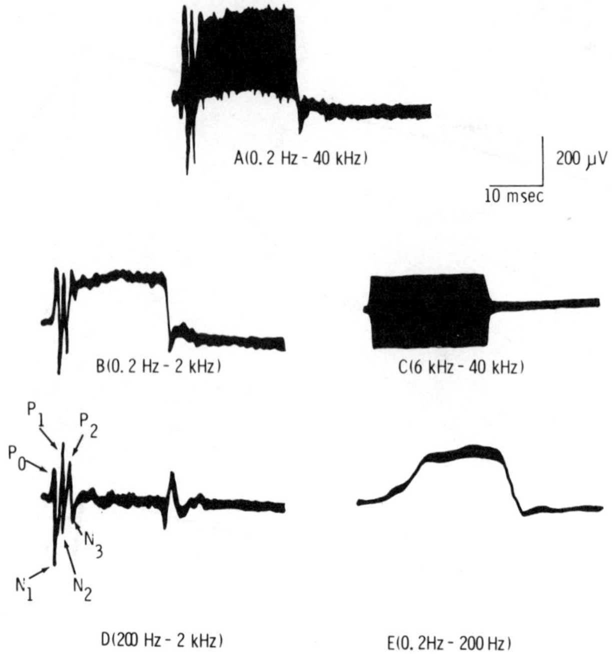

Figure 2.10 Recording of the electric response to a tone burst obtained from the scala tympani of an anesthetized guinea pig. Trace A: recording with open-filter settings. Traces B, C, D, and E: after interposition in the recording system of various filter bandpasses. Negative is down. Refer to text for further details.

intensity of the sound stimulus. The faster the rate of rise, the larger the CAP.[94] Figure 2.11 illustrates the changing N_1-P_1 magnitude and latency of N_1 with changing intensity of a click stimulus. The changing magnitude is attributed to the recruiting of all-or-none action potentials from additional neurons occurring in the volume conductor. The earlier latency is probably due to the fact that most of the additional fibers are recruited basalward to the point of maximal stimulation; that is, earlier in terms of traveling-wave travel time along the basilar membrane. (For further discussion see Dobie.[96]) The diphasic nature of the input/output function has been attributed to outer hair-cell activity (low-intensity portion) and inner hair-cell activity (high-intensity portion).[5,97] Along these same lines current suggestions attribute the low-intensity portion of N_1 to the low-intensity tips of the neural tuning curves and the high-intensity portion to the low-frequency tails and high-intensity tips of the tuning curves.

Whatever their origin, drugs, toxic substances, and treatments affect the curve in different ways. As shown in Figure 2.12, drugs such as salicylate[98] and loss of the outer hair cells[5] appear to produce curves with only the low-intensity "sensitive" portion abolished (Figure 2.12, Curve B).[57,99] On the other hand, drugs like aminooxyacetic acid,[100] ethacrynic acid,[101] and

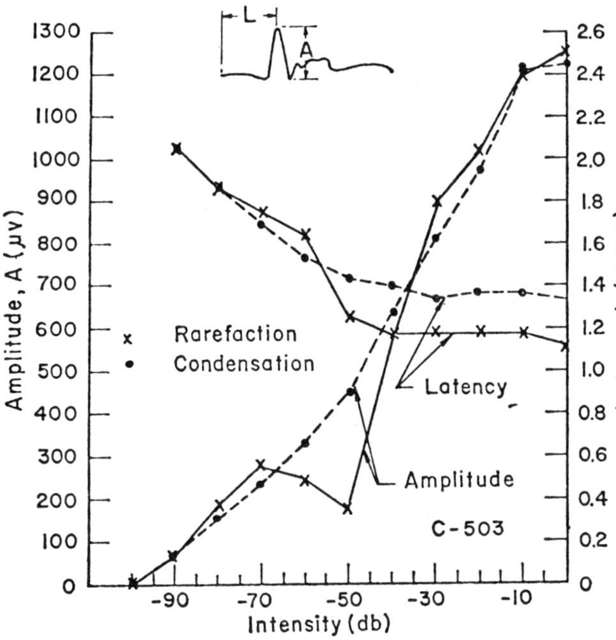

Figure 2.11 Amplitude and latency of the CAP ($N_1 - P_1$ magnitude, N_1 latency) as a function of sound (click) intensity from the cat. The solid curves represent results obtained with rarefaction clicks, the interrupted lines, results from condensation clicks. Intensity is given in terms of dB attenuation of the input voltage (2.5 V) to the earphone as in Figure 2.7. (From Peake and Kiang.[95])

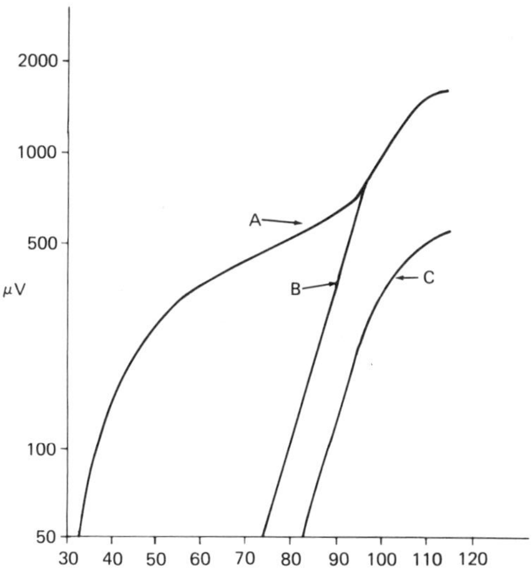

Figure 2.12 Output curves of the CAP ($N_1 - P_1$) magnitude record from the guinea pig cochlea under various conditions: normal (A), postsalicylate (B), and postaminooxyacetic acid (C). Intensity is given in terms of dB SPL (reference = 0.0002 dyne/cm²).

intense-sound damage[101] produce curves with their low- and high-intensity portions shifted (Figure 2.12, Curve C).

Several researchers have monitored the CAP as an indication of cochlear function[102,103]; however, the CAP is a monitor of synchrony and therefore an abstract indication of function; for instance, glutamate,[98] environmental noise,[104] and cyanide[38] will decrease the magnitude of the CAP, yet the effect on the primary-auditory-nerve activity is different for all three. Thus cyanide decreases primary-unit activity,[86] glutamate increases the asynchronous discharge of the primary units,[105,106] and environmental noise changes the pattern of the unit's response.[5] Caution is advised in explaining a reduced CAP magnitude in terms of nonrecorded, single-unit activity.

2.10 BRAINSTEM-EVOKED RESPONSE (BSER)

In exploring the various sound-synchronized waveforms recordable from the scalp of subjects, Jewett et al.[107,108] and Sohmer and Feinmesser[109] discovered what has come to be called the brainstem-evoked response (BSER) or brainstem response (BSR). This response is a synchronized potential that appears in a sequential manner following an auditory click stimulus that is recordable by an active electrode on the vertex, a reference near the ear, and a remote ground. The potential is small (0.1–10.0 μV) and therefore is seen above the level of the electrical noise of the scalp only by the use of a high-gain amplifier and signal averager or computer. As in the potentials recorded from the cochlea, the BSER form is dependent on the filter settings on the recording equipment. Current practice recommends a band-pass of 100 to 3000 Hz with roll offs of no more than 6 dB/octave.

Figure 2.13 illustrates a BSER recording from an anesthetized rat. The five or six waves usually seen in the BSER recording are labeled sequentially, by convention, as Waves I to VI. Wave I occurs at 1.5 to 2.0 msec after the click stimulus and the others occur at about 1-msec intervals therafter. The largest wave in man with this electrode configuration (vertex-ear) is the IV-V complex; Wave V is usually the larger of the two.

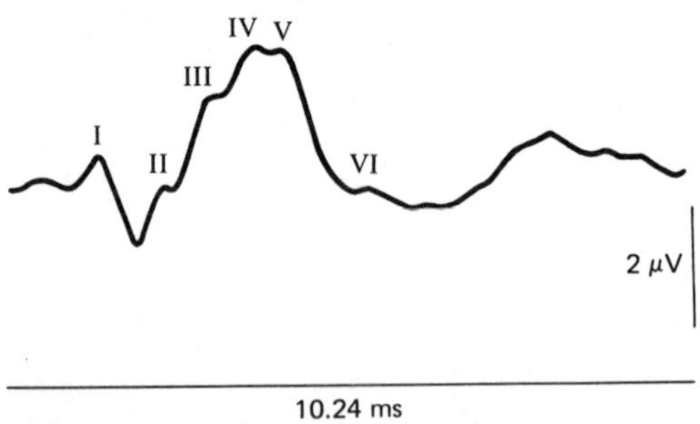

Figure 2.13 A BSER obtained from an anesthetized rat in response to a click stimulus. Shown is the sum of 256 stimuli.

The source of several of these potentials is still debated and may vary between animals and man. Ample evidence points to Wave I and II as cochlear N_1 and N_2, respectively.[110,111] Subsequent waves may represent synchronized excitatory or inhibitory postsynaptic potentials, action potentials, or a combination at various points along the auditory brainstem pathway, such as the trapezoid body, superior olive, lateral lemniscus, inferior colliculus, and medial geniculate body.[110,111]

There is now a wealth of clinical interest in these BSER waves, especially as they offer a monitor of auditory function that does not depend on a motor response from the subject.[96,112–116] The *latency* of Wave V varies with click intensity[117] and seems to be a less variable and more dependable measure across subjects than magnitude.[118] The BSER waves are dependent on the sound stimulus with fast rise time, or onset, similar to the CAP of the cochlea. This necessarily limits the frequency of pure tones used to evoke the waves to those above 1 to 2 kHz and therefore limits the information obtainable. (Information can be obtained about lower frequencies but it is necessary to use a more sophisticated approach.[114])

Marsh and Worden[119] first extended the observations of Saul and Davis[120] that a BSR evoked by a low-frequency sound could be recorded remotely, as confirmed later in the work of Moushegian and others.[121–124] This potential is called the frequency-following response (FFR) and can yield information on frequencies from 200 to 2000 Hz. Slowly, many of the origins and properties of the FFR are being worked out[125,126] and use of the FFR as a clinical tool is being explored.

2.11 MIDDLE- AND LATE-EVOKED POTENTIALS

Potentials synchronized to an auditory stimulus that appear "later" in time than the 1 to 10 msec in which the BSER components appear can be obtained with the same electrode configuration, amplifiers, and averaging techniques. Currently, they are divided into middle responses, which occur 10 to 50 msec after sound onset,[127–129] and late, slow responses, which occur with 50- to 300-msec latencies.[130,131] In contrast to the BSER the middle and late responses are susceptible to sleep stages and drug effects, although the middle components appear to be less sensitive.[132]

2.12 EFFERENT SYSTEM

Contralateral and/or homolateral olivocochlear bundles (COCB and/or HOCB) interact with most of the cochlear potentials when stimulated with electrical pulses at the floor of the fourth ventricle. The COCB has been investigated to the greatest extent and more is known concerning it. (For reviews see Klinke and Galley[133]; Desmedt[134]; Guth et al.,[135] and Chapters 1, 5, and 6).

2.12.1 Effect on Compound Action Potential of the Auditory Nerve (CAP) and Single Units

The effect of the COCB on the cochlea was first investigated in cats by Galambos.[136] He demonstrated that electrical stimulation of the COCB reduced the magnitude of the CAP and defined the optimal stimulus parameters to generate the COCB as a train of shocks presented at the rate of 100/sec for a duration of 250 to 300 msec (25 to 35 shocks). Recovery from the train of pulses for the CAP occurred within 500 msec. He also demonstrated that the COCB was most effective on a low sound-intensity-evoked CAP. The effects of changing each parameter were further defined by Desmedt[137] who also pointed out that the degree of CAP inhibition was equivalent to attenuating the sound about 20 dB. Others[138–140] confirmed that the COCB produced a smaller percentage of depression of CAP as the intensity of the sound generating the CAP increased. Thus it was suggested that "fibers with high thresholds are not influenced by COCB stimulation."[139]

A frequency selectivity for the COCB was demonstrated when it was shown that the greatest effectiveness of the COCB was on a 6- to 9-kHz-evoked CAP in guinea pig[140] and 6- to 10-kHz-evoked CAP in cat.[139]

That the inhibition of the CAP evoked by the COCB was a true inhibition of their firing and not just a result of asynchronization of cochlear nerve fibers was first demonstrated by Fex[141] and later extended by others.[142,143] Electrical stimulation of the HOCB fibers in cats has also been shown to reduce the magnitude of the CAP but to a lesser degree than the COCB when the same stimulus parameters were used.[144,145]

2.12.2 Effect on Cochlear Microphonic (CM) and Summating Potential (SP)

Fex[146] was the first to note that electrical stimulation of the COCB evoked an augmentation of the CM at frequencies of 500 Hz to 9 kHz.[141] The equivalent sound-pressure increase was 3 dB, compared with a 20-dB decrease for the CAP.[137,141,147] The HOCB produced no change in the CM of cats recorded at the round window.[145]

The interaction of the COCB and SP has been examined.[140,148,149] Fex[148] reported a summation, or occlusion, from the interaction; when the SP was recorded by the differential electrodes, however, the positive SP showed an increase for tone bursts with frequencies above 5 kHz.[140] This increase in the positive SP also paralleled the changes in the crossed olivocochlear potential, CAP, and CM with changing parameters of the COCB. Others found that, like electrical and mechanical biasing, the COCB may influence the load on the resistance in the Davis[14] model of hair-cell mechanisms by an alteration in membrane polarization.[149]

2.12.3 Crossed Olivocochlear Potential

That electrical stimulation of the COCB evokes a slow-potential change which is recordable in the cochlear fluids of cats was demonstrated by Fex.[141] As in CM and SP evoked by sound, this slow potential changes polarity across the reticular lamina.[148,150] It is largest (−2.5 m V) and negative in the scala media,[140,148] but smaller (+ 0.5 mV) and positive in the scala tympani and tunnel of Corti.[150] The magnitude of the slow potential paralleled the changes induced in the CM and CAP in onset and dissipation.[141] Flock and Russell[42] demonstrated that the negative dc resting potential of the lateral-line hair cells was increased in a negative direction (hyperpolarized) in response to efferent nerve stimulation. The hyperpolarization magnitude and duration were similar to the slow potential evoked by the COCB.

2.12.4 Central Effects

The COCB affects the sound-evoked potential not only at the round window but also in the cochlear nucleus, superior olive, and inferior colliculus.[137] The COCB affects single-unit activity in the cochlear nucleus in a complex pattern, compared with its inhibition of primary auditory afferents.[151] Thus spontaneous activity and tone-evoked activity of some units were unaffected, decreased, or increased. Other tone-evoked unit responses were decreased at low tone intensities and increased at high intensities.

2.12.5 Function of Efferents

The study of the efferents is clouded by the seemingly unphysiological stimulus parameters that are used (tetanus) and the conflicting reports of a behaviorally detectable function for the fibers. The majority of the efferent nerve endings synapse on outer hair cells which have a small afferent nerve population with unknown function. As described earlier in this chapter, the efferents may function as part of a central loop system, their activation causing alteration of the tension on the stereocilia of the outer hair cells. Evidence for this idea has recently been presented.[151a] Suggestions and evidence for the behavioral role of the efferents include improving signal-to-noise detection[152,153] and frequency discrimination,[154] and inhibiting auditory information during visual fixation.[155]

ACKNOWLEDGMENTS

Research was supported by the National Institutes of Health (Clinical Research Center Grant), USPHS NS-11647 and the Deafness Research Foundation. Laboratory facilities were provided by The Kresge Foundation. We wish to acknowledge the assistance of Pamela Burrell, Gae Decker, and Dr. Jack Cullen.

REFERENCES

1. C. I. Berlin, in J. L. Northern, Ed., *Hearing Disorders*, Little, Brown, Boston, 1976, pp. 279–296.
2. S. S. Stevens and H. Davis, *Hearing*, Wiley, New York, 1938.
3. E. A. G. Shaw, in W. D. Keidel and W. D. Neff, Eds., *Handbook of Sensory Physiology: Auditory System*, Vol. V/1, Springer-Verlag, New York, 1974, pp. 455–490.
4. E. G. Wever and M. Lawrence, *Physiological Acoustics*, Princeton University Press, Princeton, NJ, 1954.
5. P. Dallos, *The Auditory Periphery*, Academic, New York, 1973.
6. A. R. Moller, in W. D. Keidel and W. D. Neff, Eds., *Handbook of Sensory Physiology: Auditory System*, Vol. V/1, Springer-Verlag, New York, 1974, pp. 491–517.
7. G. von Bekesy and W. A. Rosenblith, in S. S. Stevens, Ed., *Handbook of Experimental Psychology*, Wiley, New York, 1951, pp. 1075–1115.
8. D. B. Webster and M. Webster, *Brain Behav. Envol.*, **4,** 310 (1971).
9. D. B. Webster and M. Webster, *Brain Behav. Envol.*, **5,** 41 (1972).
10. A. R. Moller, in W. D. Keidel and W. D. Neff, Eds., *Handbook of Sensory Physiology: Auditory System*, Vol. V/1, Springer-Verlag, New York, 1974, pp. 519–548.
11. G. von Bekesy, *Experiments in Hearing*, McGraw-Hill, New York, 1960.
12. G. von Bekesy, *J. Acoust. Soc. Am.*, **25,** 770 (1953).
13. G. von Bekesy, *J. Acoust. Soc. Am.*, **21,** 245 (1949).
14. H. Davis, *Cold Spring Harbor Symp. Quant. Biol.*, **30,** 181 (1965).
15. H. H. Lindemann, H. W. Ades, G. Bredberg, and H. Engstrom, *Acta Oto Laryngol.*, **72,** 229 (1971).
16. D. J. Lim, *Arch. Otolaryngol.*, **96,** 199 (1972).
17. C. R. Steele, in A. R. Moller and P. Boston, Eds., *Basic Mechanisms of Hearing*, Academic, New York, 1973, pp. 69–90.
18. P. Dallos, M. C. Billone, J. D. Durrant, C.-Y. Wang, and S. Raynor, *Science*, **177,** 356 (1972).
19. P. Dallos, in A. R. Moller and P. Boston, Eds., *Basic Mechanisms of Hearing*, Academic, New York, 1973, pp. 335–372.
20. J. J. Zwislocki, *Acustica*, **31,** 354 (1974).
21. P. Dallos and D. Harris, *J. Neurophysiol.*, **41,** 365 (1978).
22. I. J. Russell and P. M. Sellick, *Nature*, **267,** 858 (1977).
23. I. J. Russell and P. M. Sellick, *J. Physiol. London*, **284,** 261 (1978).
24. A. Flock and H. C. Cheung, *J. Cell Biol.*, **75,** 339 (1977).
25. R. A. Dunn and D. K. Morest, *Proc. Nat. Acad. Sci. USA*, **72,** 3599 (1975).
26. R. L. Gulley and T. S. Reese, *J. Comp. Neurol.*, **171,** 517 (1977).
27. J. Vernon and M. Meikle, in *Bioelectric Recording Techniques, Part C, Receptor and Effector Processes*, Academic, New York, 1974.
28. G. von Bekesy, *J. Acoust. Soc. Am.*, **22,** 576 (1950).
29. G. von Bekesy, *J. Acoust. Soc. Am.*, **24,** 72 (1952).
30. I. Tasaki and C. S. Spiropoulos, *J. Neurophysiol.*, **22,** 149 (1959).
31. R. Thalmann, in D. B. Tower, Ed., *The Nervous System, Vol. 3: Human Communication and Its Disorders*, Raven, New York, 1975, pp. 31–44.
32. W. Kuijpers and S. L. Bonting, *Pfluegers Arch.*, **320,** 348 (1970).

33. W. Kuijpers and S. L. Bonting, *Pfluegers Arch.*, **320,** 359 (1970).
34. R. A. Butler, *J. Acoust. Soc. Am.*, **37,** 429 (1965).
35. H. S. Sohmer, W. T. Peake, and T. F. Weiss, *J. Acoust. Soc. Am.*, **50,** 572 (1971).
36. P. Dallos, *J. Acoust. Soc. Am.*, **44,** 818 (1968).
37. F. Suga and K. W. Hattler, *Laryngoscope*, **80,** 80 (1970).
38. T. Konishi and E. Kelsey, *Acta Oto Laryngol.*, **65,** 381 (1968).
39. G. G. Harris, L. S. Frishkopf, and A. Flock, *Science*, **167,** 76 (1970).
40. A. Flock, J. M. Jorgensen and I. J. Russell, *Acta Oto Laryngol.*, **76,** 190 (1973).
41. A. Flock, M. Jorgensen, and I. Russell, in A. Moller, Ed., *Basic Mechanisms in Hearing*, Academic, New York, 1973, pp. 273–302.
41a. A. J. Hudspeth and D. P. Corey, *Proc. Nat. Acad. Sci. USA*, **74,** 2407 (1977).
42. A. Flock and I. Russell, *Nat. New Biol.*, **243,** 89 (1973).
43. M. J. Mulroy, D. W. Altmann, T. F. Weiss, and W. T. Peake, *Nature* **249,** 482 (1974).
44. T. F. Weiss, M. J. Mulroy, and D. W. Altmann, *J. Acoust. Soc. Am.*, **55,** 606 (1974).
45. T. Goto, *Transl. Beltone Inst. Hear. Res.*, **29** (February 1975).
46. R. P. Bobbin, *Arch. Otolaryngol.*, **102,** 45 (1976).
47. G. Dohlman, *Acta Oto Laryngol.*, **51,** 439 (1960).
48. I. Tasaki, in G. Rasmussen and W. F. Windle, Eds., *Neural Mechanisms of the Auditory and Vestibular Systems*, Thomas, Springfield, 1960, pp. 40–47.
49. E. G. Wever, *Physiol. Rev.*, **46,** 102 (1966).
50. L. Naftalin, *Physiol. Chem. Phys.*, **9,** 337 (1977).
50a. G. Leng, *Hear. Res.* **3,** 17 (1980).
50b. A. N. Salt and P. E. Stopp, *Exp. Brain Res.*, **36,** 87 (1979).
51. V. Honrubia and P. H. Ward, *J. Acoust. Soc. Am.*, **46,** 388 (1969).
52. D. C. Mountain, Jr., "A Comparison of Electrical Changes in the Cochlea Caused by Stimulation of the Crossed Olivocochlear Bundle and by dc Polarization," Doctoral Dissertation, Department of Electrical Engineering, University of Wisconsin, Madison, 1978.
53. D. C. Teas, D. H. Eldredge, and H. Davis, *J. Acoust. Soc. Am.*, **34,** 1438 (1962).
54. H. Davis, C. Fernandez, and D. R. McAuliffe, *Proc. Nat. Acad. Sci. USA*, **36,** 580 (1950).
55. H. Davis, I. Tasaki, and R. Goldstein, *Cold Spring Harbor Symp. Quant. Biol.*, **17,** 143 (1952).
56. H. Davis, B. H. Deatherage, D. H. Eldredge, and C. A. Smith, *Am. J. Physiol.*, **195,** 251 (1958).
57. P. Dallos and C.-Y. Wang, *Audiology*, **13,** 277 (1974).
58. R. P. Bobbin and M. I. Gondra, *Environ. Res.*, **9,** 48 (1975).
59. R. P. Bobbin and M, I. Gondra, *Ann. Otol. Rhinol. Laryngol.*, **84,** 192 (1975).
60. H. Davis, B. H. Deatherage, B. Rosenblut, C. Fernandez, R. Kimura, and C. A. Smith, *Laryngoscope*, **68,** 596 (1958).
61. N. Yoshie, in R. J. Ruben, C. Elberling, and G. Salomon, Eds. *Electrocochleography*, University Park Press, Baltimore, 1976, pp. 353–386.
62. J. N. Aran and R. C. deSauvage, *Acta Oto Laryngol.*, **83,** 153 (1977).
63. D. Robertson and G. A. Manley, *J. Comp. Physiol.*, **91,** 363 (1974).
64. D. Robertson and B. M. Johnstone, *Hear. Res.*, **1,** 31 (1978).
65. I. Tasaki, *J. Neurophysiol.*, **17,** 97 (1954).

66. N. Y.-S. Kiang, T. Watanabe, E. C. Thomas, and L. F. Clark, *Discharge Patterns of Single Fibers in the Cat's Auditory Nerve*, M.I.T. Research Monograph No. 35, M.I.T. Press, Cambridge, 1965, pp. 1–154.

67. E. F. Evans, in W. D. Keidel and W. D. Neff, Eds., *Handbook of Sensory Physiology: Auditory System*, Vol. V/2, Springer-Verlag, New York, 1975, pp. 1–108.

68. Y. Ishii, S. Matsuura, and T. Furukawa, *Jpn. J. Physiol.*, **21,** 79 (1971).

69. T. Furukawa, Y. Ishii, and S. Matsuura, *Jpn. J. Physiol.*, **22,** 617 (1972).

70. J. Fex, in W. D. Keidel and W. D. Neff, Eds., *Handbook of Sensory Physiology: Auditory System*, Vol. V/1, Springer-Verlag, New York, 1974, pp. 585–646.

71. N. Y.-S. Kiang, M. C. Liberman, and R. A. Levine, *Ann. Otol. Rhinol. Laryngol.*, **83,** 752 (1976).

72. M. C. Liberman and N. Y.-S. Kiang, *Acta Oto Laryngol.* **86,** *Suppl.* **358,** 59 (1978).

73. W. S. Rhode, *J. Acoust. Soc. Am.*, **64,** 158 (1978).

74. W. D. Keidel, *Rev. Laryngol. Otol. Rhinol.*, **95,** 463 (1974).

75. J. J. Zwislocki, in E. F. Evans and J. P. Wilson, Eds., *Psychophysics and Physiology of Hearing*, Academic, New York, 1977, pp. 125–135.

76. D. Strelioff, S. T. Sitko, and V. Honrubia, "Role of Inner and Outer Hair Cells in Neural Excitation," presented at the Research Forum of the American Academy of Ophthalmology and Otolaryngology and of the Association for Research in Otolaryngology (ARO), Dallas, Texas, September 19–20, 1975.

77. E. Zwicker, in E. Zwicker and E. Terhardt, Eds., *Facts and Models of Hearing*, Springer-Verlag, New York, 1974.

78. N.Y.-S. Kiang, E. C. Moxon, and R. A. Levine, in G. E. W. Wolstenholme and J. Knight, Eds., *Sensorineural Hearing Loss*, Churchill, London, 1970, pp. 241–268.

79. M. L. Wiederhold, *J. Acoust. Soc. Am.*, **48,** 966 (1970).

80. E. F. Evans, in E. Zwicker and E. Terhardt, Eds., *Facts and Models in Hearing*, Springer-Verlag, New York, 1974, pp. 118–129.

81. N.Y.-S. Kiang, and E. C. Moxon, *J. Acoust. Soc. Am.*, **55,** 620 (1974).

82. D. Robertson, *Science*, **186,** 153 (1974).

83. P. Dallos, A. Ryan, D. Harris, T. McGee, and O. Ozdamar, in E. F. Evans and J. P. Wilson, Eds., *Psychophysics and Physiology of Hearing*, Academic, New York, 1977, pp. 249–258.

84. R. V. Harrison and E. F. Evans, in E. F. Evans and J. P. Wilson, Eds., *Psychophysics and Physiology of Hearing*, Academic, New York, 1977, p. 259.

85. E. F. Evans, *J. Physiol. London*, **238,** 65P (1974).

86. E. F. Evans and R. Klinke, *J. Physiol. London*, **242,** 129P (1974).

87. R. Klinke and J. Smolders, in E. F. Evans and J. P. Wilson, Eds., *Psychophysics and Physiology of Hearing*, Academic, New York, 1977, pp. 109–111.

88. P. Dallos, in E. F. Evans and J. P. Wilson, Eds., *Psychophysics and Physiology of Hearing*, Academic, New York, 1977, p. 260.

89. N.Y.-S. Kiang, E. C. Moxon, and A. R. Kahn, in R. J. Ruben, C. Elberling, and G. Salomon, Eds., *Electrocochleography*, University Park Press, Baltimore, 1976, pp. 95–115.

90. W. A. Rosenblith and M. R. Rosenzweig, *J. Acoust. Soc. Am.*, **23,** 583 (1951).

91. J. D. Durrant and M. L. Ronis, *Ann. Otol. Rhinol. Laryngol.*, **84,** 88 (1975).

92. A. C. Coats and J. R. Dickey, *Ann. Otol. Rhinol. Laryngol.*, **79,** 844 (1970).

93. J. K. Cullen, Jr., M. S. Ellis, C. I. Berlin, and R. J. Lousteau, *Acta Oto Laryngol.*, **74,** 15 (1972).

94. M. H. Goldstein and N.Y.-S. Kiang, *J. Acoust. Soc. Am.*, **30,** 107 (1958).

95. W. T. Peake and N.Y.-S. Kiang, *Biophys. J.*, **2,** 23 (1962).

96. R. A. Dobie, in R. W. Keith, Ed., *Audiology for the Physician*, Williams and Wilkins, Baltimore, 1980, pp. 110–142.

97. H. Davis, in W. A. Rosenblith, Ed., *Sensory Communication*, Wiley, New York, 1961, pp. 119–141.

98. R. P. Bobbin and M. H. Thompson, *Ann. Otol. Rhinol. Laryngol.*, **87,** 185 (1978).

99. C.-Y. Wang and P. Dallos, *J. Acoust. Soc. Am.*, **52,** 1678 (1972).

100. R. P. Bobbin and M. I. Gondra, *Neuropharmacology*, **12,** 1005 (1973).

101. D. L. Kisiel, "Interaction of Intense Sound with Aminooxyacetic Acid and Ethacrynic Acid," Doctoral Dissertation, Memphis State University, Memphis, May 1979.

102. P. Dallos, D. Harris, O. Ozdamar, and A. Ryan, *J. Acoust. Soc. Am.*, **64,** 151 (1978).

103. C. H. Norris, J. Garcia-Quiroga, and P. S. Guth, *Toxicol. Appl. Pharmacol.*, **43,** 317 (1978).

104. A. J. Derbyshire and H. Davis, *Am. J. Physiol.*, **133,** 476 (1935).

105. R. P. Bobbin, *Exp. Brain Res.*, **34,** 389 (1979).

106. R. P. Bobbin and D. N. Morgan, "Actions of Glutamate, Aspartate, and Related Substances on the Spontaneous Activity of Afferent Nerves in the Toad (*Xeonpus laevis*)," presented at the Association for Research in Otolaryngology (ARO), St. Petersburg Beach, Florida, January 22–24, 1979.

107. D. L. Jewett, M. N. Romano, and J. S. Williston, *Science*, **167,** 1517 (1970).

108. D. L. Jewett and J. S. Williston, *Brain*, **94,** 681 (1971).

109. H. Sohmer and M. Feinmesser, *Isr. J. Med. Sci.*, **6,** 219 (1970).

110. A. Lev and H. Sohmer, *Arch. Klin. Exp. Ohren. Nasen. Kehlkopfheilk.*, **201,** 79 (1972).

111. J. S. Buchwald and C.-M. Huang, *Science*, **189,** 382 (1975).

112. K. Hecox and R. Galambos, *Arch. Otolaryngol.*, **99,** 30 (1974).

113. J. K. Cullen, Jr., C. I. Berlin, M. I. Gondra, and M. L. Adams, *Arch. Otolaryngol.*, **102,** 482 (1976).

114. H. Davis, *Ann. Otol. Rhinol. Laryngol.* **85,** Suppl. 28, 1 (1976).

115. C. I. Berlin and R. A. Dobie, in W. F. Rintelmann, Ed., *Hearing Assessment*, University Park Press, Baltimore, 1979, pp. 425–458.

116. C. I. Berlin, in F. N. Martin, Ed., *Pediatric Audiology*, Prentice-Hall, Englewood Cliffs, NJ, 1978, pp. 113–173.

117. T. J. Meunier, Jr., and J. G. May, *Am. Speech Hear. Assoc.*, **18,** 658 (1976).

118. R. P. Bobbin, J. G. May, and R. L. Lemoine, *Arch. Otolaryngol.*, **105,** 467 (1979).

119. J. T. Marsh and F. G. Worden, *Laryngoscope*, **78,** 1149 (1968).

120. L. J. Saul and H. Davis, *Arch. Neurol. Psychiatry*, **28,** 1104 (1932).

121. G. Moushegian, A. L. Rupert, and R. D. Stillman, *Electroencephalogr. Clin. Neurophysiol.*, **35,** 665 (1973).

122. G. M. Gerken, G. Moushegian, R. D. Stillman, and A. L. Rupert, *Electroencephalogr. Clin. Neurophysiol.*, **38,** 379 (1975).

123. D. M. Daly, R. J. Roeser, and G. Moushegian, *Electroencephalogr. Clin. Neurophysiol.*, **40,** 132 (1976).

124. R. D. Stillman, G. Moushegian, and A. L. Rupert, *Audiology*, **15,** 10 (1976).

125. J. Gardi, "The Scalp-Recorded Frequency Following Response: Its Origins, Its Frequency Specificity, and Its Clinical Applicability," Doctoral Dissertation, University of California, San Francisco, Velobind, Inc., San Francisco, 1978.

126. S. C. Bledsoe, Jr., "The 500 Hertz Frequency-Following Potential in Kangaroo Rat (*Dipodomys Spectabilis*): An Analysis of Its Frequency Specificity," Doctoral Dissertation, University of Texas Health Science Center of Dallas, 1979.

127. C. C. McRandle, M. A. Smith, and R. Goldstein, *Ann. Otol. Rhinol. Laryngol.*, **83,** 695 (1974).

128. R. Goldstein and C. C. McRandle, in S. K. Hirsch, D. H. Eldredge, I. J. Hirsh, and S. R. Silverman, Eds., *Hearing and Davis: Honoring Hallowell Davis*, Washington University Press, St. Louis, 1976, pp. 445–456.

129. M. I. Mendel, C. D. Adkinson, and L. A. Harker, *Ann. Otol. Rhinol. Laryngol.*, **86,** 293 (1977).

130. R. Goldstein and D. C. Kendall, *J. Speech Hear. Disord.*, **28,** 331 (1963).

131. H. Davis, P. A. Osterhammel, C. C. Wier,and D. B. Gjerdingen, *Electroencephalogr. Clin. Neurophysiol.*, **33,** 537 (1975).

132. M. I. Mendel, E. C. Hosick, T. R. Windman, H. Davis, S. K. Hirsh, and D. F. Dinges, *Electroencephalogr. Clin. Neurophysiol.*, **38,** 27 (1975).

133. R. Klinke and N. Galley, *Physiol. Rev.*, **54,** 316 (1974).

134. J. E. Desmedt, in W. D. Keidel and W. D. Neff, Eds., *Handbook of Sensory Physiology: Auditory System*, Vol V/2, Springer-Verlag, New York, 1975, pp. 219–246.

135. P. S. Guth, C. H. Norris, and R. P. Bobbin, *Pharmacol. Rev.*, **28,** 95 (1976).

136. R. Galambos, *J. Neurophysiol.*, **19,** 424 (1956).

137. J. E. Desmedt, *J. Acoust. Soc. Am.*, **34,** 1478 (1962).

138. H. S. Sohmer, *Acta Oto Laryngol.*, **60,** 59 (1965).

139. M. L. Wiederhold and W. T. Peake, *J. Acoust. Soc. Am.*, **40,** 1427 (1966).

140. T. Konishi and J. Z. Slepian, *J. Acoust. Soc. Am.*, **49,** 1762 (1971).

141. J. Fex, *Acta Physiol. Scand.*, **55,** Suppl. **189,** 1 (1962).

142. M. L. Wiederhold and N.Y.-S. Kiang, *J. Acoust. Soc. Am.*, **48,** 950 (1970).

143. D. C. Teas, T. Konishi, and D. W. Nielsen, *J. Acoust. Soc. Am.*, **51,** 1256 (1972).

144. J. E. Desmedt and V. LaGrutta, *Nature*, **200,** 472–474 (1963).

145. H. S. Sohmer, *Acta Oto Laryngol.*, **62,** 74 (1966).

146. J. Fex, *Acta Oto Laryngol.*, **50,** 540 (1959).

147. J. E. Desmedt and P. Monaco, *Nature,* **192,** 1263 (1961).

148. J. Fex, *J. Acoust. Soc. Am.* **41,** 666 (1967).

149. J. D. Durrant and D. Gans, *Acta Oto Laryngol.*, **80,** 13 (1975).

150. J. Fex, in A. V. S. de Reuck and J. Knight, Eds., *Ciba Foundation Symposium on Hearing Mechanisms in Vertebrates*, Churchill, London, 1968, pp. 169–181.

151. A. Starr and A. S. Wernick, *J. Neurophysiol.*, **31,** 549 (1968).

151a. J. H. Siegel and D. O. Kim, *Neurosci. Abstr.*, **6,** 41 (1980).

152. J. H. Dewson, III, *J. Neurophysiol.*, **31,** 122 (1968).

153. C. Trahiotis and D. N. Elliott, *J. Acoust. Soc. Am.*, **47,** 592 (1970).

154. M. J. Capps and H. W. Ades, *Exp. Neurol.*, **21,** 147 (1968).

155. L. C. Oatman, *Exp. Neurol.*, **32,** 341 (1971).

CHAPTER 3

Cochlear Biochemistry

ARTHUR MICHAEL FELDMAN, M.D., Ph.D.

Clinical Instructor of Otolaryngology
Louisiana State University
School of Medicine in Shreveport
Department of Otolaryngology
Shreveport, Louisiana

CONTENTS

3.1 INTRODUCTION

In the last decade our knowledge of the biochemical pathways on which the cochlea depends for normal cell functioning has increased dramatically. The level of knowledge of cochlear biochemistry, however, is well behind that of other organ systems. Because the small cochlear tissues are sequestered in a dense bony capsule, it is difficult to apply the techniques developed for the study of biochemical phenomena in more accessible secretory and neural tissues such as the kidney and brain. Despite these experimental difficulties, recent advances in technique and methodology have led to many promising results. This chapter is designed to provide the reader with a broad perspective of the accomplishments in the field of cochlear biochemistry, especially that of the cochlear membrane, and to provide a basis for the discussions in the succeeding chapters. A brief review of the biochemical pathways involved in each area is included and, wherever appropriate, more comprehensive reviews of specific areas of cochlear biochemistry have been cited.

3.2 BIOCHEMICAL METHODOLOGY IN THE COCHLEA

To appreciate fully and to analyze biochemical studies in the cochlea it is important to have a conceptual idea of the techniques available and of their limitations and advantages. There are three types of experimental approaches to the study of cochlear biochemistry:

1. Indirect studies.
2. Histochemistry.
3. Quantitative histochemistry and microchemical analysis.

3.2.1 Indirect Studies

Initially only indirect studies were applied to the study of the cochlea. These studies were based on the correlation between measurable physiological parameters and specific biochemical pathways known to be responsible for the maintenance of these parameters; for example, because it was well established that the endolymphatic potential (EP) was dependent on a high metabolic activity, any agent that decreased EP was thought to block cochlear metabolism. Because of advancing technology, however, most physiological parameters of the cochlea can now be measured. The techniques which have been well described include measurements of electrophysiological potentials such as the cochlear action potential (CAP), cochlear microphonics (CM), the endocochlear dc potential (EP),[1] fluid electrolyte concentrations,[2] fluid production,[3] and cochlear hydrostatic pressure.[4]

Pharmacologic agents for probing the role of specific enzyme systems in cochlear physiological systems have become available (see the review by Brown and Feldman[18]). The obvious limitation of this type of indirect approach is its lack of specificity; for example, although a fall in EP may well be due to a block in cellular metabolism, it can also be caused by a mechanical injury, changes in cell permeability, ischemia, changes in pH, or accumulation of toxic substances. Therefore indirect studies must be accompanied by measurements obtained by a different approach in order to substantiate the results.

3.2.2 Histochemical Studies

A popular model for the study of cochlear biochemistry has been the application of histochemical techniques to localize and quantify cochlear enzymes. The advantage of the technique, when used on a light or electron microscopic level, has been that it allows visualization of the chemical characteristics of individual cells without the disruption and fractionation methods of more classical biochemistry. The difficulties inherent in the technique are that cell structure must be maintained with fixatives without altering the characteristics of the enzyme system. In most cases compromises must be made between maintaining cellular structure and enzyme function.

Histochemical techniques have been applied extensively in the ear to study cochlear dehydrogenases.[5] This is done with electron acceptors that, on reduction, become insoluble and highly colored. The most popular electron acceptors in the study of the dehydrogenases are derivatives of tetrazolium salts that precipitate as insoluble, highly colored formazans. Steps in the experimental process include isolation of the cochlea, fixation (although the tissues are sometimes studied fresh), incubation with appropriate substances and electron acceptors, and preparation for light or electron microscopy. Scarpelli[6] has reviewed the advantages and disadvantages of the current methods of ultrastructural histochemistry. Accurate localization of enzymatic products depends on the following:

1. The nature and distribution of the substances.
2. The nonspecific binding of the electron acceptor.
3. The characteristics of the enzyme.
4. The solubility and visibility of the final reaction product.

In addition, successful results are dependent on homogeneous diffusion of fixative and substrate, minimal nonenzymatic hydrolysis of the substrate, and rapid reaction time.[5]

3.2.3 Quantitative Histochemical and Microchemical Analysis

One of the most productive techniques on the study of cochlear biochemistry has been the quantitative histochemical and cytochemical method developed by Thalmann and his coworkers.[7–8] This method, which is a modification of microanalytical techniques first described by Lowry,[9] has been reviewed more recently.[7] It consists of six basic steps:

1 The cochlea are rapidly frozen *in situ* with liquid Freon-12B or by placing the temporal bone in the coolant immediately after removal.
2 The temporal bone, if frozen *in situ,* is removed in a cryostat and burr holes are made in the cochlear shell and vestibule.
3 The cochleas are lyophilized for 24 hr.
4 Microdissection of the lyophilized samples is carried out at room temperature under conditions of low humidity. At this point morphological evaluations can be performed on representative sections to ensure the accuracy of the technique.
5 The amount of tissue recovered is quantitated by measuring the weight of the freeze-dried sample on a quartz fiber balance. It is also possible to measure the size of the sample by assaying for the concentration of tissue protein.
6 Chemical analysis can be performed on the cochlear samples. One method links enzymatic activity with the oxidation or reduction of pyridine nucleotides (NADT and NADPT). The changes in fluorescence are then measured directly or after enzyme cycling, which increases the quantity of the end product and the sensitivity of the assay. New radioimmunoassays developed by Hodgen and Falk[10] for cyclic AMP and cyclic GMP can also be applied to these samples. These techniques allow measurements in the femtomolar range and have been used to study cyclic AMP accumulation in small tissue samples such as the choroid plexus[93] and in small tissue slices.[10]

Although numerous techniques are available with which to study cochlear biochemistry, the investigator must keep several important points in mind:

1 Because of the bony encapsulation and small size of the membranous labyrinth, standard techniques must be modified for use in the ear.
2 Any technique represents a compromise between advantageous and disadvantageous qualities.
3 Because of the problems peculiar to inner-ear biochemistry, information must be gathered by several methods to ensure the reliability of the results.

3.3 STRUCTURAL COMPONENTS OF THE COCHLEA

Since the early studies of Danielli[11] in the 1950s it has been generally accepted that the plasma membranes of cells are composed of a lipid–protein "mosaic." The lipids isolate the cell from its environment and act as a two-dimensional solvent for the macromolecules. The proteins reinforce the lipid bilayer, promote selective interchange between the cell and its environment, act as receptors, and provide polar pathways through which substances can be transported across the thickness of the membrane. The Danielli model consists of two lipid layers arranged tail to tail and surrounded on both sides by layers of bound protein which penetrate the lipids in some places. On the outside surface of the bound protein is a layer of loosely attached, absorbed protein that acts to buffer the membrane against stresses and also serves as a receptor site. More recently Singer[12] visualized the proteins as being folded up and embedded by a hydrophobic end in the interior of the lipid bilayer and having a hydrophilic end projecting into the aqueous medium surrounding the membrane (Figure 3.1). In some cases the protein can have two hydrophilic ends projecting on either side of the membrane and a hydrophobic middle to hold it in place; these proteins could facilitate transport through membrane protein channels. Research to date indicates that this model is compatible with known membrane functions and physiology. The protein portion of the membrane is probably composed of numerous different proteins whose isolation is currently of great interest to researchers who are studying membrane structure and transport across membranes. Membrane lipids are composed of a three-carbon glyceryl framework. Attached to the carbons are two long-chain fatty acids and a polar group. The two primary classifications of membrane lipids are the phospholipids and the sphingolipids. The phospholipids contain two fatty-acid chains linked by ester bonds (usually a saturated and an unsaturated) and a polar group that contains phosphate. The sphingolipids differ in that the first fatty-acid chain always contains 15 carbons and is linked by a carbon-carbon bond, whereas the second chain, which can be one of a

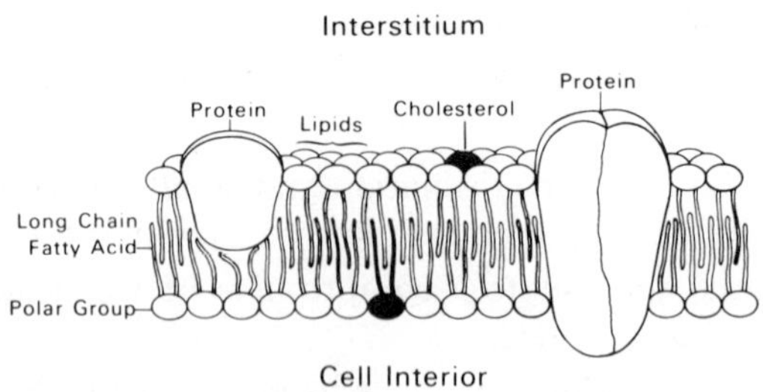

Figure 3.1 Three-dimensional illustration of the membrane model as described by Singer.[12] Large globular proteins protrude from the membrane. Those that pass through the membrane contain transport pores, whereas those that are embedded in the membrane serve as "active sites." (Redrawn from Singer.[12])

number of fatty acids, is linked by an amide bond. The polar group of the sphingolipids may be a phosphate-plus-choline structure (sphingomyelin), a simple hydroxyl (ceramides), a simple sugar (cerebrosides), or a complex polysaccharide (gangliosides).[13] Various membranes contain different combinations of lipids. Lipid membranes do not appear to be rigid in nature and the fatty-acid chains appear to have considerable mobility. Therefore, rather than a crystalline gel, lipids take the form of a liquid crystal. The fluidity in the lipid membrane is controlled by several variables, including temperature and fatty-acid composition, the fluidity being greater at higher temperatures and shorter chain lengths. It is evident that protein function and membrane permeability are dependent on the fluidity of the membrane and that the lipid fluidity can be altered by the polar group binding of ions (Na^+, K^+, and Ca^{2+}), proteins, or drugs.[13]

3.3.1 Phospholipids

Recent studies have been directed toward the role of membrane phospholipids, in particular of the phosphoinositides in the cochlea.[14] Current research on phosphoinositol has been reviewed by Hawthorne and White,[15] and it is generally accepted that the secretory functions of a wide variety of cells is accompanied by an increased turnover in phosphotidylinositol and phosphatidic acid but not in the other phospholipids (Figure 3.2). This increase in activity is most often seen as an increase in ^{32}P labeling. After perfusing the perilymphatic compartment of the cochlea with ^{32}P orthophosphate (which is converted *in vivo* to ^{32}P ATP) Stockhorst and Schacht[14] found that the phosphoinositides incorporated ^{32}P more rapidly than any other phospholipids and that the highest rate of labeling occurred in the stria vascularis, followed by the organ of Corti and the spiral ligament. Perfusion of the perilymphatic channels with 10^{-4}–$10^{-2}M$ neomycin caused a dose-related decrease in ^{32}P incorporation into phosphotidylinositol diphosphate in the stria vascularis and organ of Corti[14] and had a similar effect when for three weeks[16] the drug (100 mg/kg) was administered subcutaneously. In addition, neomycin inhibited the binding of Ca^{2+} to the phosphoinositides,[17] which would imply that the ototoxicity of neomycin could be the result of interference with membrane Ca^{2+} uptake. Low concentrations of neomycin *in vitro* form a complex with polyphosphoinositides and it is possible that this is the mechanism of neomycin ototoxicity. To conclude a causal relationship,[14,16,17] however, it must be determined whether cochlear drug concentrations used in the experimental studies are reached in clinical situations.[18]

3.3.2 Proteins

Although the proteins of the whole guinea pig cochlea have been electrophoretically separated,[19] little biochemistry has been applied to their iso-

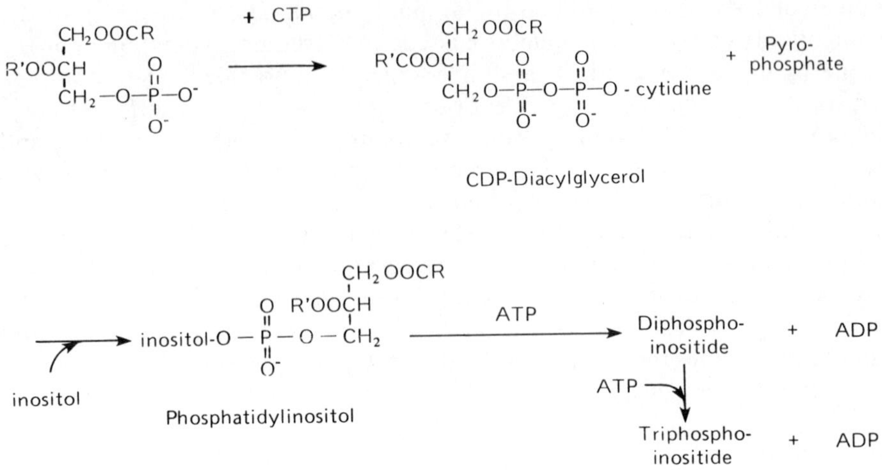

Figure 3.2 Biosynthesis of the phosphoinositides.

lation and characterization. Stockhorst and Schacht[14] and their coworkers were able to separate and measure proteins from the organ of Corti, spiral ligament, and stria vascularis with disk electrophoresis and ^{35}S-methionine, ^{3}H-methionine, and ^{3}H-leucine to mark the proteins. Considerable variation was seen in the peaks from the different cochlear structures, and neomycin treatment appeared to have no effect on amino acid incorporation into the cochlear proteins.

3.3.3 Mucopolysaccharides

The epithelial cells of most secretory membranes are covered by an outer cell coat which looks "fuzzy" when the cell membrane is viewed with an electron microscope. This coat consists of three major components:

1. The carbohydrate moities of glycolipids, particularly the cerebrosides and gangliosides.
2. Glycoproteins.
3. Acid mucopolysaccharides.[20]

The acid mucopolysaccharides have interested otolaryngologists because of the high frequency of deafness in cases of mucopolysaccharidosis. Although the exact role of mucopolysaccharides in physiologic and pathophysiologic conditions has not yet been established, it has been proposed that they function to control electrolyte and water in the extracellular spaces.[21] The two most abundant mucopolysaccharides are hyaluronic acid, a linear polymer composed of repeating units of D-glucuronic acid and *N*-acetyl-D-glucosamine, and chondroitin, which differs from hyaluronic acid in that it contains *N*-acetyl-D-galactosamine instead of *N*-acetyl-D-glucosamine. The sulfate ester derivatives of chondroitin, chondroitin sulfate A and C, are major components of connective tissue. Saito and Daly[22] found that the tectorial membrane and Reissner's membrane contained 0.1% of acid mucopolysaccharides per dry weight, whereas the stria vascularis and the basilar membrane contained 0.6%. Using a more sensitive method, electrophoretic microanalysis, Saito et al.[21] found that the lateral wall of the cochlea contained the highest concentration of mucopolysaccharides. Of the total mucopolysaccharide measured 75% was chondroitin sulfate B, 12% was chondroitin sulfate A, and 13% was hyaluronic acid. The major components in the cochlear wall differed from those in kidney, brain, and liver and the total quantity of mucopolysaccharides was higher than in other organs. Saito and Daly[23] found that kanamycin-induced ototoxicity in guinea pigs was associated with a decrease in the quantities of mucopolysaccharides in the stria vascularis and spiral ligament. They proposed that the decrease was due to the formation of drug-mucopolysaccharide complexes, which were then digested by fibroblasts, and to inhibition of mucopolysaccharide synthesis. The role of the decreased mucopolysaccharides in the etiology of kanamycin-induced ototoxicity remains an interesting problem.

3.4 REVIEW OF ANAEROBIC AND AEROBIC METABOLISM

The life of the cell, and therefore the physiological functioning of all organ systems, depends on the ability of the cell to convert substrates into energy aerobically and anaerobically in the form of ATP or phosphocreatine (Figure 3.3). When ATP stores are exhausted by molecular synthesis or active transport, phosphocreatine yields its Pi to ADP to form ATP and creatine, a reaction catalyzed by creatine phosphokinase. Although the biochemical reactions involved in cellular energy production have been described by Lehninger[20] and others,[24,25] it would seem appropriate to review the major steps in metabolism briefly before discussing current theories in cochlear energy production and use.

Anaerobic metabolism, or glycolysis, occurs in two major stages. In the first glucose is enzymatically phosphorylated by ATP to glucose-6-phosphate and changed to fructose-6-phosphate (by the action of phosphohexose isomerase), which is phosphorylated to form fructose-1,6-diphosphate. Fructose-1,6-diphosphate is then cleaved to form two molecules of glyceraldehyde-3-phosphate. Glucose residues of glycogen and starch can also enter the glycolytic chain at this point by the enzymatic activity of glycogen phosphorylase and phosphoglucomutase. In the second stage of glycolysis glyceraldehyde phosphate is oxidized to 1,3-

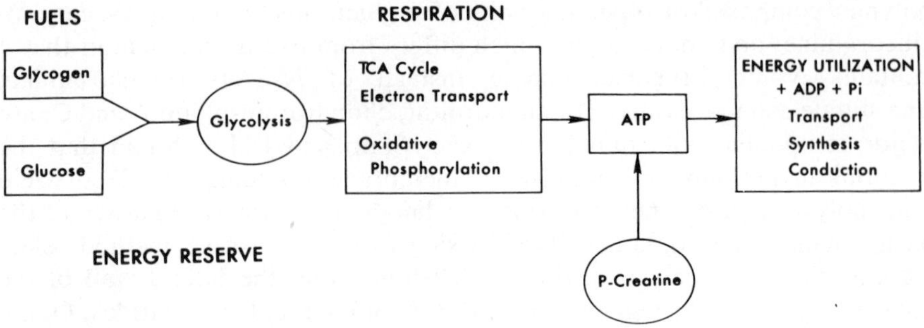

Figure 3.3 A diagrammatic model of normal energy production and utilization.

diphosphoglycerate, with the result that NADH is formed from NAD, and on to pyruvate through a sequence of reactions. The NADH is reconverted to NAD in the last step of glycolysis when pyruvate is reduced to lactate by lactate dehydrogenase. Although two molecules of ATP are required to prime glycolysis, four ATPs are formed by glycolysis to give a net yield of two ATPs. The rate-limiting step in glycolysis is the phosphorylation of fructose 6-phosphate to fructose 1,6-diphosphate by phosphofructokinase.

In aerobic metabolism pyruvate is converted into acetyl CoA and shunted through the mitochondrial tricarboxylic acid cycle. The overall rate is controlled by the isocitrate-dehydrogenase reaction. During the cycle the pyridine-linked isocitrate, α-ketoglutarate dehydrogenase, and flavin-linked succinate dehydrogenase, catalyze the transfer of H^+ to NAD, NADP, and FAD, respectively, and result in the formation of NADH, NADPH, and FADH. In a series of reactions pairs of electrons flow down a chain of electron carrier enzymes, a process that conserves energy because of the successively lower energy level of each step. This chain is referred to as the electron transport system and the free energy that is conserved results in the coupled phosphorylation of ADP to ATP by a process called oxidative phosphorylation. This sequence of events results in the net production of 35 ATP molecules from one molecule of glucose.

3.5 COCHLEAR METABOLISM

Since Bekesy's[26] early calculations were made it has been apparent that the sensory response of the inner ear depends on an abundant energy supply obtained from metabolic activity and it was suggested that energy might be produced by metabolic activity in the stria vascularis.[27] Wever et al.[28] found that extreme oxygen deprivation caused a rapid decrease in cochlear potentials and Kimura and Perlman[29] observed similar results with hypoxia, anoxia, and occlusion of the arterial supply to the cochlea.

3.5.1 Respiratory Enzymes

Early studies in which light and electron microscopic histochemical techniques were used showed the presence of respiratory enzymes in the stria vascularis and organ of Corti; deficiencies in these techniques, however, led to results that were difficult to interpret[30–33]. For example, little succinic dehydrogenase or lactic dehydrogenase activity was seen in the stria vascularis, probably because of the failure of the incubation medium to penetrate the stria.[33] Stack and Webster[34] found that, at rest, tricarboxylic acid cycle enzymes were present in the sensory epithelium, stria vascularis, spiral ligament, and external spiral sulcus. Sowinski[35] demonstrated histochemically that the intracellular location of the dehydrogenases was identical in the inner and outer hair cells, stria vascularis, and spiral ligament. Quantitatively, activities of these enzymes are highest in the stria vascularis and higher in the outer than in the inner hair cells. This work is supported by the elegant *in vitro* studies of Thalmann and coworkers[36–40] (see Table 3.1). In the first application of their technique these investigators found no difference between levels of the pyridine nucleotides NAD, NADH, NADP, and NADPH in the organ of Corti compared with the stria vascularis. After ischemia the NADH/NAD ratio increased in both tissues.[36] In subsequent studies they found that levels of enzymes of glycolysis and the pentose-phosphate pathway were almost the same in the organ of Corti and stria vascularis but were an order of magnitude lower in Reissner's membrane.[41] Enzymes of the tricarboxylic acid cycle were two to three times higher in stria vascularis than in the organ of Corti and the activity in Reissner's membrane was even lower than in the organ of Corti. Activities of these enzymes in the stria vascularis and organ of Corti were not differentially graded from base to apex of the cochlea. These findings are generally consistent with earlier studies[42] based on the Cartesian Diver method which showed that oxygen consumption in the stria vascularis was high when compared with the liver and kidney, whereas oxygen consumption in the spiral ligament and organ of Corti was low (Table 3.2). Although this report suggests that the energy supply of the organ of Corti and stria vascularis depends largely on oxidative metabolism, it appears that the organ of Corti has a greater dependence on glycolysis than the stria vascularis, but the stria has an abundance of respiratory enzymes consistent with its high metabolic rate and secretory function. Furthermore, it is believed that much of the energy supply needed by the hair cells for electrical transduction is provided by the stria vascularis.[37,43]

3.5.2 Energy Production and Use

Thalmann and his coworkers[37–40] have provided considerable evidence to show variations between energy production and use in the stria vascularis

Table 3.1 *In vitro* Activity of Cochlear Metabolic Enzymes from Thalmann[37] [a]

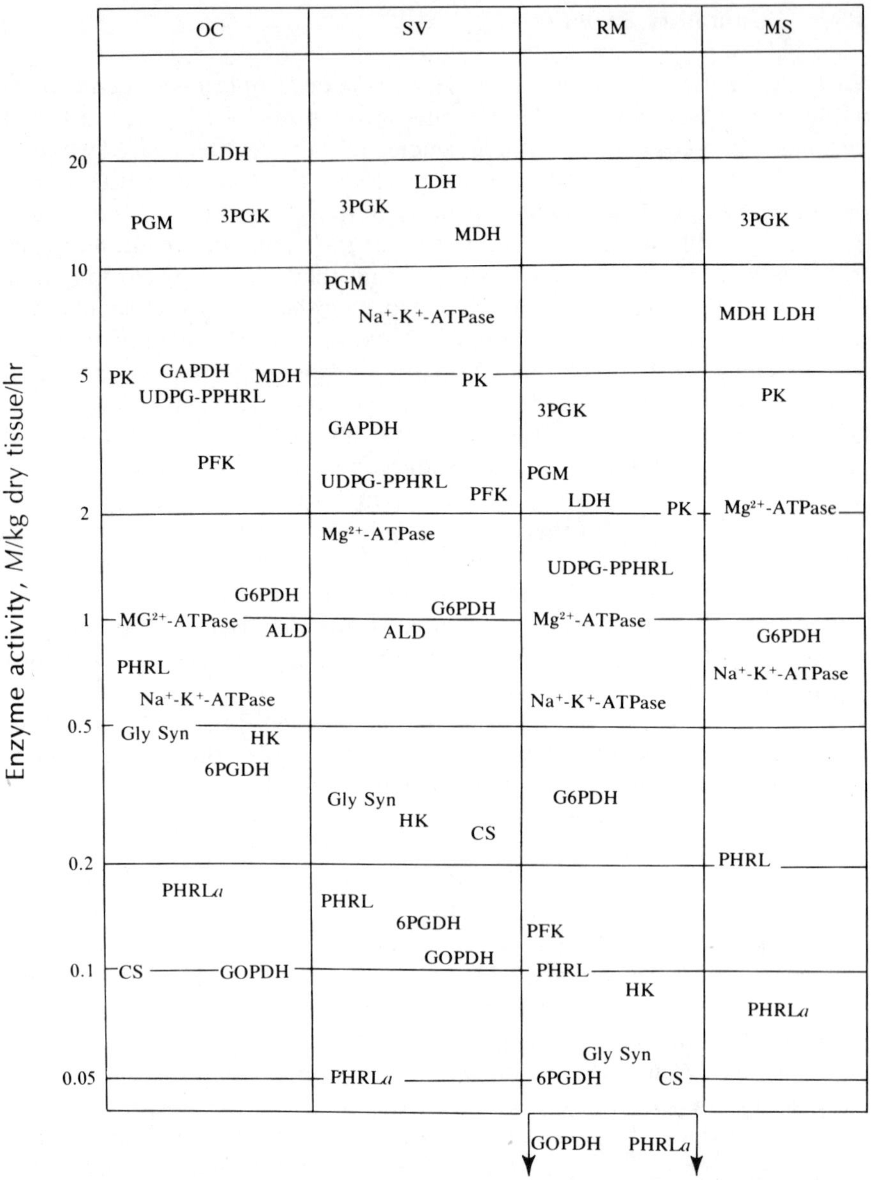

[a]ALD—aldolase. CS—citrate synthetase, GAPDH—glyceraldehyde-P-dehydrogenase, Gly Syn — glycogen synthetase, GOPDH — glycerol-l-P dehydrogenase, G6PDH—glucose-6-P-dehydrogenase, HK—hexokinase, LDH—lactate dehydrogenase, MDH—malate dehydrogenase,PFK—phosphofructokinase, 6PGDH—6-P-gluconate dehydrogenase, 3PGK—3-P-glycerate kinase, PGM—phosphoglucomutase, PHRL—phosphorylase, PHRL*a*—phosphorylase *a*, PK—pyruvate kinase, UDPG-PPHRL—UDPG-pyrophosphorylase, OC—organ of Corti, SV—stria vascularis, RM—Reissner's membrane, MS—macula sacculi, MU—macula utriculi. CA—crista ampullaris, AW—ampullar wall, SCC—semicircular canal.

Table 3.1 (Continued)

MU	CA	AW	SCC	
				20
3PGK				10
LDH MDH PK	LDH MDH	3PGK LDH		5
	G6PDH PK	MDH	LDH MDH PK	2
Mg^{2+}-ATPase G6PDH	Mg^{2+}-ATPase	Mg^{2+}ATPase	Mg^{2+}-ATPase	1
Na^+-K^+-ATPase	Na^+-K^+–ATPase	Na^+-K^+-ATPase G6PDH	G6PDH	0.5
PHRL	PHRL		Na^+-K^+-ATPase	0.2
				0.1
PHRL*a*	PHRL*a*			0.05

Table 3.2 Oxygen Consumption of Guinea Pig Cochlear Tissues Adapted From Chou and Hughes.[42]

Tissue	Oxygen consumption $\mu l\ O_2$/mg dry wt/hr ± SE
Stria vascularis	10.1 ± 0.9
Spiral ligament	0.8 ± 0.5
Organ of Corti	0.9 ± 0.2
Sacculus wall	3.8 ± 0.7
Utriculus wall	0.7 ± 0.1
Liver	2.4 ± 0.3
Kidney	6.7 ± 0.7

and the organ of Corti. In experimentally induced anoxia or ischemia CM falls and the EP reverses polarity.[40] These changes are closely associated with decreases in ATP levels in the stria vascularis, despite accelerated glycolysis and phosphorylation out of the phosphocreatine pool (Figure 3.4). In the organ of Corti there is only a slow decline in ATP levels in individual outer hair cells and in the organ as a whole. It appears that the decline in CM parallels the decline in EP and these declines are due to exhaustion of energy supplies in the stria vascularis.[37] Although the decline in EP is rapid, it should be noted that the revival of the stria vascularis is slow. Thalmann and his coworkers[37,44] also found that the energy-use rate in the stria vascularis was high, although its energy reserve was comparatively low. Paradoxically, the organ of Corti, which has a much lower energy-use rate, had much higher energy reserves. Thalmann and coworkers proposed that the dependence of the organ of Corti on glycogen metabolism is functionally correlated. Although the efficiency of the glycolytic pathway is poor, it can be rapidly activated in the presence or absence of oxygen and is therefore well adapted to the sudden changes in work load that occur in the sensory apparatus of the ear. The poor efficiency of the system predicates a large reserve of high-energy stores; however, it is also possible that the predominance of glycolysis in the organ of Corti is an adaptation to low levels of tissue oxygen. This theory is supported by the finding that when the perilymphatic space is perfused with iodoacetate, a potent inhibitor of glycolysis, there is a rapid reduction in CM and in the ATP levels in the organ of Corti.[43] The reduction in ATP is greatest in the apical turns of the cochlea, the portion that contains the highest concentration of glycogen and might depend the most on glycolysis.

3.5.3 Energy Sources

Studies of the energy sources of the cochlea have yielded interesting results, some of which are unexplained as well as controversial. Thalmann and his coworkers[37,39,41] proposed that glycogen serves as the primary energy reserve in the organ of Corti. Although both the organ of Corti and the stria

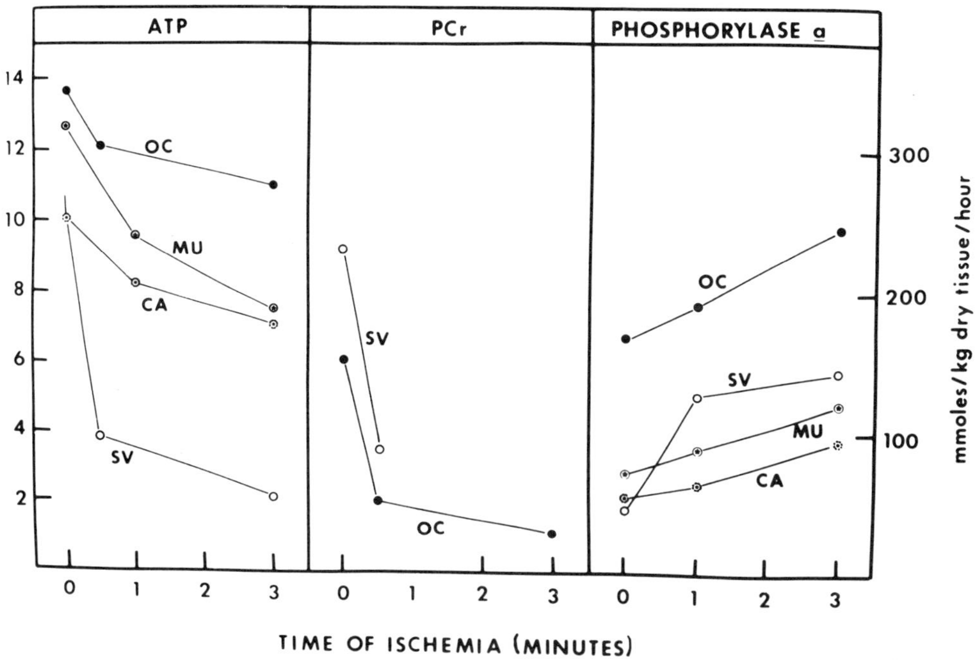

Figure 3.4 Influence of short-term ischemia on levels of ATP, phosphocreatine (PCr), and phosphorylase *a* in the guinea pig inner ear. (From Thalmann.[8]) Left ordinate = mmole/kg dry weight/hr ATP and PCr; right ordinate = mmole/kg dry weight/hr PHOSPHORYLASE *a*. (CA – crista ampullaris, MU – macula utriculi, OC – organ of Corti, SV – stria vascularis.)

vascularis of the guinea pig contain substantial amounts of glycogen, the levels of glycogen in the organ of Corti increase progressively from the basal to the more apical turns (Figure 3.5). The largest glycogen stores were found in the outer hair cells; lower levels occurred in the inner hair cells and in the Hensen and Deiters cell layers.[37,41] Ishii et al.[45] found that the histochemical localization of glycogen was species-dependent. The greatest amount of glycogen was contained in the Deiters' cells of the mouse and the outer hair cells of the guinea pig but was not seen at all in the cat. They also found that exposure to noise decreased the amount of glycogen in the outer hair cells. Aminoglycoside-induced ototoxicity has also been associated with glycogen concentrations. In guinea pigs treated with tobramycin the most susceptible outer hair cells were those that contained the smallest amount of glycogen.[46] Glycogen content also decreases after ischemia in the organ of Corti.[40] Another study that confirmed the role of glycogen in cochlear energy production was the histochemical work of Duvall and Hukee,[47] who discovered that glycogen appeared in the form found in tissues that need a continuous supply of energy, such as the kidney and cardiac muscle, rather than in the form associated with storage and seen in the liver. Glycolysis appears to be of little significance in the stria vascularis aside from its role in producing pyruvate for entry into the tricarboxylic acid cycle. Although it is generally

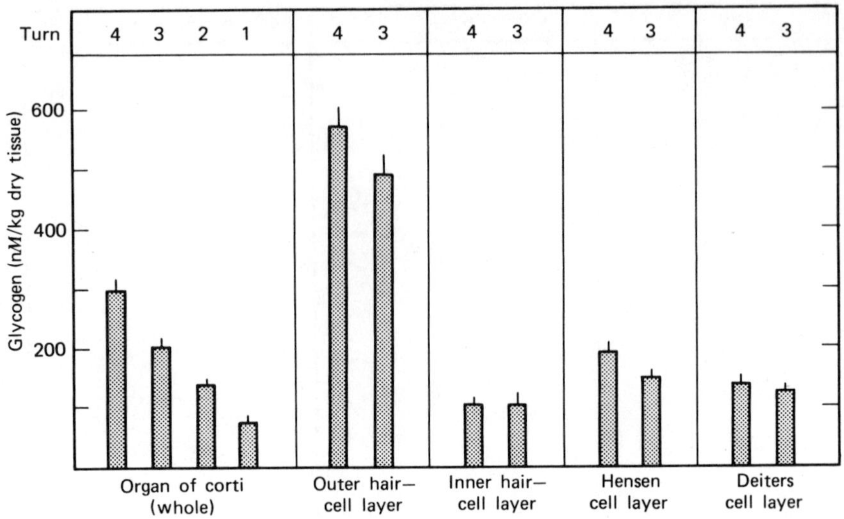

Figure 3.5 Glycogen levels in different turns of the cochlea and cell layers of the organ of Corti. (From Thalmann et al.[127])

accepted that EP is maintained by aerobic metabolism, Thalmann et al.[43] found in preliminary investigations that glycolysis might support the EP under certain conditions.

Tachibana et al.[48] demonstrated that drug-induced inhibition of glycolysis in the organ of Corti could account for the ototoxicities of some pharmacologic agents. The aminoglycoside kanamycin caused a decrease in the activities of the Embden-Meyerhof pathway in the organ of Corti but had no effect on its hexose-monophosphate pathway or the Embden-Meyerhof and hexose-monophosphate pathways in the stria vascularis. Similar results were produced in the kidney (which is susceptible to kanamycin-induced toxicity) but not in the liver or brain. Furthermore, kanamycin suppresses respiratory and possibly ATPase activity in the organ of Corti.[18,49,50]

The metabolism of phosphocreatine in the cochlea has also been studied by Thalmann and his coworkers.[38,51] Although phosphocreatine shows a concentration gradient within the cochlear turns, its concentration decreases in higher turns rather than increasing as glycogen does. Levels in the first two turns of the organ of Corti are higher than those found in the stria vascularis, whereas concentrations in the third and fourth turn of the organ of Corti and in Reissner's membrane are lower than those in the stria vascularis.[38,51] ATP levels were higher in the organ of Corti than in the stria vascularis, but they did not show an activity gradient along the length of the cochlea in either of these structures.[38,39,52] Although the organ of Corti depends primarily on glycolysis for its energy need and the stria vascularis on oxidative metabolism, it is evident that the physiological functioning of the cochlea is dependent on the integrity of both organ of Corti and stria vascularis metabolic pathways.

It has been proposed that the loop diuretics cause hearing loss by interrupting normal energy production as well as energy use in the stria vascularis,[49,53,54] but because they also affect membrane transport systems they are discussed in the next section of this chapter.

Early investigators felt that the endolymph provided the nourishment for the cells of the organ of Corti. It is now generally accepted, however, that the rich vascular supply provides the stria vascularis with metabolic substrates, whereas the cells of the organ of Corti receive their supplies from the perilymph through the cortilymph[55a] or by diffusion from the capillaries of the basilar membrane.[55b]

The organ of Corti and the stria vascularis contain significant quantities of amino acids[52]; the organ of Corti also contains lipid deposits in the Hensen cells. Thalmann et al.,[43] on the basis of their calculations of the respiratory quotients, proposed that carbohydrates serve as the primary energy source in the stria vascularis and organ of Corti. They also stated that a shortage of fuel plays no role in cochlear pathophysiology; this, however, has been disputed. Koide et al.[56] first reported a decrease in the CM of hypoglycemic cats. Later Juhn and Young[57,58] found that perilymph glucose levels closely reflected plasma glucose levels in the hyperglycemic and hypoglycemic states. Makimoto and Silverstein[59] found that although perilymph glucose levels decreased in hypoglycemia no effect could be seen on endolymph glucose concentrations or on CM. These results are in conflict with those of an earlier study which had shown an increase in the Na^+/K^+ ratio in the endolymph during hypoglycemia.[60] It is interesting that blood glucose changes were reflected in CSF and in the perilymph, whereas thyrocalcitonin induced hypocalcemia without a change in CSF or perilymph Ca^{2+} levels.[58]

Because studies to date have shown varied results, it would seem that further investigations are needed to clarify the relationship between substrate availability and cochlear function. The potential importance of this work is illustrated by several clinical studies which have shown a correlation between metabolic disorders, particularly hypoglycemia and diabetes mellitus, and fluctuant hearing loss.[55a,61] In addition, alterations in thyroid secretion have been associated clinically with changes in audition.[62]

3.6 SECRETORY ENZYMES IN THE COCHLEAR MEMBRANE

Na/K ATPase, carbonic anhydrase, and adenylate cyclase are known to be associated with electrolyte transport and fluid secretion in various organ systems. These three enzymes have begun to attract the interest of cochlear biochemists.

3.6.1 Adenosine Triphosphatase (ATPase)

Since its first description by Skou[63], ATPase has been studied in numerous tissues. These investigations have been reviewed by Skou[64] and Dahl and Hokin.[65] ATPase catalyzes the hydrolysis of ATP to ADP and Pi. Two types of enzyme have been studied. One is stimulated by magnesium ions and is known as magnesium ATPase; the other is stimulated by sodium and potassium as well as magnesium and is designated Na/K ATPase. The latter enzyme is inhibited by ouabain. It has been proposed that Na/K ATPase plays a role in active ion transport which is necessary for the maintenance of ion gradients in single cells, transport of salt and water across epithelial cells, and nerve and muscle repolarization.[65,66] Kuijpers et al.[67] and Bonting[68] found that Na/K ATPase is present and highly active in the cochlea and that it can be inhibited by perilymphatic perfusion with ouabain. This inhibition, however, was not visible after systemic administration of the drug. Subsequent studies[69] revealed that the enzyme is present in the stria vascularis and that its kinetics are similar to those in other tissues. Enzyme activity was not found in appreciable quantities in other portions of the cochlea, especially Reissner's membrane,[69] but Nakai and Hilding[70] demonstrated some activity on the outer surface of the cells of the organ of Corti. Activity in the stria vascularis decreased from base to apex,[69] and enzyme activity in the rat reached adult levels 19 to 25 days postpartum, a time that coincided with the functional maturity of the cochlea.[71]

Ouabain not only inhibited strial Na/K ATPase but it also decreased the EP and CM.[69,72,73] The relationship between the inhibition curves for Na/K ATPase and ouabain-induced decreases in endolymph K^+ and EP[68,69,72,73] was close. On the basis of these data it was suggested that the Na/K ATPase system of the stria vascularis was responsible for the maintenance of cochlear cation gradients, EP, and CM.[68] The Na^+/K^+ ratio in the endolymph, however, is not dramatically altered after ouabain inhibition of Na/K ATPase.[72] Furthermore, Brusilow and Gordes[74] showed that EP and the maintenance of the endolymphatic Na^+/K^+ gradient were not linked.

Because the loop diuretic ethacrynic acid decreases the EP in the guinea pig,[18] it was thought that it acted by an effect on Na/K ATPase. In the rat[74] inhibition of EP with ethacrynic acid failed to alter the endolymphatic Na^+/K^+ ratio except in high doses. Thalmann et al.[43,75] found that ethacrynic acid inhibits Na/K ATPase activity only at high concentrations (Figure 3.6) and that the stria vascularis does not accumulate this drug. Another loop diuretic, furosemide, has no effect on Na/K ATPase activity.[43] Therefore ATPase inhibition cannot account for the initial drop in EP.

The cochlear effect of ouabain does not appear to be due solely to an inhibition of Na/K ATPase. Thalmann et al.[43] found that when EP was maximally reduced by ouabain ATP levels were unchanged and phosphocreatine levels were increased in the stria vascularis. When ischemia was superimposed over the treatment with ouabain, a slow, rather than rapid,

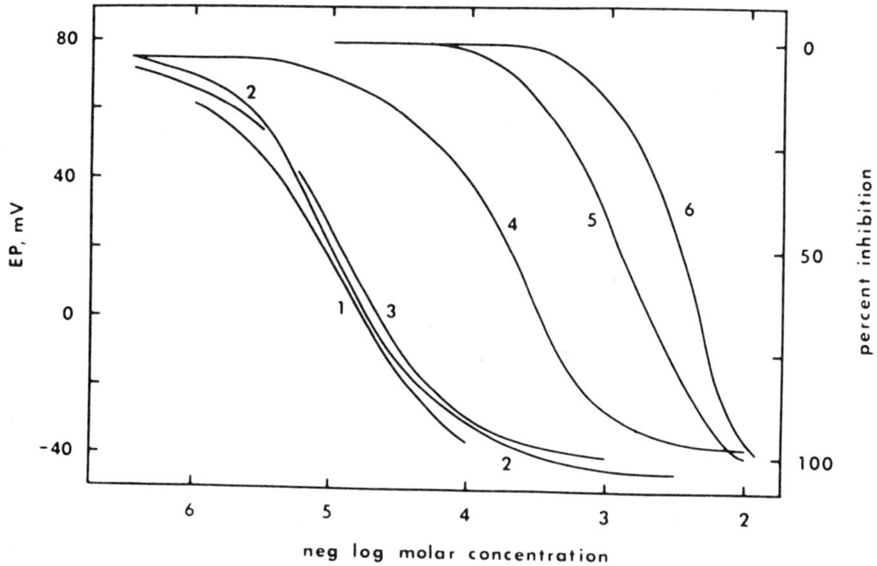

Figure 3.6 Inhibition curves for EP, strial Na/K ATPase and strial adenylate cyclase after exposure to loop diuretics from Thalmann et al.[43] Curves two and three, respectively, are the inhibition curves of the endolymphatic potential (left ordinate) and strial adenylate cyclase (7 min preincubation; right ordinate) with respect to ethacrynic acid. Curves four and one, respectively, are inhibition curves of the endolymphatic potential (left ordinate) and strial adenylate cyclase (15 min preincubation; right ordinate) with respect to furosemide. Curves five and six, respectively, represent the inhibition of strial Na/K ATPase *in vitro* with regard to ethacrynic acid with and without 30 min of preincubation.

decline in ATP and phosphocreatine levels was apparent. These results indicate that ouabain had a dramatic effect on cochlear energy use. Therefore it seems that linking Na/K ATPase activity with the maintenance of EP as well as the endolymphatic Na^+/K^+ ratio is probably an oversimplification of the mechanisms of fluid and electrolyte transport in the cochlea, especially when EP and the Na^+/K^+ ratio appear to be mutually independent. In the remainder of this chapter some of the other systems that might well participate in electrolyte transport and/or fluid secretion in the cochlea are discussed.

3.6.2 Carbonic Anhydrase

Since the initial description of carbonic anhydrase by Meldrum and Roughton[76] in 1932 this enzyme has been thoroughly studied; its chemistry and physiology have been extensively reviewed by Maren.[77] It has been found throughout the biologic community and in most mammalian organs. Carbonic anhydrase is defined as any enzyme that catalyzes the following reaction: $CO_2 + H_2O \leftrightharpoons H_2CO_3$. Subsequently H_2CO_3 is converted to HCO_3^- + H^+ by an uncatalyzed reaction. Although carbonic anhydrase is fundamental to the functioning of the bicarbonate buffering system, it might function also in anion, cation, and fluid secretion into the cerebrospinal fluid.[78,79,80] This theory is supported by the fact that administration of acetazolamide, an inhibitor of carbonic anhydrase activity, results in a 60% decrease in cerebrospinal fluid production.[81] Acetazolamide has also proved efficacious in the treatment of the excessive ocular fluid secretion associated with glaucoma. In addition, one group of investigators found that depression of proximal tubular reabsorption of electrolytes and water is facilitated by inhibition of carbonic anhydrase activity[82]; however, attempts to reproduce these data in another laboratory were unsuccessful.[83] Furthermore, gastric acid secretion in the gut has been associated with carbonic anhydrase stimulation.[84]

Erulkar and Maren[85] first measured carbonic anhydrase activity in the ear of the cat and found that its activity was high, greater than the activity found in whole blood. This activity increased in the apical portions of the cochlea. Drescher[86] purified carbonic anhydrase from the membranous lateral wall of the guinea pig cochlea which made up approximately 1% of the total protein in the membranous lateral wall; its activity was about twice that in whole blood. Although Erulkar and Maren[85] found that acetazolamide lowered potassium levels in the endolymph, Maren has questioned the results[87] and Silverstein and Yules[88] were unable to find alterations in the Na^+/K^+ ratio after systemic administration of acetazolamide. Also, acetazolamide is not efficacious in the treatment of endolymphatic hydrops (see discussion of this disease in Chapter 4). In studies of ion movements from plasma to endolymph in the dog fish Maren et al.[89] found that carbonic anhydrase inhibition decreased the rate of HCO_3^- accumulation, probably by reducing the hydration of tissue and plasma CO_2. They proposed that endolymph formation is the result of HCO_3^- formation linked with K^+ transport, the two reactions depending on catalysis by carbonic anhydrase and Na/K ATPase. This theory is supported by studies in the guinea pig in which carbonic anhydrase inhibition retarded the accumulation of HCO_3^- in endolymph (Saul Brusilow, personal communication of unpublished observations). Carbonic anhydrase clearly plays an important role in strial functioning; however, its specific function and relationship to endolymph secretion can only be speculated. Because the proposals for a secretory role of carbonic anhydrase are based primarily on experimental results obtained after inhibiting carbonic anhydrase with acetazolamide, the validity of this theory can be substantiated only after ascertaining that acetazolamide does not affect other secretory processes in these cells. Rodriquez et al.[90] found that not only did acetazolamide inhibit renal carbonic anhydrase but it also caused a significant increase in cyclic AMP accumulation, a substance associated with renal fluid and electrolyte movement. In the choroid plexus acetazolamide inhibited carbonic anhydrase and CSF production but had no effect on cyclic AMP production (Feldman, unpublished results). This is particularly significant in that cyclic AMP mediates CSF production.[91–93]

3.6.3 Adenylate Cyclase and Cyclic Nucleotides

The role of cyclic AMP in expressing the action of various hormones was first elucidated by Sutherland in the early 1960s.[94] Since these studies the cyclic nucleotides have been studied actively in a number of laboratories and the work has been reviewed extensively.[94–96] Cyclic AMP, found in every tissue studied, serves numerous and diverse functions. It mediates TSH stimulation of the thyroid gland, the renal response to parathyroid hormone, the effect of epinephrine, glucagon, and TSH on lipolysis in the fat depots, and the release of insulin by the pancreas.[95] Cyclic AMP is also thought to govern the secretory action of many epithelial cells. It initiates secretion of the anterior pituitary trophic hormones in response to hypothalamic releasing factors, absorption of water in the kidney in response to vasopressin, and calcium homeostasis in response to parathyroid hormone. The actions and enzymes involved in the adenylate cyclase-cyclic AMP system have been thoroughly studied in the epinephrine and glucagon-induced regulation of glycogen breakdown and synthesis.

It has been demonstrated that hormones bind to specific receptor sites located on the blood vascular side of a cell (Figure 3.7). The interaction of the hormone and the receptor initiates the stimulation of the membrane-bound adenylate cyclase with which it is associated. It appears that this activation might not occur directly but in the activation of an unknown compound called a transducer.[96] Adenylate cyclase catalyzes the formation of cyclic AMP from ATP. Cyclic AMP can then be metabolized by phosphodiesterase to the inactive 5′ AMP or bound to a specific protein kinase. The protein kinase then facilitates the phosphorylation of a membrane-bound or cytoplasmic protein.[96]

Ahlstrom et al.[97] first identified cyclic AMP in the stria vascularis and organ of Corti of the guinea pig cochlea. Base activities were comparable to those seen in other secretory epithelia but were lower than levels seen in the brain. Cyclic AMP *in vitro* had no effect on glycogen phosphorylase or Na/K ATPase. Perfusion of the perilymph with dibutyryl cyclic AMP, a derivative that crosses cell membranes more easily, produced a significant increase in the EP. In addition, catecholamines have been closely associated with adenylate cyclase activity in a number of tissues.[95,98] Therefore Ahlstrom[97] studied the effects of the α-adrenergic blocking agent phentolamine and found that it produced an initial increase and secondary decrease in the EP. As a consequence they proposed a possible role for catecholamines in endolymph production. Feldman and Brusilow (unpublished results) were unable to demonstrate a change in cyclic AMP levels in the stria vascularis after systemic administration of α- and β-adrenergic agents. It is noteworthy that the β-adrenergic agonist, isoproterenol, caused a small but significant increase in the EP. These data would seem to be more consistent with the results obtained after phentolamine administration because α- and β-

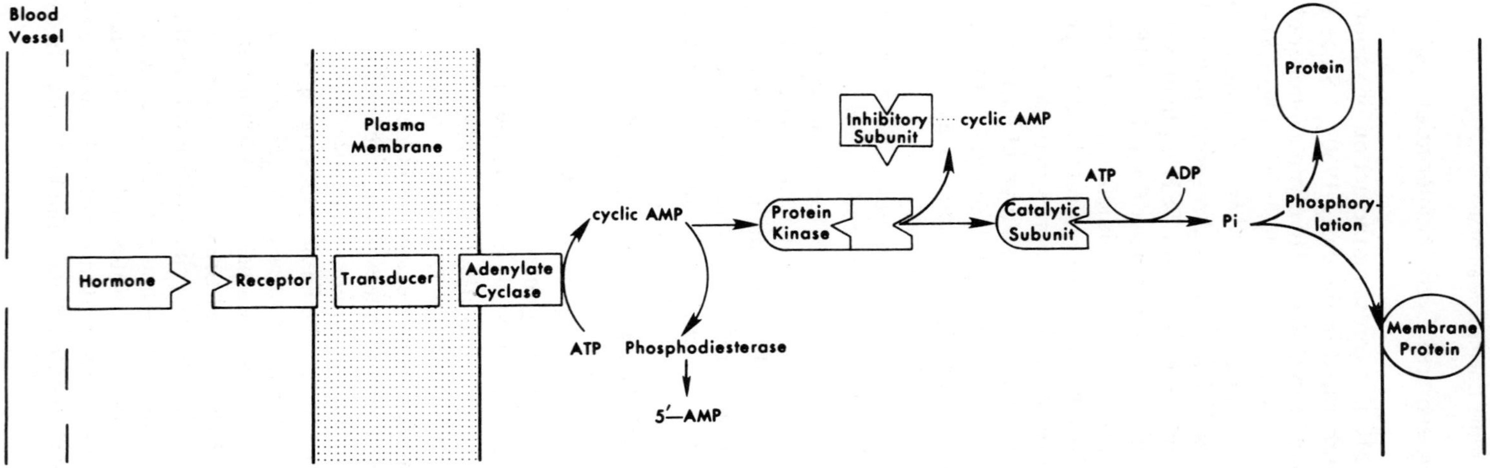

Figure 3.7 A schematic diagram of the adenylate cyclase–cyclic AMP system.

adrenergic agents often exert opposite effects. It is also possible that we did not measure an increase in cyclic AMP accumulation because we were unable to inhibit phosphodiesterase, a standard procedure in *in vitro* studies. The cyclic AMP that accumulated in excess and was not bound to a protein kinase could have been rapidly metabolized by phosphodiesterase and therefore was not recovered in our analytical procedure.

To probe the adenylate cyclase–cyclic AMP system of the cochlea purified cholera toxin was injected into the scala media.[3] Cholera toxin has been shown to improve fluid and electrolyte transport in the gut,[99,100] the kidney,[101,102] and the choroid plexus[91-93] by the stimulation of the adenylate cyclase–cyclic AMP system. It has also been demonstrated that cholera toxin is able to cross the luminal membrane of epithelial cells, bind to the adenylate cyclase enzymes on the anteluminal side of the cell (regardless of the specificity of their accompanying receptor site), and initiate a dramatic increase in cyclic AMP production.[103,104] In the cochlea, cholera toxin caused a significant increase in endolymph production (Figure 3.8), measured with an inulin dilution technique.[3] This increase was not associated with changes in EP or endolymph electrolyte concentrations. These investigations were consistent with studies of CSF production and gut secretion after cholera toxin challenge. In both, the secretion after cholera toxin challenge was isotonic with respect to normal secretory constituents. Studies in the gut showed that the massive secretion of fluid associated with cholera toxin challenge in that tissue was due to inhibition of sodium transport and stimulation of an outwardly directed chloride pump.[105,106] When endolymphatic pressures were measured after challenge with cholera toxin there was a significant increase in hydrostatic pressure in the scala media, which supports the results obtained with the inulin dilution technique.[4]

Paloheimo and Thalmann[75] have shown that the loop diuretics, furosemide and ethacrynic acid, inhibit adenylate cyclase in the organ of Corti and stria vascularis (see Figure 3.6). Although inhibition of adenylate cyclase may be the primary site of diuretic action, the exact etiology of the ototoxicity and the fall in EP remains unclear. The mercurial diuretic, mersalyl, inhibits adenylate cyclase and Na/K ATPase *in vitro* but requires a much higher concentration to affect the EP *in vivo*.[43] The discrepancy between the *in vivo* and *in vitro* results makes the data difficult to interpret.

Cyclic GMP exists in numerous tissues, including brain, liver, and kidney; it is synthesized by the enzyme, guanylate cyclase, which is found in the cytosolic and membrane fractions of the cell.[96] Cyclic GMP is present in cells in concentrations much smaller than those of cyclic AMP. Goldberg and his coworkers[96] found that acetylcholine could increase myocardial concentrations of cyclic GMP while slightly depressing cyclic AMP concentrations. Conversely, isoproterenol depressed cyclic GMP levels and at the same time stimulated cyclic AMP levels. From this study and subsequent studies with other cyclic GMP-linked hormones they proposed the Yin-Yang theory of cyclic AMP–cyclic GMP,[107] which is based on the supposition that

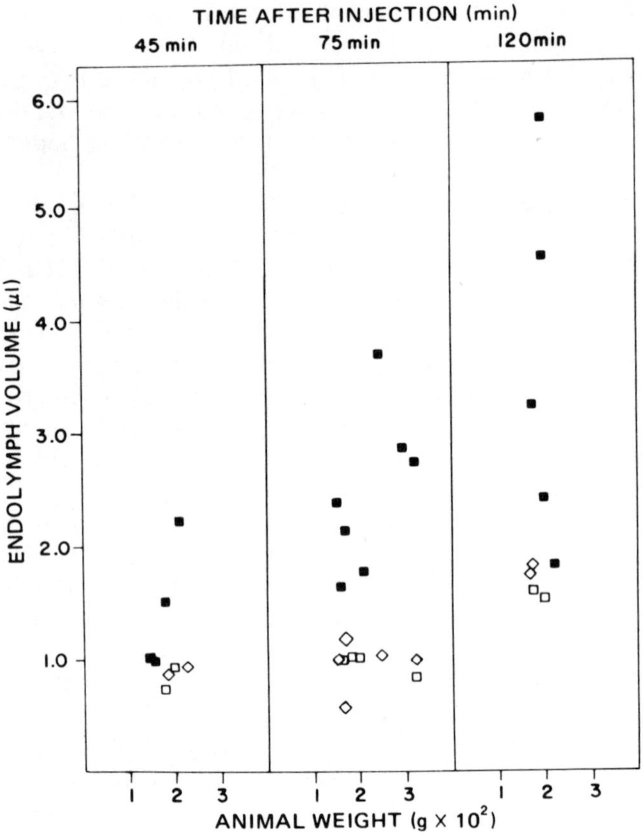

Figure 3.8 Endolymph volume at various times after injection of active cholera toxin (■), deactivated cholera toxin (□), or 0.15 *M* KCl (◇). Each point represents an individual animal. (From Feldman and Brusilow.[3])

cyclic AMP and cyclic GMP mediate opposing cellular functions. This theory has been supported by subsequent studies.[107] β-Adrenergic responses are mediated by cyclic AMP, whereas α-responses are mediated by cyclic GMP. Prostaglandin E_2, which relaxes vascular smooth muscle by stimulating cyclic AMP production, apparently can initiate contraction by stimulating cyclic GMP. Evidence indicates that both cyclic AMP and cyclic GMP may act to mediate the expression of substances that enter the cell as well as those that bind to membrane receptor sites.[107]

Guanylate cyclase and cyclic GMP were measured in the guinea pig cochlea by Guth and Stockwell.[108] Although they were able to record the presence of cyclic GMP in the cochlea, they were unable to observe any changes in cyclic GMP levels or in enzyme activity after administration of kanamycin or ethacrynic acid. Technical difficulties may have accounted for these results. Obviously further studies of cyclic GMP in the cochlea should provide important information about cochlear biochemistry.

Prostaglandins

Prostaglandins are naturally occurring fatty acids that make up a family of closely related derivatives of prostanoic acid; the first member of the family was described by Bergstrom and his coworkers in 1962.[109] Subsequently it was shown that the prostaglandins were synthesized from arachidonic acid and linolenic acid, both of which are derived from dietary linoleic acid. The physiology, pharmacology, and biosynthesis of the prostaglandins have been thoroughly reviewed by Horton,[110] Pickles,[111] Bergstrom and Samuelson,[112] and others. Prostaglandins influence fluid and electrolyte movements in a number of secretory epithelia, including the toad bladder,[113,114] the gut,[115] the kidney,[116,117] and the choroid plexus.[92,93] These actions are mediated by a stimulatory or inhibitory effect on cyclic AMP production[99,100,113,114,115]. For example, prostaglandin E_1 stimulates sodium transport by stimulation of adenylate cyclase and inhibits vasopressin-induced water flow by inhibiting adenylate cyclase.[113] These studies have led to the hypothesis that there is intracellular compartmentalization of various cyclic AMP pools,[114] a theory supported by studies in the choroid plexus (Feldman, unpublished results). It has also been shown that cholera toxin-induced secretions in the gut as well as in the ventricles of the brain could be significantly reduced by pretreatment with indomethacin, a potent inhibitor of prostaglandin synthesis.[92,118] Paradoxically, when indomethacin alone was given to the animals there was an increase in CSF production and in fluid reabsorption in the gut. It is obvious that the various prostaglandins have a complex function in secretory tissues and that simultaneous inhibition of synthesis of all the prostaglandins yields confusing results.

Although no studies have been performed to date on the role of prostaglandin synthesis in the cochlea, tinnitus, vertigo, and, in some cases, temporary hearing loss have been associated with the clinical use of nonsteroidal anti-inflammatory agents, such as the salicylates, indomethacin, naproxen, fenoprofen, and ibuprofen,[119–121] to block prostaglandin synthesis. Experimentally, salicylate causes an initial depression of the CAP which is followed by a reduction in CM.[122,123]

The well-documented relationship among prostaglandins, cyclic AMP accumulation, and cell secretion in the choroid plexus, kidney, and gut and the evidence that cyclic AMP plays a role in endolymph production tend to assign an important role for postaglandins in the cochlear epithelia. A systematic study of the role of the prostaglandins in the cochlea would provide valuable information on the mechanisms of the anti-inflammatory drugs and help to fill some of the gaps in our knowledge of cochlear secretion.

3.7 CONCLUSIONS

Despite a great increase in our knowledge of cochlear biochemistry in the last decade, our pool of information is analogous to a jigsaw puzzle in that many pieces are missing and some of those we have still do not fit. This can be demonstrated by looking at what is known about the effects of the ototoxic loop diuretics, ethacrynic acid and furosemide, on biochemical pathways and physiological parameters of the cochlea. The effect of ethacrynic acid on endolymph composition appears to be species specific. In dogs ethacrynic acid causes a fall in potassium concentration and a rise in sodium concentrations[74]; however, no changes in endolymph ionic composition are seen in the rat or the guinea pig.[53] Ethacrynic acid decreases the EP in all of these species (except at low doses in the dog) and the effect is dose-dependent. Because of the significant fall in EP at appropriate doses, it was earlier assumed that the primary site of action was Na/K ATPase, the enzyme thought to be responsible for the maintenance of EP. This drug, however, also inhibits strial adenylate cyclase, the enzyme that may be responsible for endolymph secretion. Although *in vitro* results may not accurately reflect *in vivo* situations, the studies in the ear are consistent with those in other organs in that ethacrynic acid also inhibited adenylate cyclase activity in the kidney.[124] Furthermore, ethacrynic acid reverses cyclic AMP-mediated intestinal secretion following cholera toxin challenge by selectively inhibiting the active chloride pump.[125] Brusilow[126] found that furosemide in the guinea pig caused a fall in EP as well as a rise in the Na^+/K^+ ratio. The electrolyte changes, but not the change in EP, could be prevented by pretreating the animals with propranalol and it was proposed that propranalol acted by inhibiting adenylate cyclase. This work supported earlier findings that EP and the endolymph Na^+/K^+ ratio were mutually independent. An additional piece of information was the finding by Thalmann[127] that ethacrynic acid inhibited normal energy use in the cochlea. Although the effects of ethacrynic acid on cochlear physiology and biochemistry have been well studied, it is obvious that important pieces of the puzzle are still missing and must be found before it can be put together and a workable model of loop diuretic ototoxicity established.

From data accumulated in the last decade it is known that the cochlea depends on structural integrity, metabolic enzymes, and secretory enzymes for physiological functioning. To obtain a better understanding of cochlear pathophysiology, however, we must define the relationship among adenylate cyclase, Na/K ATPase, and EP, learn more about the characteristics of the adenylate cyclase and fluid transport systems, and define the role of prostaglandins in cell metabolism and secretion. In addition, we must attempt to learn the relationship of clinical problems, such as fluctuant hearing loss and Meniere's disease, to biochemical pathways in the cochlea.

ACKNOWLEDGMENTS

I thank Dr. Saul W. Brusilow for his helpful critique and Mrs. Tommie Lue Maddox and Ms. Susie Fessler for preparation of the manuscript.

REFERENCES

1. M. Lawrence, in C. A. Smith and J. A. Vernon, Eds., *Handbook of Auditory and Vestibular Research Methods*, Charles C Thomas, Springfield, 1976, pp. 181–207.
2. H. Silverstein, in C. A. Smith and J. A. Vernon, Eds., *Handbook of Auditory and Vestibular Research Methods*, Charles C Thomas, Springfield, 1976, p. 420.
3. A. M. Feldman and S. W. Brusilow, *Proc. Nat. Acad. Sci. USA*, **73,** 1761 (1976).
4. A. M. Feldman, H. R. Bittner, and S. W. Brusilow, submitted for publication.
5. D. A. Hilding and A. Sugiura, in M. M. Paparella, Ed., *Biochemical Mechanisms in Hearing and Deafness*, Charles C Thomas, Springfield, 1970, pp. 137–147.
6. D. G. Scarpelli, in M. M. Paparella, Ed., *Biochemical Mechanisms in Hearing and Deafness*, Charles C Thomas, Springfield, 1970, pp. 125–135.
7. R. Thalmann, in C. A. Smith and J. A. Vernon, Eds., *Handbook of Auditory and Vestibular Research Methods*, Charles C Thomas, Springfield, 1976, pp. 359–418.
8. R. Thalmann, Acta Oto Laryngol., **73,** 160 (1972).
9. O. H. Lowry, *Harvey Lect.*, **58,** 1 (1963).
10. G. O. Hodgen and R. T. Falk, *Int. J. Appl. Radiat. Isot.*, **22,** 492 (1971).
11. J. F. Danielli, in G. Weissmann and R. Claiborne, Eds., *Cell Membranes: Biochemistry, Cell Biology and Pathology*, H. P. Publishing Co., New York, 1975, pp. 3–12.
12. J. Singer, in G. Weissmann and R. Claiborne, Eds., *Cell Membranes: Biochemistry, Cell Biology and Pathology*, H. P. Publishing Co., New York, 1975, pp. 35–44.
13. D. Chapman, in G. Weissmann and R. Claiborne, Eds., *Cell Membranes: Biochemistry, Cell Biology and Pathology*, H. P. Publishing Co., New York, 1975, pp. 13–23.
14. E. Stockhorst and J. Schact, *Acta Oto Laryngol.*, **83,** 401 (1977).
15. J. N. Hawthorne and D. A. White, *Vitam. Horm.* NY, **33,** 529 (1975).
16. J. Schacht, *J. Acoust. Soc. Am.*, **59,** 940 (1976).
17. A. Orsulakova, E. Stockhorst, and J. Schacht, *J. Neurochem.*, **26,** 285 (1976).
18. R. D. Brown and A. M. Feldman, *Ann. Rev. Pharmacol. Toxicol.*, **18,** 233 (1978).
19. D. M. Neville, *Biochem. Biophys. Acta*, **133,** 68 (1967).
20. A. L. Lehninger, *Biochemistry: The Molecular Basis of Cell Structure and Function*, Worth, New York, 1970.
21. H. Saito, A. Nakamura, and T. Iida, *Ann. Otol. Rhinol. Laryngol.*, **214,** 149 (1976).
22. H. Saito and J. F. Daly, *Acta Oto Laryngol.*, **69,** 333 (1970).
23. H. Saito and J. F. Daly, *Acta Oto Laryngol.*, **71,** 22 (1971).
24. A. White, P. Handler, and E. L. Smith, *Principles of Biochemistry*, McGraw-Hill, New York, 1968.
25. R. H. Mahler and E. H. Cordes, *Biological Chemistry*, Harper and Row, New York, 1966.
26. G. Bekesy, *J. Acoust. Soc. Am.*, **23,** 576 (1951).
27. H. Davis, *Physiol. Rev.*, **37,** 1 (1957).
28. E. G. Wever, M. Lawrence, R. W. Hemphill, and C. B. Straut, *Am. J. Physiol.*, **159,** 199 (1949).
29. R. Kimura and H. B. Perlman, *Ann. Otol. Rhinol. Laryngol.*, **67,** 5 (1958).
30. K. H. Vosteen, *Laryngoscope*, **70,** 351 (1960).
31. Y. Nakai, *Ann. Otol. Rhinol. Laryngol.*, **74,** 326 (1965).
32. Y. Koide, Y. Yoshikawa, and M. Mosimoto, *Ann. Otol. Rhinol. Laryngol.*, **71,** 96 (1962).
33. H. H. Spoendlin and K. Balogh, Jr., *Laryngoscope*, **73,** 1061 (1963).

34. C. R. Stack and D. B. Webster, *Acta Oto Laryngol.*, **72,** 28 (1971).
35. H. Sowinski, *Folia Morphol. Warsaw*, **35,** 231 (1976).
36. F. M. Matschinsky and R. Thalmann, *Laryngoscope*, **77,** 292 (1967).
37. R. Thalmann, T. Miyoshi, J. Kusakari, and I. Ise, *Otolaryngol. Clin. N. Am.*, **8,** 313 (1975).
38. R. Thalmann, T. Miyoshi, J. Kusakari, and I. Thalmann, *Audiology*, **12,** 364 (1973).
39. R. Thalmann, I. Thalmann, and T. H. Comegys, *Laryngoscope*, **82,** 2059 (1972).
40. R. Thalmann, T. Miyoshi, and I. Thalmann, *Laryngoscope*, **82**(12), 2249 (1972).
41. I. Thalmann, F. M. Matschinsky, and R. Thalmann, *Ann. Otol. Rhinol. Laryngol.*, **79,** 12 (1970).
42. J. T. Y. Chou and D. E. Hughes, in S. Rauch, Ed., *Biochemie des Hororgans*, G. Thieme Verlag, Stuttgart, 1964, p. 446.
43. R. Thalmann, I. Thalmann, I. Ise, and S. Paloheimo, *Laryngoscope*, **87,** 699 (1977).
44. R. Thalmann, J. Kusakari, and T. Miyoshi, *Laryngoscope*, **83,** 1690 (1973).
45. D. Ishii, T. Takahashi, and K. Balogh, *Acta Oto Laryngol.*, **67,** 573 (1969).
46. P. S. Postma, J. C. Pecorak, J. Prazma, S. S. Logue, and N. D. Fischer, *Arch. Otolaryngol.*, **102,** 154 (1976).
47. A. J. Duvall, III, and M. J. Hukee, *Ann. Otol. Rhinol. Laryngol.*, **85,** 234 (1976).
48. M. Tachibana, O. Mizukoshi, and K. Kuriyama, *Biochem. Pharmacol.*, **25,** 2297 (1976).
49. Y. Kaku, J. L. Farmer, Jr., and W. D. Hudson, *Arch. Otolaryngol.*, **98,** 282 (1973).
50. Y. Koide, A. Hata, and R. Hando, *Acta Oto Laryngol.*, **61,** 332 (1966).
51. J. Krzanowski, Jr., and E. M. Matschinsky, *J. Histochem. Cytochem.*, **19,** 321 (1971).
52. R. Thalmann, in D. Henderson, R. Hamernik, J. Mills, and D. S. Dosanjh, Eds., *The Effects of Noise on Hearing: Critical Issues*, Raven, New York, 1976, pp. 111–127.
53. P. M. Sellick and B. M. Johnstone, *Prog. Neurobiol.*, **5,** 337 (1974).
54. P. M. Sellick and B. M. Johnstone, *Pfluegers Arch.*, **352,** 339 (1974).
55a. H. B. Goldman, *Otolaryngol. Clin. N. Am.*, **8,** 369 (1975).
55b. B. Kellerhals, ORL, **38,** 193 (1976).
56. Y. Koide, T. Shigeo, Y. Makota, and M. Konno, *Ann. Otol. Rhinol. Laryngol.*, **69,** 1083 (1960).
57. S. K. Juhn and J. N. Youngs, *Arch. Otolaryngol.*, **96,** 556 (1972).
58. S. K. Juhn and J. N. Youngs, *Laryngoscope*, **86,** 273 (1976).
59. K. Makimoto and H. Silverstein, *Laryngoscope*, **84,** 722 (1974).
60. M. Mendelsohn and J. Roderique, *Laryngoscope*, **82,** 1533 (1972).
61. A. E. Kitabchi and J. J. Shea, *Otolaryngol. Clin. N. Am.*, **8,** 357 (1975).
62. W. L. Meyerhoff, *Laryngoscope*, **86,** 483 (1976).
63. J. C. Skou, *Biochem. Biophys. Acta*, **23.** 394 (1957).
64. J. C. Skou, *Physiol. Rev.*, **45,** 596 (1965).
65. J. L. Dahl and L. E. Hokin, *Ann. Rev. Biochem.*, **43,** 327 (1974).
66. S. L. Bonting and L. L. Caravaggio, *Arch. Biochem. Biophys.*, **101,** 37 (1963).
67. W. Kuijpers, A. C. Vander Vleuten, and S. L. Bonting, *Science*, **157,** 949 (1967).
68. S. L. Bonting, *Curr. Probl. Clin. Biochem.*, **3,** 231 (1971).
69. W. Kuijpers and S. L. Bonting, *Biochem. Biophys. Acta*, **173,** 477 (1969).
70. Y. Nakai and D. A. Hilding, *Acta Oto Laryngol.*, **64,** 477 (1967).
71. W. Kuijpers, *Acta Oto Laryngol.*, **78,** 341 (1974).
72. T. Konishi and M. Mendelsohn, *Acta Oto Laryngol.*, **69,** 192 (1970).

73. W. Kuijpers, *Acta Oto Laryngol.*, **67,** 200 (1969).
74. S. W. Brusilow and E. Gordes, *J. Clin. Invest.*, **52,** 2517 (1973).
75. S. Paloheimo and R. Thalmann, *Arch. Otorhinolaryngol. NY*, **217,** 347 (1977).
76. N. U. Meldrum and F. J. W. Roughton, *J. Physiol. London*, **80,** 113 (1933).
77. T. H. Maren, *Physiol. Rev.*, **47,** 595 (1967).
78. T. H. Maren and L. E. Broder, *J. Pharmacol. Exp. Ther.*, **172,** 197 (1970).
79. T. H. Maren, *Am. J. Physiol.*, **222,** 885 (1972).
80. B. P. Vogh and T. H. Maren, *Am. J. Physiol.*, **228,** 673 (1975).
81. H. Davson, *Physiology of the Cerebrospinal Fluid*, Churchill, London, 1967, p. 134.
82. N. P. Beck, J. S. Kim, M. Wolak, and B. B. Davis, *J. Clin. Invest.*, **55,** 149 (1975).
83. L. C. Garg, *Biochem. Pharmacol.*, **24,** 437 (1975).
84. S. Narumi and Y. Maki, *Biochem. Biophys. Acta*, **311,** 90 (1973).
85. S. D. Erulkar and T. H. Maren, *Nature*, **189,** 459 (1961).
86. D. G. Drescher, *Proc. Nat. Acad. Sci. USA*, **74,** 892 (1977).
87. T. H. Maren, in V. B. Mountcastle, Ed., *Medical Physiology*, Mosby, St. Louis, 1974, pp. 1116–1141.
88. H. Silverstein and R. B. Yules, *Laryngoscope*, **81,** 873 (1971).
89. T. H. Maren, E. R. Swenson, and A. D. F. Addink, *Ann. Otol.*, **84,** 847 (1975).
90. H. J. Rodriquez, J. Walls, J. Yates, and S. Klahr, *J. Clin. Invest.*, **53,** 122 (1974).
91. M. H. Epstein, A. M. Feldman, and S. W. Brusilow, *Science*, **196,** 1012 (1977).
92. A. M. Feldman, T. Smith, M. H. Epstein, and S. W. Brusilow, *Brain Res.*, **142,** 379 (1978).
93. A. M. Feldman, M. H. Epstein, and S. W. Brusilow, *Brain Res.*, **167,** 119 (1979).
94. E. W. Sutherland, *Science*, **177,** 401 (1972).
95. G. A. Robison, R. W. Butcher, and E. W. Sutherland, *Cyclic AMP*, Academic, New York, 1971.
96. N. D. Goldberg, in G. Weissmann and R. Claiborne, Eds., *Cell Membranes: Biochemistry, Cell Biology and Pathology*, H. P. Publishing Co., New York, 1975, pp. 185–202.
97. P. Ahlstrom, I. Thalmann, R. Thalmann, and I. Ise, *Laryngoscope*, **85,** 1241 (1975).
98. N. P. Beck, S. W. Reed, H. V. Murdaugh, and B. B. Davis, *J. Clin. Invest.*, **51,** 939 (1972).
99. D. V. Kimberg, M. Field, J. Johnson, A. Henderson, and E. Gershon, *J. Clin. Invest.*, **50,** 1218 (1971).
100. G. W. G. Sharp and S. Hynie, *Nature*, **229,** 266 (1971).
101. R. M. Friedler, K. Kurokawa, J. W. Coburn, and S. G. Massry, *Kidney Int.*, **7,** 77 (1975).
102. K. Kurokawa, R. M. Friedler, and S. G. Massry, *Kidney Int.*, **7,** 137 (1975).
103. N. P. Pierce, C. C. J. Carpenter, and W. B. Greenough III, *Bacteriol. Rev.*, **35,** 1 (1971).
104. N. Sahyoun and P. Cuatrecasas, *Proc. Nat. Acad. Sci. USA*, **72,** 3428 (1975).
105. M. Field, *Am. J. Physiol.*, **221,** 992 (1971).
106. M. Field, D. Fromm, R. Al-Awgati, and W. B. Greenough, III, *J. Clin. Invest.*, **51,** 796 (1972).
107. N. D. Goldberg, M. K. Haddox, E. Dunham, C. Lopez, and J. W. Hadden, in B. Clarkson and R. Baserga, Eds., *The Cold Spring Harbor Symposium on the Regulation of Proliferation in Animal Cells*, Cold Spring Harbor Laboratory, New York, 1974, pp. 609–626.
108. P. S. Guth and M. Stockwell, *J. Neurochem.*, **28,** 263 (1977).

109. S. Bergstrom, R. R. Yhage, B. Samuelson, and J. Sjovall, *J. Biol. Chem.*, **238,** 3555 (1963).
110. E. W. Horton, *Physiol. Rev.*, **49,** 122 (1969).
111. V. R. Pickles, *Biol. Rev.*, **42,** 614 (1967).
112. S. Bergstrom and B. Samuelsson, Eds., *Prostaglandins*, Almqvist and Wiksell, Stockholm, 1968.
113. L. C. Lipson and G. W. G. Sharp, *Am. J. Physiol.*, **220,** 1046 (1971).
114. J. Flores, P. A. Witkum, B. Beckman, and G. W. Sharp, *J. Clin. Invest.*, **56,** 256 (1975).
115. R. Al-Awgati and W. B. Greenough, *Nature (New Biol.)*, **238,** 26 (1972).
116. N. P. Beck, T. Kaneko, U. Zor, J. B. Field, and B. B. Davis, *J. Clin. Invest.*, **50,** 2461 (1971).
117. J. J. Grantham and J. Orloff, *J. Clin. Invest.*, **47,** 454 (1968).
118. A. Wald, G. S. Gotterer, G. R. Rajendra, N. A. Turjman, and T. R. Hendrix, *Gastroenterology*, **72,** 106 (1977).
119. H. F. H. Hill, A. G. S. Hill, A. G. Mowat, B. M. Anse, II, J. A. Mathews, M. H. Seifert, J. M. Gumpel, and A. G. Christie, *Ann. Rheum. Dis.*, **33,** 12 (1974).
120. K. Brune, M. Glatt, and P. Graf, *Gen. Pharmacol.*, **7,** 27 (1976).
121. H. S. Diamond, *J. Rheumatol.*, **3** (Suppl. 2), 67 (1976).
122. D. L. McPherson and J. F. Miller, *Arch. Otolaryngol.*, **99,** 304 (1974).
123. J. E. Hawkins, in W. D. Keidel and W. D. Neff, Eds., *Handbook of Sensory Physiology*, Vol. V/3, Springer, New York, 1976, pp. 707–748.
124. L. D. Barnes, Y. S. E. Hill, and T. P. Dousa, *Life Sci.*, **16,** 255 (1975).
125. Q. Al-Awqati, M. Field, and W. B. Greenough, III, *J. Clin. Invest.*, **53,** 687 (1974).
126. S. W. Brusilow, *Can. J. Physiol. Pharmacol.*, **54,** 42 (1976).
127. R. Thalmann, I. Thalmann, and T. H. Comegys, *Laryngoscope*, **80,** 1619 (1970).

CHAPTER 4

Cochlear Fluids: Physiology, Biochemistry, and Pharmacology

ARTHUR M. FELDMAN, M.D., Ph.D.

Clinical Instructor in Otolaryngology
Louisiana State University
School of Medicine in Shreveport
Department of Otolaryngology
Shreveport, Louisiana

CONTENTS

4.1 INTRODUCTION

The cochlear fluids are dependent on the biochemical pathways of the cochlea for their secretion. At the same time they provide the environmental milieu necessary for normal cochlear function. Significant auditory deficits result from small changes in the normal parameters of the cochlear fluids produced by pharmacological, pathophysiological, or morphological manipulations. The cochlear fluids are generally considered to have four major functions[1]:

1. To provide nutrients and remove catabolic wastes from the cells lining the cochlear duct.
2. To interface ossicular chain vibrations with the sensory apparatus of the organ of Corti.
3. To control pressure distribution within the cochlea.
4. To provide an appropriate chemical environment for energy transformation.

The biochemical mechanisms involved in the secretion of the cochlear fluids were discussed in Chapter 3. We now consider the composition of the cochlear fluids, the sources of endolymph and perilymph, physiological parameters of the cochlear fluids, and the effects of pharmacologic agents and pathophysiological disturbances on fluid composition and distribution.

4.2 THE COMPOSITION OF COCHLEAR FLUIDS

4.2.1 Sodium and Potassium Levels in the Cochlear Fluid

Analytical Methods

The morphology of the cochlea was discussed in Chapter 1 and it will be remembered that two types of fluid are found in the cochlea: perilymph, which fills the scala tympani and scala vestibuli, and endolymph, which is found in the scala media. It is generally accepted that perilymph resembles extracellular fluid and is isotonic with respect to Na^+, whereas endolymph resembles intracellular fluid and is isotonic with respect to K^+ (Figure 4.1). Considerable controversy has developed in regard to the exact electrolyte composition of these two fluids, due primarily to the different techniques used to measure it. Although a discussion of the mechanics of the techniques of microanalysis of inner ear fluid is beyond the scope of this chapter, it is important to have some concept of the commonly used methods. As one would imagine, the primary difficulty in obtaining cochlear fluids is related to exposing the encapsulated fluid compartments and withdrawing adequate

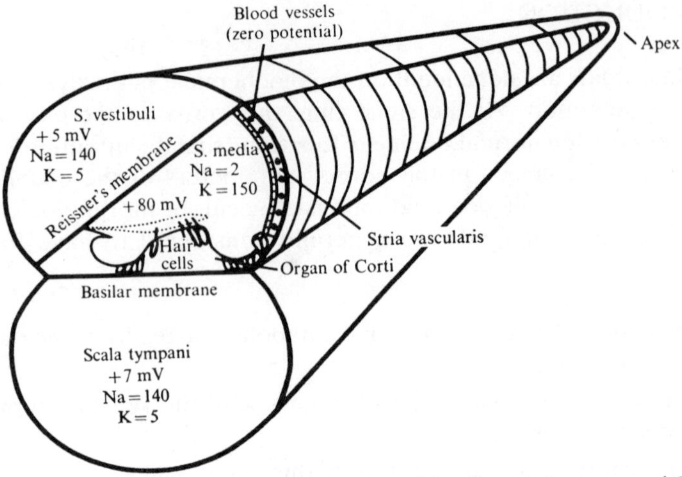

Figure 4.1 Schematic representation of the cochlea from Johnstone and Sellick.[4]

fluid samples without contaminating endolymph with perilymph or perilymph with blood. Two popular methods involve the removal of samples with calibrated micropipettes or *in situ* measurements with ion sensitive microelectrodes.

Microanalytical techniques to measure inner ear fluid concentrations have been described by Silverstein,[2] who used cats and humans, and by Brusilow and Gordes,[3] who used dogs and guinea pigs. Basically, samples of fluid are removed with double-barreled micropipettes, which have one side filled with oil for sample withdrawal; the other side is filled with KCl and connected to an electrometer for the measurement of EP (to ensure proper placement of the pipette). After transfer with calibrated transfer pipettes the fluid samples are analyzed with a flame photometer. Obviously the primary hazard of this technique is the contamination of the fluid sample by perilymph, blood, or endolymph.

Johnstone and Sellick[4,5] have demonstrated the efficacy of using ion-specific electrodes for the determination of cochlear fluid concentrations. The major pitfall of this technique is that the electrodes are interfered with by EP, which must then be considered in calculating the electrolyte concentration. Flock[6] determined relative ion distribution in the inner ear by using an energy dispersive X-ray spectrometer in conjunction with a scanning electron microscope. This technique supported earlier work and allowed analysis of areas previously inaccessible.

That perilymph is isotonic with respect to extracellular Na^+ and endolymph is isotonic with respect to intracellular K^+ has been known since the early studies of Smith et al.[7] in 1954. The exact ionic concentration of these electrolytes is still in doubt, however. The variation between endolymph and perilymph measured by the two techniques described is not significant in experiments performed to measure the effects of drugs on fluid ion concentrations as long as the values obtained in a particular laboratory produce mean values with a small standard error in repeated trials. An exact knowledge of endolymph ion concentrations is required to determine the active transport of Na^+ into and out of the scala media. Sellick and Johnstone[5] have calculated that if Na^+ is at equilibrium its concentration in endolymph is 7 meq/L when the EP is +80 m V, but if it is above or below this value an active transport mechanism must be present.

Perilymph

Perilymph can be measured in experimental situations because uncontaminated samples can be obtained with ease. Bosher and Warren[8] found that perilymph in the rat closely resembled plasma or spinal fluid; it had a Na^+ concentration of 138 meq/L and a K^+ concentration of 7 meq/L. Makimoto and Silverstein[9] showed that perilymph in the cat scala vestibuli possesses a Na^+ concentration of 147 meq/L and the scala tympani has a Na^+ concentration of 157 meq/L. Potassium concentrations were 10.5 and 3.8 meq/L in the scala vestibuli and scala tympani, respectively. Because these compartments are contiguous at the helicotrema, it is difficult to interpret these data, although it supports the theory (discussed later in this chapter) that perilymph is formed from the vascular plexus of the cochlea and not from the CSF.

Endolymph

Because the exact values of the endolymph electrolytes are controversial (Table 4.1), it is appropriate to mention values obtained with both techniques. Sellick and Johnstone[5] found that endolymph Na^+ concentrations in the guinea pig ranged from 0.1 to 2.7 meq/L when measured with Na^+-specific microelectrodes. The EP, measured simultaneously, was subtracted from the Na^+ potential; however, this potential did not incorporate all the EP

Table 4.1 Endolymph Electrolyte Concentrations (meq/L)

Investigator	Cochlear Duct Na^+	Cochlear Duct K^+	Utricle Na^+	Utricle K^+
Smith et al., 1954[7]	38	—	15.8	144
Silverstein, 1966[14]	25	161	40	127
Bosher and Warren, 1968[8]	0.91	154	—	—
Mendelsohn and Konishi, 1969[38]	5.4	147	—	—
Silverstein and Yules, 1970[19]	4.5	160	—	—
Sellick and Johnstone, 1972[5]	0.1–2.7	—	14.3	—
Makimoto and Silverstein, 1974[9]	6.1	171	14.9	155

and "electrical contamination" had to be calculated. These experiments were supported by the use of an *in vivo* calibration curve obtained by perfusing the scala media with known concentrations of electrolytes while the EP was normal and the Na^+ electrode was in the scala media.

Makimoto and Silverstein,[9] who used the endolymph withdrawal technique in the cat, found Na^+ values of 6.07 meq/L and K^+ concentrations of 171 meq/L. It should be noted that while *in vivo* control was not used, the standard error within a population of greater than 40 animals was insignificant. Furthermore, these values were supported by the experiments of Brusilow and Gordes,[3] who used a similar technique in guinea pigs.

Cortilymph

In addition to the fluids found in the scala vestibuli, scala tympani, and scala media, the organ of Corti contains an interstitial fluid called cortilymph which is believed to be continuous with the perilymph of the scala tympani.[10] Therefore, interference with active transport of nutrient materials into perilymph or the ionic composition of perilymph could affect the hair cells and afferent nerve endings.

Sodium and Potassium and Cochlear Function

The upper portion of the hair cell is in contact with the K^+-rich endolymph and is therefore affected by changes in endolymphatic electrolyte gradients. The importance of the endolymphatic ion gradient in cochlear functioning is demonstrated by the fact that when the scala media is perfused with perilymph there is a remarkable depression of cochlear potentials.[11] In addition, when the scala media is perfused with NaCl the potentials are again depressed. Therefore the high K^+ concentration in the endolymph appears to be indispensible for maintaining cochlear function. When a small quantity of KCl is injected into the perilymph, there is a moderate decrease in the CM and CAP but no change in EP.[12] The investigators proposed that fatigue may be related to a leakage of K^+ from endolymph to cortilymph.

A detailed discussion of the circulation of the labyrinthine fluids is beyond the scope of this chapter. One should keep in mind, however, that the cochlear perilymph is contiguous with the fluids that bathe the perilymphatic portion of the vestibular apparatus, whereas the cochlear endolymph is anatomically separated from and chemically different than the vestibular endolymph.

4.2.2 Other Natural Constituents of Cochlear Fluids

Although investigators have been interested primarily in inner ear Na^+ and K^+ concentrations, numerous other components of the cochlear fluids have been studied (Figure 4.2). Bosher and Warren[13] found an endolymph Ca^{2+}

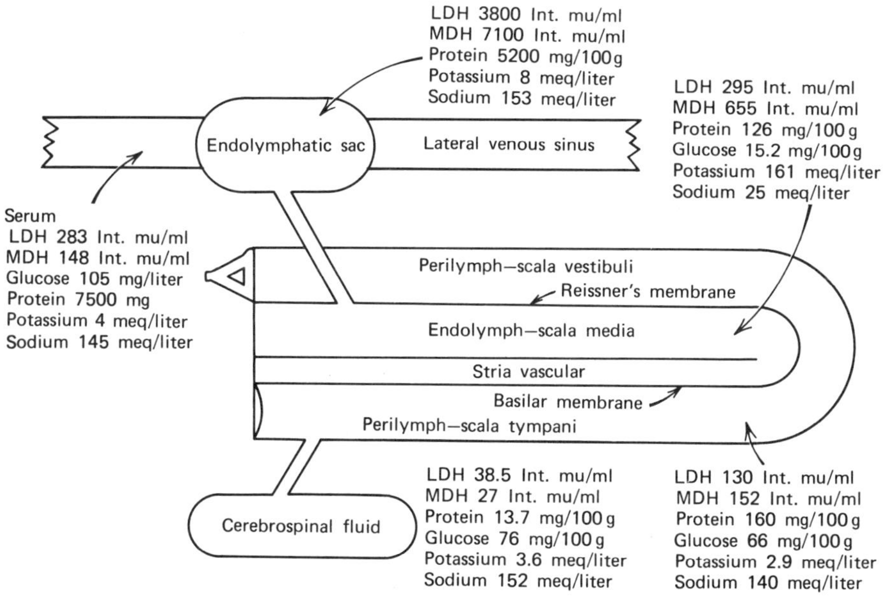

Figure 4.2 Cochlear fluid constituents from Silverstein.[14] It should be noted that some of the electrolyte values have been changed in more recent studies. (See Table 4.1.)

concentration of $3 \times 10^{-5}M$ in the rat, the ion occurring almost completely in the noncomplexed state. This value was well below the usual extracellular concentraton. Endolymph Mg^{2+} concentration was 1×10^{-3} M in the scala vestibuli and $0.68 \times 10^{-3}M$ in the scala tympani. The chloride ion (Cl^-) appears to be present in both endolymph and perilymph at a concentration of 115 meq/L.[6]

Silverstein[14] measured the concentrations of malic dehydrogenase, lactic dehydrogenase, protein, and glucose in the perilymph, endolymph, and CSF. Figure 4.2 shows that protein concentration was similar in endolymph and perilymph, considerably higher in the endolymphatic sac, and lower in the CSF. Glucose concentration was low in endolymph and greater in perilymph and CSF. Lactic dehydrogenase (LDH) and malic dehydrogenase (MDH) levels could be described as follows: endolymphatic sac > endolymph > perilymph > CSF. The values in the endolymphatic sac support its role as a metabolic sink for the absorption of endolymph.

Although considerable attention has been given to the constituents of the cochlear fluids, particularly Na^+ and K^+, the pH has been measured in only a few studies. Ledoux[15] found that the pH of endolymph and perilymph was 7.82 and 7.87, respectively. If we assumed that the pCO_2 of these fluids is similar to that of plasma (40 mm Hg), the calculated HCO_3^- concentration would be 62.9 and 70.7 mM, respectively (Brusilow, personal communication). Misrahy et al.,[16] however, determined the pH of endolymph to be 7.44

and of perilymph to be 7.88, which would suggest HCO_3^- concentrations of 26.2 and 72.3 mM, respectively. Although these data are conflicting, they do suggest that the bicarbonate concentration in cochlear fluids may be higher than plasma levels. This is supported by the studies of Erulkar and Maren,[17] who found that the tissues of the inner ear had a high concentration of carbonic anhydrase and that ^{14}C HCO_3^- accumulated in endolymph less readily when carbonic anhydrase was inhibited. The administration of the carbonic anhydrase inhibitor, acetazolamide, does not appear to have any effect on the concentrations of Na^+ or K^+ in the cochlear fluids.[18,19] No recent attempt has been made to measure the pH or HCO_3^- concentration of endolymph. With the advent of pH and ion-sensitive microelectrodes such measurements should be made; they would contribute important information about cochlear fluid physiology.

4.2.3 Drugs as Constituents of Cochlear Fluids

When considering the constituents of the cochlear fluids, it is also important to remember that just as physiologically occurring substances appear to be able to enter the cochlear fluids, iatrogenic agents can also appear in the perilymph and endolymph. Unfortunately the means by which most ototoxic agents enter the cochlear fluids is uncertain. Attempts to elucidate this mechanism have been made in several studies. Watanabe et al.[20] obtained postmortem samples of perilymph and endolymph after intramuscular administration of the ototoxic aminoglycoside, kanamycin, to guinea pigs. They found that kanamycin appeared rapidly in the perilymph and remained detectable even after blood levels were no longer measurable. Perilymph levels remained measurable for 18 hr in acute experiments, whereas plasma levels were measurable for only 8 hr. It is interesting that kanamycin could not be detected in endolymph in acute experiments, but it could be recovered from the endolymph after two weeks of intramuscular administration. These studies are supported by preliminary investigations in our laboratory which demonstrated that acute gentamicin administration resulted in the detection of gentamicin within the perilymph but not in the endolymph (observations on unpublished data).

Salicylate, another well known ototoxic drug,[21] will penetrate the perilymph[22a]; however, no measurements have been made in the endolymph. Obviously our knowledge of the penetration of drugs into the cochlear fluids is severely limited and this provides a fertile area of investigation, particularly for the young investigator interested in studying cochlear pharmacology.

Two possible major mechanisms that could account for the penetration of potentially ototoxic drugs into cochlear fluids are passive diffusion and active transport. To determine which of these mechanisms is functioning, we must know the concentrations of the drugs within the perilymph, endolymph, and serum as well as the pH values of the particular fluids. Most of the ototoxic agents are weak organic acids or bases. Therefore, if the actual drug concentration ratio (cochlear fluid/serum) approximates that predicted from the pH values of the cochlear fluid and serum and the pK_a of the drug by using the equations related to pH partitioning and ion trapping,[22b] we could conclude that the drug penetrates the membrane passively. If the concentration ratio were greater than that predicted, active transport could be involved. On the other hand, if the ratio were less than the predicted value, it would indicate that the fluid compartment was selectively impermeable to the drug or that the transfer rate constant for removal of the drug was much greater than the one associated with transfer of the drug into that compartment. Obviously a systematic study of the permeability characteristics of cochlear membranes to a variety of drugs of varying size, pK_a, and lipid solubility would add greatly to our knowledge of the cochlear fluids.

4.3 SOURCES OF PERILYMPH AND ENDOLYMPH

4.3.1 Perilymph

The site of perilymphatic fluid production is controversial. Two hypotheses have been proposed; (1) the perilymph originates from the cerebrospinal fluid (CSF); (2) it is an ultrafiltrate of the perilymphatic capillaries. The CSF theory is based on experiments in which various substances appear in the perilymph following subarachnoid space injection.[23-25] The physiological significance of these experiments must be questioned, however, because unphysiological pressure gradients between the two compartments may be produced by the opening of a subarachnoid cistern and by the introduction of various substances into the CSF. Furthermore, although the cochlear aqueduct of guinea pigs has a large open lumen, the communication in primates appears to be more tortuous and the connection may not always be patent.[26] Studies with patients by Ritter and Lawrence[27] showed that dye and radioactive protein failed to get into the perilymph. In contrast, occasional reports have described the escape of excessive CSF from the oval window during stapes surgery.[1] If, however, in a particular individual or species there were communication between the CSF and the perilymph, the two fluid pressures might equilibrate without flow of fluid.[10]

If flow occurred between CSF and perilymph, we would expect perilymph to resemble CSF closely in composition; however, it appears to resemble an ultrafiltrate of blood. The protein content of perilymph is much lower than that found in blood but is still considerably higher than in CSF (Figure 4.2). In addition, if the serum glucose level were altered by administration of insulin, there would be a corresponding change in perilymph glucose concentrations but not in CSF glucose levels.[10] Furthermore, Choo and Tabowitz[28,29] found that when electrolytes were parenterally administered to cats the electrolytes appeared in the CSF at a slightly slower rate than in the perilymph. If the CSF supplied the perilymph, we would expect that the electrolytes would appear in the CSF before entering the perilymph. The blood ultrafiltration theory is further supported by the finding that surgical obstruction of the cochlear aqueduct in cats produced neither histologic changes nor functional alterations in hearing.[30] Schnieder[10] proposed that the ultrafiltration mechanism was composed of a mesh of perilymphatic connective tissue that contained an extensively ramified capillary network with a large surface facing the perilymphatic space. Small molecular weight substances could then pass through the capillary membranes in both directions, their mobility being inversely related to their size. Diffusion velocity would be a function of the concentration gradient and size of the substance. This theory has been slightly modified by Juhn et al.,[31] who found that the entrance of Na^+ into perilymph was a slow process. Ultrastructural studies of the perilymphatic vessels showed that the capillaries were surrounded by layers of pericytes and fibrocytes and that the endothelial cells have a lack of fenestration. The ultrastructure could account for the slow diffusion of substances into perilymph and might constitute a blood-labyrinth barrier.

Although the ultrafiltration theory appears to be compatible with most of the data collected to date, it is important to mention the double-perilymph-origin model proposed by Kellerhals.[32] The theory is based on experiments in which the appearance of dyes in the CSF and perilymph was monitored over time after injection of tracer into the CSF. Kellerhals[32] found that local perilymph production with the cochlea exceeded the influx of CSF by a ratio of about 2:1 in the guinea pig. Therefore part of the perilymph might be derived from the perilymphatic capillary network, whereas the remainder would come from the CSF. The contribution of either perilymph source could vary according to the individual situation, the species being studied, and the particular location within the cochlear duct. This theory appears attractive and has been supported by recent studies.[32a]

4.3.2 Endolymph

Although the site of perilymph production seems embroiled in controversy, it is generally accepted that the site of endolymph production in the cochlea is the stria vascularis and that endolymph reabsorption occurs in the endolymphatic sac. That the stria vascularis is the secretory membrane is supported by morphological as well as biochemical evidence. As discussed in Chapter 3, the stria vascularis contains a large number of oxidative enzymes for glucose metabolism and for fueling the active transport systems. In addition, the stria vascularis has high concentrations of Na/K ATPase, adenylate cyclase, and carbonic anhydrase, all of which have been implicated as having some role in the maintenance of normal fluid production and composition in the cochlea. Furthermore, ultrastructural studies have shown that the structure of the stria vascularis is correlated with a secretory function[33,34] and hearing deficits are often correlated with a deficiency in the quality of the endolymph.[35] Morphological changes in the stria vascularis have been associated with pathological changes, evidenced by the strial atrophy which, at times, accompanies the sensorineural deafness of aging.[35]

4.3.3 Effects of Drugs on the Ionic Composition of the Cochlear Fluids

Alteration of the ionic constituents of the endolymph or perilymph or changes in the active transport associated with the formation of cochlear fluids can affect the physiological functioning of the auditory apparatus and result in loss of hearing. Because of the increased awareness of the importance of the cochlear fluids in normal auditory functioning, researchers have begun to study the effects of ototoxic agents on cochlear fluid constituents. The ototoxic drugs and their mechanisms of action have been reviewed by Brown and Feldman[21] and the biochemical pathways affected by many of these agents were discussed in Chapter 3. In the context of this chapter, however, the effects of some of these agents on cochlear fluid production and composition are reviewed briefly.

The loop diuretic, ethacrynic acid, has a well-known ototoxic liability; its effect on cochlear fluids appears to be species-specific. In the dog there is a complete reversal of the high K^+, low Na^+ concentrations in endolymph in response to low doses. In contrast, in the cat and rat only minimal changes in endolymph composition occur, whereas in the guinea pig there is no change after ethacrynic acid administration. Furosemide, another loop diuretic, changes endolymph ionic composition in all the species studied.[21]

The administration of ouabain, a potent Na/K ATPase inhibitor, into the perilymphatic space of guinea pigs results in a rise in endolymphatic Na^+ and a fall in endolymphatic K^+.[37] Similar changes become apparent when guinea pigs are exposed to anoxia.[38] These observations support the concept that endolymphatic Na^+ and K^+ concentrations are maintained by active ion transport.

When the concentrations of Na^+ and K^+ are altered in the blood by peritoneal dialysis with NH_4Cl and glucose there is no significant change in perilymph Na^+ or K^+.[39] These results indicate the independence of perilymph from systemic alterations and/or the presence of a homeostatic control, but when the serum osmolality is changed by injecting glycerine a parallel change in perilymphatic osmolality shows after a short time lag.[40] Therefore the blood-perilymph barrier appears to be permeable to glycerin and water, hence susceptible to osmotic changes. This may explain the reduction in perilymphatic fluid pressure following the intravenous administration of glycerol.[41]

Nakashima and his coworkers[42-44] have recently reported that intense acoustic stimulation causes a decrease in K^+ concentration and an increase in Na^+ concentration in the endolymph of the normal guinea pig when measured with cation-sensitive electrodes. The site of these endolymphatic cationic changes has, to date, eluded determination. Finally, the administration of a single oral dose of ethyl alcohol to guinea pigs slows the movement of Na^+ into the perilymph.[36] The relevance of this study to human subjects is not known.

4.4 Cochlear Hydrostatic Pressures

The measurement of the hydrostatic fluid pressures of the cochlear compartments has been the subject of several investigations. Values for perilymphatic pressure have ranged from greater than 14 cm of H_2O[45,46] to less than 5 cm H_2O,[47] and estimates of endolymphatic pressures have ranged from 14 cm of H_2O[45] to less than 3 cm of H_2O.[47] Several studies have demonstrated that the hydrostatic pressure of the endolymphatic compartment was less than that of the perilymphatic space[46,47]; however, newer data have contradicted these findings.[45] We[48] recently attempted to resolve these differences by using a specially designed, highly sensitive measuring device. The advantages of our technique are the following:

1. Small pipette tips (2.0–20μ) are used for measurements.
2. Rapid response time exists in the transducer.
3. The transducer can be equilibrated in situ.
4. The instrument is validated and calibrated *in vivo* (Figure 4.3).

With this technique perilymphatic measurements were made through the round window membranes in animals in which the ossicular structures had been removed and in those in which the middle-ear structures were intact. Endolymphatic pressures were measured after removal of the ossicular

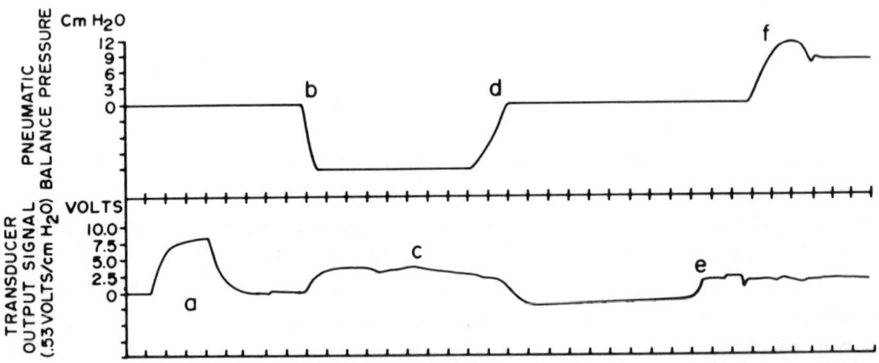

Figure 4.3 Representative measurement of the hydrostatic pressures of the perilymphatic space through the round window membrane showing: (a) external calibration, (b) pneumatic back pressure, (c) placement of pipette on round window membrane, (d) release of back pressure and equilibration of pipette at membrane, (e) zeroing transducer, and (f) membrane puncture and pneumatic nulling of resultant transducer output signal (from Feldman et al.[48]).

Table 4.2 Hydrostatic Fluid Pressures in the Cochlear Compartments[a]

	Fluid Pressures ($cm\ H_2O$)
	Mean Pressure ± SEM (N)
Endolymph[b]	
Basilar membrane	0.12 ± .08 (9)
Spiral ligament	3.34 ± .57 (5)
Perilymph	
Radical approach	2.47 ± .22 (11)
Intact ossicles	4.70 ± .36 (5)

[a]From Feldman et al.[48]

[b]It should be noted that all endolymph measurements were made after the radical surgical approach had been used; that is, the ossicles were disrupted. Therefore the endolymph values measured through the spiral ligament should be compared with perilymph values, using the radical approach. Endolymph values measured through the basilar membrane were obtained after removal of the round window membrane. The result was loss of perilymphatic pressure and a consequent decrease in endolymphatic pressure.

chain structures by penetration through the spiral ligament and stria vascularis or the basilar membrane. (In the case of penetration through the basilar membrane the perilymphatic compartment was disrupted.) The results of these experiments can be seen in Table 4.2. It should be noted that a significant difference existed between perilymphatic pressures in the presence and absence of intact ossicular chain structures. In addition, the integrity of the perilymphatic system is a prerequisite for normal endolymphatic structures and pressure. No significant differences appeared between endolymphatic and perilymphatic pressures when measured by the same surgical approach. Furthermore, the administration of purified cholera toxin, which had been shown to increase CSF production (presumably by stimulation of adenylate cyclase), resulted in a significant increase in endolymphatic pressure (from 0 ± 0 cm H_2O to 1.59 ± 0.8 cm H_2O, according to the basilar membrane approach[48]).

4.5 CLINICAL ASPECTS OF THE COCHLEAR FLUIDS

Schuknecht and his coworkers[49] first demonstrated the usefulness of biochemical analysis of the inner ear fluid in the diagnosis of difficult clinical problems. Samples were removed from postmortem specimens, patients undergoing surgical procedures, and from patients with diagnostic labyrinthotomies. Care was taken to avoid contamination of the samples with blood or tissue fluid and values obtained from a population of cats was considered as a norm. Patients with otosclerosis showed normal perilymphatic values for Na^+, K^+, and protein and others undergoing transmeatal labyrinthectomy for Meniere's disease had values for endolymph consistent with those of normal mammalian endolymph. Patients with proved acoustic neuromas, however, showed marked increases in perilymphatic protein values which were consistent with the finely granular acidophilic staining precipitate seen histologically in the cochleas of some patients with acoustic neuromas.

4.5.1 Overproduction of the Cochlear Fluids

Meniere's disease, idiopathic endolymphatic hydrops, is illustrative of our sparcity of knowledge of the physiology of the cochlear fluids. Since the first description by Prosper Meniere in 1861 of a series of patients presenting with episodic vertigo, sensorineural hearing loss, and tinnitus little progress has been made in determining the etiology of the disease. This is due to several problems: the lack of an animal model or natural occurrence of a similar disease in animals; the difficulty in obtaining information and specimens from the patient; and our incomplete understanding of fluid balance in the normal ear.[50] Theories of the etiology of the disease abound and are based on abnormalities in vascular function, vasodilation or vasoconstriction, autonomic dysfunction, abnormal histamine release, allergic reactions, abnormal hypothalamic impulses, adrenocortical dysfunction, hypoglycemia, hypothyroidism, and endolymphatic sac ischemia. Godlowski[51] has recently proposed that Meniere's disease is due to a generalized molecular disease of proteins that results in the accumulation of hydrophylic hyaluronate mucopolysaccharides in the endolymph. It has also been pointed out by Harker and McCabe[50] that most patients with this disease are in excellent health.

Despite this obvious confusion three experimental approaches have provided new insight into Meniere's disease and the cochlear fluids. Kimura[52] found that when the endolymphatic sac was obliterated in the cat histologic observation revealed consistent hydrops, demonstrated by convexity of Reissner's membrane (Figure 4.4). The pathologic specimens removed from experimental animals in which hydrops was induced closely resembled the morphologic changes seen in human temporal bone specimens. Although Meniere's disease could be attributed solely to changes in the morphology of the endolymphatic duct and sac, Kimura and Schuknecht[53] postulated that it could also be due to oversecretion or changes in endolymph concentration, unrelated to changes in the endolymphatic sac.

As discussed in Chapter 3, studies in our laboratory have shown that the stimulation of stria vascularis cyclic AMP production with the adenylate

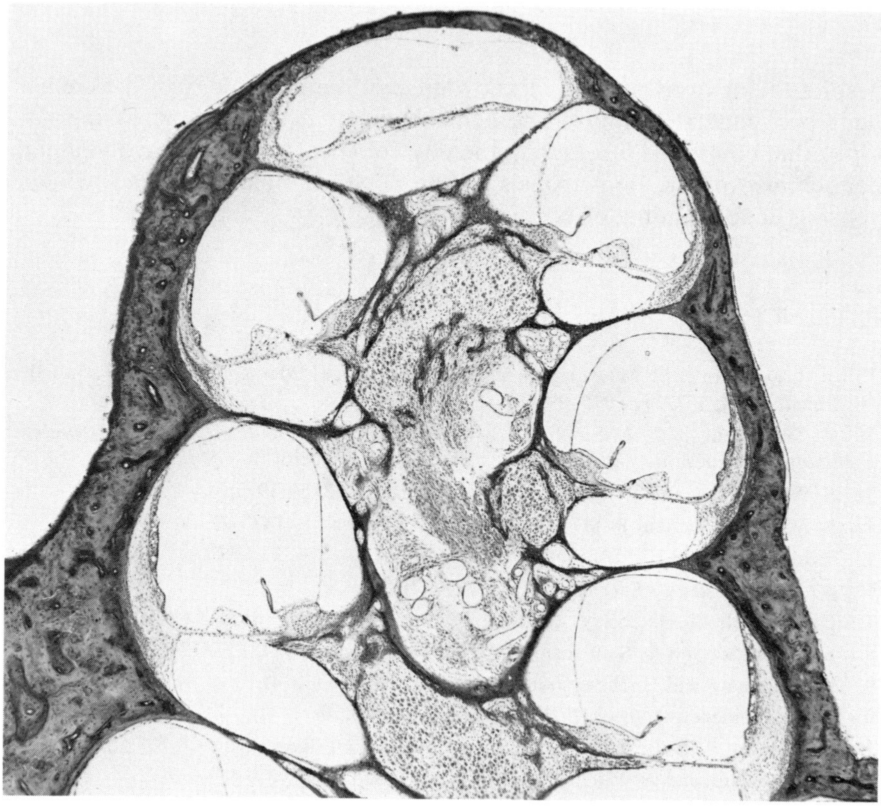

Figure 4.4 Photomicrograph of cochlea in which the cochlear and vestibular aqueducts were obliterated. Extensive hydrops can be seen in the swelling of the Reissner's membrane. Atrophy of the neurosensory elements and the stria vascularis is seen in the apical turns (from Kimura et al.[30]).

cyclase stimulant cholera toxin resulted in a significant increase in endolymph production. That an increase in cyclic AMP stimulated endolymph production could result in the production of an endolymphatic hydrops was further demonstrated by the fact that the introduction of cholera toxin into the scala media also resulted in a significant increase in hydrostatic pressure.[48]

Support for a viral causation of Meniere's disease has been provided in studies by Davis and Johnson.[54] Direct inoculation of the inner ear of neonatal hamsters demonstrated that influenza virus infected mesenchymal cells of the perilymphatic channels of the cochlea, mumps virus infected endolymphatic structures, herpes simplex virus infected, primarily, the sensory cells of the labyrinth, and rubeola and vaccinia infected both perilymphatic and endolymphatic cells. It would seem possible that a viral entity could be responsible for changes in reabsorption in the endolymphatic sac or secretion from the stria vascularis.

4.6 PERSPECTIVE

Despite the obvious paucity of knowledge of the physiology of the cochlear fluids our understanding of these mechanisms is rapidly increasing. It is hoped that continued research in the physiological processes involved in the maintenance of the homeostasis of the cochlear fluids will lead to an increasing understanding of cochlear pathology.

REFERENCES

1. M. Lawrence, in M. M. Paparella and D. A. Shumrick, Eds., *Otolaryngology*, Saunders, Philadelphia, 1973, pp. 275–298.
2. H. Silverstein, in C. A. Smith and J. A. Vernon, Eds., *Handbook of Auditory and Vestibular Research Methods*, Charles C Thomas, Springfield, Ill., 1976, p. 420.
3. S. W. Brusilow and E. Gordes, *J. Clin. Invest.*, **52,** 2517 (1973).
4. B. M. Johnstone and P. M. Sellick, *Q. Rev. Biophys.*, **5,** 1 (1972).
5. P. M. Sellick and B. M. Johnstone, *Pfluegers Arch.*, **336,** 11 (1972).
6. A. Flock, *Acta Oto Laryngol.*, **83,** 239 (1977).
7. C. A. Smith, O. H. Lowry, and M. L. Wu, *Laryngoscope*, **64,** 141 (1954).
8. S. K. Bosher and R. S. Warren, *Proc. R. Soc. London*, **171,** 227 (1968).
9. K. Makimoto and H. Silverstein, *Ann. Otol.*, **83,** 174 (1974).
10. E. A. Schnieder, *Ann. Otol. Rhinol. Laryngol.*, **83,** 76 (1974).
11. T. Konishi, E. Kelsey, and G. T. Singleton, *Acta Oto Laryngol.*, **62,** 393 (1966).
12. J. P. Legouix and A. Pierson, *Audiology*, **16,** 453 (1977).
13. S. K. Bosher and R. L. Warren, *Nature*, **273,** 377 (1978).
14. H. Silverstein, *Ann. Otol. Rhinol. Laryngol.*, **75,** 48 (1966).
15. A. Ledoux, *Bull. Soc. R. Sci. Liege,* **12,** 254 (1943).
16. G. A. Misrahy, K. M. Hildreth, L. C. Clark, and E. W. Shinabarger, *Am. J. Physiol.,* **194,** 393 (1958).
17. S. D. Erulkar and T. H. Maren, *Nature*, **189,** 459 (1961).
18. M. Mendelsohn and J. Mittelman, *Ann. Otol. Rhinol. Laryngol.*, **80,** 186 (1971).
19. H. Silverstein and R. B. Yules, *Laryngoscope*, **81,** 873 (1971).
20. Y. Watanabe, R. Nukajina, R. Oda, M. Uno, and T. Naito, *Med. J. Osäka Univ.*, **21,** 257 (1971).
21. R. D. Brown and A. M. Feldman, *Ann. Rev. Pharmacol. Toxicol.*, **18,** 233 (1978).

22a. H. Silverstein, J. M. Bernstein, and G. Davies, *Ann. Otol. Rhinol. Laryngol.*, **76,** 118 (1967).

22b. L. Schanker, in J. R. DiPalma, Ed., *Drill's Pharmacology in Medicine*, 4th ed., McGraw-Hill, New York, 1971, pp. 21–35.

23. L. Gisselsson, *Acta Oto Laryngol.*, **37,** 268 (1949).
24. J. Arvnvig, *Acta Oto Laryngol. Suppl.* No. 96 (1951).
25. F. Altman and J. G. Waltner, *Laryngoscope*, **60,** 727 (1950).
26. D. H. Moscouitch, R. P. Gannon, and C. A. Laszlo, *Ann. Otol.*, **82,** 53 (1973).
27. F. N. Ritter and M. Lawrence, *Laryngoscope*, **75,** 1224 (1965).
28. Y. B. Choo and D. Tabowitz, *Ann. Otol.*, **73,** 92 (1964).

29. Y. B. Choo and D. Tabowitz, *Ann. Otol.*, **74,** 140 (1965).

30. R. S. Kimura, H. F. Schuknecht, and C. Y. Ota, *Acta Oto Laryngol.*, **77,** 1 (1974).

31. S. K. Juhn, J. Pearce, and J. Guzowski, *Arch. Otorhinolaryngol. NY*, **212,** 213 (1976).

32. B. Kellerhals, *ORL*, **38,** 193 (1976).

32a. B. Kellerhals, *Acta Oto Laryngol.,* **87,** 370 (1979).

33. R. L. Johnson and H. H. Spoendlin, *Ann. Otolaryngol.*, **75,** 127 (1966).

34. E. Reale, L. Luciano, K. Franke, E. Pannese, G. Wermster, and S. Iurato, *J. Ultrastruct. Res.*, **53,** 284 (1975).

35. H. F. Schuknecht, K. Watanuki, T. Takahashi, A. A. Belal, R. S. Kimura, D. D. Jones, and C. Y. Ota, *Laryngoscope*, **84,** 1777 (1974).

36. J. Pietroski, *Acta Oto Laryngol.*, **71,** 494 (1971).

37. T. Konishi and M. Mendelsohn, *Acta Oto Laryngol.*, **69,** 192 (1970).

38. M. Mendelsohn and T. Konishi, *Ann. Otol.*, **78,** 65 (1969).

39. S. K. Juhn, *Arch, Otolaryngol.,* **93,** 384 (1971).

40. S. K. Juhn, *Arch. Otolaryngol.,* **102,** 683 (1976).

41. C. Angelborg and B. Agerup, *Acta Oto Laryngol.*, **79,** 81 (1975).

42. T. Nakashima, N. L. Meiring, and J. B. Snow, Jr., *Arch. Otolaryngol.*, **94,** 109 (1971).

43. J. E. Leonard, T. Nakashima, and J. B. Snow, Jr., *Arch. Otolaryngol.*, **94,** 541 (1971).

44. F. Suga, T. Nakashima, and J. B. Snow, Jr., *Life Sci.*, **9,** 163 (1970).

45. B. I. J. Beentjes, *Acta Oto Laryngol.*, **73,** 112 (1972).

46. F. I. Weille, H. G. O'Brien, L. Clark, P. Rahn, and G. Jako, *Ann. Otol.*, **70,** 528 (1961).

47. D. McN. Martinez, *Acta Oto Laryngol. Suppl.*, **238,** 1 (1968).

48. A. M. Feldman, H. R. Bittner, and S. W. Brusilow, *Neurolog. Res.,* **1,** 11 (1979).

49. H. F. Schuknecht, W. L. Griffin, Jr., G. Davies, and H. Silverstein, *Acta Oto Laryngol.,* **65,** 169 (1968).

50. L. A. Harker and B. F. McCage, in M. M. Paparella and D. A. Shumrick, Eds., *Labyrinthine Disorders, Otolaryngology*, Saunders, Philadelphia, 1973, 439–449.

51. Z. Godlowski, *Acta Oto Laryngol.* Suppl. No. 299 (1972).

52. R. S. Kimura, *Otolaryngol. Clin. N. Am.*, **1,** 457 (1968).

53. R. S. Kimura and H. F. Schuknecht, *Pract. Oto-Rhino-Laryngol.*, **27,** 343 (1965).

54. L. E. Davis and R. T. Johnson, *Lab. Invest.*, **34,** 349 (1976).

5.1 INTRODUCTION

The literature of sensory pharmacology is pitifully thin. Sensory processes simply have not been of classical concern to pharmacologists. There is no clear reason for this except that those scientists who have influenced neuropharmacological thought have concerned themselves with the central nervous system and its peripheral efferent connections rather than its afferent or sensory input. As a result none of the primary afferent transmitters is known, with the arguable exceptions of substance P and adenosine triphosphate.

Chemical neurotransmission and its associated processes seem to be favorite sites of action of drugs that influence nervous function. Whether this is the cause or the effect of all the interest in transmission by pharmacologists is hard to determine. Nevertheless, it can be said that the understanding of transmission and its associated processes is important to an understanding of drug mechanisms. It is absolutely essential for the development of new drugs designed to act at new sites, such as the inner ear.

One can only guess at the clinical applications of the information gained from basic studies of transmission in the auditory system. Afferent transmitter antagonists could be used to treat incapacitating tinnitus (if not of central origin), or motion sickness, if the primary transmitters of vestibular and auditory hair cells are the same. It may be possible to enhance the effect of the transmitter by slowing the rate at which its action is terminated; or it might be possible to stimulate the hair cells to produce more transmitter by providing more of the transmitter precursor. These last two stratagems might prove useful in the treatment of sensorineural deafness in which some functioning hair cells remain. One can only guess where knowledge and ingenuity will lead us.

5.2 TRANSMISSION AT THE PRIMARY AFFERENT SYNAPSE

5.2.1 Ultrastructure

The structural characteristics of the hair cell-VIII nerve synapse are similar to those of other chemically mediated synapses. Although the specific features vary from species to species, a synaptic cleft of 20-nm (200-Å) width filled with filamentous material is typical. The postsynaptic membrane is generally thickened and electron-dense. Presynaptically, the hair cell exhibits specializations in the form of localized membrane thickenings and an electron-dense body, rod-shaped or spherical and 0.1 to 0.4 μ in height or diameter, which is surrounded by a relatively small number of electron-transparent vesicles of 30-to-50 nm (300–500 Å) diameter. There is no morphological evidence of electrotonic junctions between the hair cell and the VIII nerve fibers.

Smith and Sjostrand[1,2] first described the ultrastructural features of the afferent synapse in inner and outer hair cells of the guinea pig cochlea. Presynaptically, the synapse is characterized by the presence of a relatively large osmiophilic mass, rodlike in shape and surrounded by a single layer of synaptic vesicles, called a synaptic body. The synaptic body varies in height from 0.17 to 0.4 μ and has no apparent limiting membrane. Several of these structures are visible at some nerve endings, although at others none is apparent. The inner hair cells also exhibit a narrow, localized thickening beneath the synaptic body and an indentation of the postsynaptic membrane, but these characteristics are not obvious at the outer hair cell synapse.

Similar synaptic features have been described in the cochlea of the newborn mouse,[3] the monkey,[4] the rabbit,[5] and man.[6] In the outer hair cells of the cat,[6–8] however, the synaptic body is not visible and synaptic vesicles are not obvious. The synaptic cleft is 10 to 20 nm wide and slight presynaptic projections of the presynaptic density are present.[6] The synaptic cleft contains some dense material and the synapse is often invaginated into the presynaptic membrane.[7] The structure of the inner hair cell afferent synapse in the cat is similar to that described in the guinea pig. The electron-dense synaptic bodies appear as bars, rings, round masses, or ribbons surrounded by a layer of vesicles. Longitudinal striations are present in the synaptic cleft.[7] The outer hair cells of the chinchilla apparently do not demonstrate the electron-dense synaptic body, although they are present in the inner hair cells.[9]

Freeze-fracture studies of the chinchilla cochlea have further elucidated the anatomical characteristics of the afferent synapse.[10] Presynaptically, the inner hair cell has a well-delineated aggregate of particles at the region of the membrane near the synaptic body. The particle aggregates at the outer hair cell synaptic region are diffusely distributed. The postsynaptic membrane of the radial nerve afferent terminals on inner hair cells has an aggregate of large particles on its external membrane leaflet, whereas the outer spiral afferent nerve terminals of the outer hair cells (where synaptic bodies are not present) have their particle aggregates on the cytoplasmic leaflet and the individual particles are smaller. Although the synaptic structure, revealed by freeze fracture in the inner and outer hair cells, resembles those of chemically transmitting synapses, the authors[10] suggest that the difference in structure between the inner and outer hair cells may mean that the two populations of hair cells release different transmitters or have different transmitter mechanisms. Such a suggestion is also put forth by Dunn and Morest[6] who observed a difference in synaptic anatomy at the inner and outer hair cells of the cat cochlea.

In the mammal the presence of the synaptic body is not a consistent feature of the hair cell-receptoneural junction. As Smith and Sjostrand[1,2] have pointed out, at some hair cell-VIII nerve synapses the synaptic body is not visible. In the cat and chinchilla the synaptic body is not evident at all in the outer hair cells. In the acoustico-lateralis organs of submammalian vertebrates the presence of the synaptic body surrounded by a layer of vesicles is a more consistent feature of the afferent synapse. In addition, studies of the synapse in these animals have yielded detailed characterizations of the ultrastructural features associated with the synaptic body.

In the lateral line organ the hair cells exhibit a synaptic body adjacent to the afferent nerve which is ovoid or spherical in shape and had a diameter that ranges from 0.1 to 0.3 μ. The structure is surrounded by a "halo" of electron-transparent vesicles which are 30 to 60 nm in diameter. A 20-nm synaptic cleft separates the thickened pre- and postsynaptic membranes.[11-17] Similar synaptic structures are found in the electric receptors in Amiurus,[18] the goldfish saccular macula, which serves as an acoustic receptor,[19] the amphibian papilla of the newt,[20] the basilar papilla of the pigeon,[21] the basilar papilla of the bullfrog (*Rana catesbeiana*),[22] and the basilar papilla of the lizard.[23] They are also found in the vestibular hair cells of the rat,[24] the bullfrog (*Rana catesbeiana*),[25] the lamprey (*Lampetra fluviatilis*),[26] and the frog (*Rana temporaria*).[27] The electron-dense presynaptic thickening often takes the form of a rodlet and is thus termed the synaptic rodlet. In the goldfish saccular macula the presynaptic thickenings take the form of conical projections. The rodlets or conical projections seem to connect to the synaptic body by filamentous connections.[16,18,19,25] Filamentous connections between the synaptic body and vesicles have also been described.[14,21,26]

The presence of a synaptic body is not unique to the hair cells of the acousticolateralis organs. Similar structures, termed synaptic ribbons or lamellae, have been demonstrated at other sensory synapses such as the retinal rod cells,[28] the photoreceptive cells of the pineal gland,[29] and vertebrate taste buds.[30] The function of the synaptic body is at present unknown, but several hypotheses concerning its function have been proposed. Osborne and Thornhill[25] suggest that the synaptic body, in connection with the synaptic rodlets, serves to store the afferent transmitter, which is formed in the synaptic vesicles. The suggestion is based on their finding that pretreatment of frogs with various drugs known to interfere with monoamine storage mechanisms produced similar changes in the synaptic body and rodlets. An alternate proposal is that the synaptic body functions to localize and regulate the release of transmitter from synaptic vesicles.[18,31] Although there is little direct anatomical evidence to suggest that the vesicle contents are released by exocytosis (such as the demonstration of omega figures), coated vesicles, presumed to be a remnant of the vesicular membrane, have been demonstrated in the hair cells of the pigeon basilar papilla[21] and in goldfish saccular macula.[32] On the other hand, Osborne and Thornhill[25] suggest that the afferent transmitter is released from the synaptic rodlets, where it may be stored, into the synaptic cleft by a gating mechanism rather than by exocytosis.

In developing organs the synaptic body can be demonstrated in the cytoplasm[26] and surrounded by vesicles.[15,17] These findings suggest that the synaptic body develops at some distance from the synaptic membrane and migrates to that structure. In an interesting experiment Jorgensen and Flock[17] amputated the tails of larval salamanders and continually transected the nerves to the regenerating lateral line organs. This enabled them to study the development of the ultrastructural characteristics of the noninnervated lateral line organ. They found that synaptic bodies and vesicles developed in the cytoplasm and in some cases migrated to the presynaptic membrane where membrane specialization, complete with pre-"synaptic" rodlets and synaptic vesicles, occurred. This suggests that the innervation of the afferent synapse is controlled by the hair cell itself.

The anatomical evidence supports the hypothesis that transmission at the afferent synapse is chemically mediated. The hypothesis is also supported by evidence that no gap junctions appear between the hair cells and the afferent nerve fibers in the cat,[6] guinea pig,[33] and chinchilla,[34,35] but the paucity of vesicles at the receptoneural junction (Yamanda[14] has calculated 200 to 300 synaptic vesicles to a synaptic body) suggests that if the hair cells release transmitters from vesicles the stimulation of the postsynaptic receptors by transmitter molecules must be extremely effective. Perhaps the receptors are exquisitely sensitive to the transmitter (i.e., the affinity of the receptor for the transmitter is high and the transmitter has an extremely high degree of efficacy) or the mechanisms for termination of the action of the transmitter are not effective. The paucity of vesicles could also be due to a high rate of synthesis of the transmitter coupled with a high turnover rate of vesicular contents. (This is not an unreasonable suggestion because the ear is *constantly* bombarded with acoustic stimuli.)

The suggestion has been made that the inner and outer hair cells of the cat and chinchilla may release different transmitters, based on their differential ultrastructural anatomy.[6,10] Although this is indeed a possibility, Smith and Sjostrand's findings[1,2] that at some of the afferent synapses in the guinea pig the synaptic body was not evident must be considered. The implication made by this differential transmitter hypothesis, at least in the guinea pig, would be that different outer hair cells in the same cochlea and perhaps different synapses in the same hair cell release different transmitters. A more conservative explanation may be that different mechanisms are present for transmitter release at these differing synapses, as proposed by Dunn and Morest[6] and Gulley and Reese.[10]

Still another possible site of afferent transmission in the cochlea bears mentioning. In his efforts to discover evidence of synaptic coupling between the outer and inner hair cell systems Bodian[35b] found clefts between pairs of presynaptic afferent fibers. These clefts suggest the possibility of dendrodendritic interaction. These contacts, however, seem to be confined to the outer hair cell system. The function of this contact site can only be wondered at. The variety of junctions in the cochlea now includes adrenergic afferents, the cholinergic efferents of the olivo-cochlear bundle, the inner and outer hair cell receptoneural junctions, and a dendro-dendritic site. The cochlea continues to provide us with challenging puzzles.

5.2.2 Physiology

In 1961 Davis[36] proposed that the following series of events is involved in the transmission of sensory stimuli: sensory stimulation produces a graded receptor potential in the sensory receptor cell which then, by an unknown mechanism, causes the transfer of information to the dendrites of the afferent nerve fibers. If threshold is reached, propagated action potentials are generated. At the time of Davis' proposal this sequence of events had not been demonstrated. The question whether transmission was electrically or chemically mediated had not been settled. Since then, however, evidence has accumulated to indicate that Davis' hypothesis does apply to the hair cell–receptoneural junction.

The cochlear microphonics (CM; cochlear ac potential), first described by Wever and Bray,[37] has been considered a reflection of the receptor potential.[38] The CM is an extracellular, volume-conducted ac potential that is essentially the same in its temporal structure as the waveform of the acoustic stimulus. This potential is not generated in the absence of hair cells[39] and the energy contained in the CM is greater than the energy in the stimulus waveform. The CM is considered a "gross" potential; that is, it is a summed response of a large number of individual hair-cell receptor potentials.[38]

The intracellular response of the hair cells to acoustic stimulation has been measured. Harris et al.[40] obtained intracellular recordings from identified hair cells in the lateral line organ of the mudpuppy (*Necturus maculosus*) and measured their response to stimulation by a pulsating jet of water. The hair cells responded to the stimulus by generating an ac response that was as high as 0.8 mV, which could be abolished by the injection of methylene blue through the recording pipette. In some of the hair cells of a single neuromast of the *Necturus* lateral line organ the receptor potentials were 180° out of phase with the stimulus waveform, whereas in others the receptor potential was in phase with the waveform. These data were consonant with an anatomical study that demonstrated that different hair cells in these sense organs have their kinocilia oriented in opposite directions. It had been demonstrated that the microphonic potential in these organs had a double harmonic component in the potential; that is, the frequency of the microphonic potential is at twice the frequency of the stimulus waveform.[12] It appeared that the orientation of the kinocilia determined the phase relationship of the microphonic potential to the stimulus waveform. The finding that the hair cells could be divided into two populations according to their intracellular response to stimulation supports the suggestion that the CM is an extracellularly recorded receptor potential. The experiments of Harris et al.[40] indicate that a receptor potential in the hair cells is generated in response to appropriate stimulation and that the CM is apparently an extracellular field potential generated as a result of the summation of many individual receptor potentials. The fact that the receptor potentials were obtained only in hair cells and not in supporting cells strengthens these conclusions.

Mulroy et al.[41] have substantiated some of the findings of Harris et al.[40] and have made an additional interesting observation in measuring the intracellular response to acoustic stimulation in hair cells and supporting cells of the basilar papilla of the alligator lizard (*Gerrhonotus multicarinatus*). The basilar papilla of the lizard is similar in structure to the cochlea and may be considered a homologous organ. In response to sound stimulation the hair cells produced dc and ac potentials. The dc potential was reminiscent of another extracellularly measured potential, the dc summating potential, which occurs simultaneously with the microphonic potential.[42,43] The intracellular dc potential observed was always in the depolarizing direction and, like the ac response, varied with the intensity of the stimulus. Harris et al.[40] were able to observe similar responses to tone bursts in supporting cells of the basilar papilla and suggested that they may also play a role in the transduction process.

Sand et al.[44] produced evidence that the receptor potential is responsible for the liberation of transmitter and the consequent depolarization of the VIII nerve dendrites. Recording the intracellular response of hair cells of the lateral line organ of the mudpuppy (*Necturus maculosa*), they repeated the observations of Harris et al.[40] that sinusoidal stimulation produced an ac potential of less than 1 mV. They also measured action potentials in the lateral line nerve and found that they were synchronized with the stimuli. They were able to mimic the mechanically evoked response by injecting sinusoidal current into the hair cell with a recording electrode. An increase in the probability of occurrence of spikes was obtained in the outward phase of current injection, which indicated that the intracellular potential of the hair cell determines the process of transmitter release and consequent action-potential generation.

Russell and Sellick[45] recorded the intracellular response to acoustic stimulation in hair cells of the guinea pig cochlea but were unable to record a component of the "receptor potential" that corresponded to the CM because their microelectrode high-frequency cutoff did not permit such recordings. They were able, however, to record a dc potential in response to sound that appeared to correspond to the summating potential and which ranged between 1.6 and 17 mV.

Action potentials have not generally been observed in the hair cells.[40,41,44,46,47a,b] In support of this statement Flock et al.[46] demonstrated that membrane resistance in the hair cells of the lateral line of the burbot (*Lota lota*) varied linearly with the membrane potential. There did not appear to be a regenerative component to resistance with depolarization of the hair cell. Similar results were reported in cochlear hair cells by Russell and Sellick.[47c] An exception is Hudspeth and Corey's[47d] observation of action potentials during the recording of intracellular potentials in the hair cells of the sacculus in *Rana catesbeiana*, although it is difficult to determine from their article whether they eliminated the possibility that the recordings were made from VIII nerve dendrites.

Principally because of the technical difficulties of obtaining intracellular recordings from VIII nerve dendrites in the cochlea, direct electrophysiological evidence that transmission at the hair cell–receptoneural junction is chemically mediated has come from studies in lower vertebrates. A series of experiments by Furukawa et al.[48] on the VIII nerve of the goldfish have characterized the postsynaptic responses during transmission at the hair cell–receptoneural junction. In the goldfish the sacculus serves as an auditory organ. This preparation has the particular advantage that some of the VIII nerve fibers are large enough (15μ in diameter) to allow intracellular penetration with a microelectrode.[49] Furukawa and Ishii[49] first described the presence of excitatory postsynaptic potentials (EPSPs) in the VIII nerve. The EPSP preceded the generation of the action potential. Later publications were devoted to characterizing the postsynaptic responses to acoustic stimulation. Furukawa et al.[48] studied the time course of the postsynaptic potentials in response to sinusoidal acoustic stimuli. A microphonic potential can be obtained from the goldfish saccule in response to acoustic stimulation. This potential was also considered a reflection of the receptor potential and the potential preceded the corresponding EPSP by 0.5 to 0.6 msec. A correlation existed between the width of the EPSP and that of the microphonic potential. Lower frequency stimuli produced EPSPs of longer duration than higher frequency stimuli. At a given frequency of stimulation an increase in the intensity of stimulation produced a prolongation of the EPSP. The observation that the time course of the EPSP corresponds to the time course of the sinusoidal wave of the acoustic stimulus and that of the microphonic potential is interesting, although not completely unexpected. This observation may be interpreted to imply that the release of transmitter from the hair cells is graded according to the waveform of the receptor potential. Another explanation may be that the longer duration of the EPSP with lower frequency stimuli is accounted for by an increased scatter in the timing of transmitter release.

In the same article the authors report the observation of spontaneous miniature excitatory postsynaptic potentials (mEPSPs), most of which were of shorter duration than the EPSPs. The authors propose that the EPSP is composed of a number of mEPSPs evoked with a slightly different timing. Finally, the authors cooled the preparation and found that the synaptic delay time was markedly increased, whereas an increase in the duration of the EPSP was less marked.

Ishii et al.[50] applied a Poisson analysis to the EPSPs in the goldfish VIII nerve. Generally, when data for Poisson analyses are obtained, the quantal content of the EPSP is reduced, as is the EPSP size, by lowering the calcium content of the medium or by raising the magnesium content. In their studies

Ishii et al.[50] reduced the EPSP size by decreasing the intensity of the acoustic stimulus. With the application of weak sounds, the EPSPs showed marked fluctuations in size. Even weaker sounds showed more marked fluctuations. The fluctuations of EPSP size at the neuromuscular junction which result when the concentrations of calcium and/or magnesium are altered have been shown to obey Poisson's law,[51,52] thus indicating that the EPSP is formed from a large number of contributing units. The Poisson relation was applicable to the EPSPs of the VIII nerve of the goldfish in response to weak sounds, although discrepancies were found in its application to the EPSPs that resulted from a strong acoustic signal. The authors conclude that transmission between the hair cells and the VIII nerve involves quantal release of transmitter. They postulate tentatively that there are multiple release sites in hair cells, each with a different sensitivity to a given depolarizing stimulus (i.e., the receptor potential), and that transmitter is released when threshold is reached for that particular site. Although such an hypothesis is tenable, it is equally tenable to propose that the number of quantal packets released at a given site is directly dependent on the level of depolarization rather than on the "threshold" of individual release sites. The latter hypothesis would be consistent with the findings of Furukawa et al.[48] that the time course of the EPSP is dependent on the waveform of the stimulus.

The input-output relations of the EPSP were studied by Ishii et al.,[53] who found that the microphonic potential amplitude was related to the EPSP amplitude in the sigmoidal fashion, whereas the microphonic potential amplitude was related to the sound stimulus intensity in a saturable linear fashion. The sigmoidal relationship between the microphonic potential and the EPSP is reminiscent of the pharmacological dose-response relationship and may be interpreted as an indication that the afferent transmitter release is related to the level of depolarization of the receptor potential, the transmitter binding to the postsynaptic receptors according to the laws of mass action kinetics and generating a sigmoidal response pattern to increasing quantities of transmitter.

The EPSPs to a given sinusoidal stimulus decreased rapidly at each peak of the waveform. In addition, the input-output functions of the EPSPs, were less steep with successive EPSPs. An examination of their input-output function curves for the first, second, and third EPSPs shows that the maximal amplitude of each EPSP obtained was identical for all, although at low stimulus intensities the successive EPSPs were smaller than those that preceded. On the basis of these results the authors suggest that the process of adaptation might be due to a partial depletion of transmitter.

Furakawa et al.[48] were able to obtain a reversal potential for the EPSP. They injected current into the VIII nerve dendrites through the intracellularly placed recording electrodes. When a weak hyperpolarizing current was applied an increase occurred in the amplitude of both spikes and EPSPs. When the intensity of the currents was increased the blocked spike potentials left enormous EPSPs. The EPSPs were also increased in duration, thus leading to a summation of successive EPSPs. An injection of current in the depolarizing direction made the EPSP smaller. When the current intensity was strong enough the EPSP was reversed in sign. Such reversals were observed in three of 25 trials. More commonly, the EPSPs were simply abolished. The reversal potential for the EPSP was calculated to have about 0 mV membrane potential. The presence of a reversal potential for the EPSP is further evidence that transmission at this synapse is chemically mediated.

Flock and Russell[47b] observed the presence of excitatory postsynaptic potentials in the afferent nerve terminals of the lateral line nerve of the burbot (*Lota lota*). Sand et al.[44] observed spontaneous EPSPs in the afferent terminals of the lateral line nerve of the mudpuppy (*Necturus maculosa*).

Thus the hypothesis that there is a chemically mediated component of hair cell–neural transmission has been unequivocally demonstrated on electrophysiological grounds. Whether the findings of Furukawa et al.[48] in the goldfish VIII nerve and those of Sand et al.[44] and Flock and Russell[47b] in the lateral line nerve will be applicable to the organ of Corti remains to be seen. Anatomical evidence points to the similarity of synaptic structure in all hair cell–receptoneural synapses. Therefore such characterizations may be universally applicable to the hair cell–receptoneural junction.

5.2.3 Pharmacology of the Afferent Synapse

Criteria Required of Transmitter

A number of chemical substances have been proposed, with little evidence, as the transmitter released by the hair cell in response to sensory stimulation. To prove that a given substance is a transmitter at a chemically mediated synapse it is generally considered necessary to fulfill the following criteria:

1. It must be demonstrated that the presynaptic cell of a given synapse is capable to synthesizing the putative transmitter.
2. A mechanism of storage of the potential transmitter substance must be demonstrated.
3. A mechanism of termination of action of the suspected transmitter should be demonstrated.
4. Administration of the putative transmitter substance should mimic the action of presynaptic stimulation.
5. Pharmacologic agents should have the same action on the effects produced by the administered transmitter candidate as they have on presynaptic stimulation.
6. It is most important that it be shown that the putative transmitter is released during presynaptic stimulation.

In investigations into the identity of the afferent transmitter (the transmitter released by the hair cells in response to sensory stimulation) the tacit assumption is made that all hair cells of the acousticolateralis system release the same transmitter. This assumption is based on the common evolutionary origin of these two organs. It should be noted, however, that Glenn[54] has rejected this assumption on the fossil evidence that the earliest vertebrates had both organs and that the innervations of both systems in fishes are completely separate in the central nervous system. Therefore the applicability of any given finding must be tempered with an acknowledgment of the possibility that there may be species differences in the identity of the afferent transmitter and that synapses exhibiting differential structural characteristics may use different transmitters. In addition, in the interpretation of pharmacological data obtained from the cat and guinea pig it is important to note that any effects of drugs or putative transmitters on the compound action potential (CAP) probably reflect the effects of those agents on the synapses of the inner hair cells because 95% of the afferent fibers in the cat and 85 to 90% in the guinea pig innervate the inner hair cells.[55,56]

It is a possibility that distinct differences may exist in receptor (pharmacological) sensitivity or in the transmitter release mechanism between the inner and outer hair cells. The data of Gulley and Reese,[10] discussed earlier, suggest that the macromolecular configuration of the postsynaptic receptor, and perhaps its susceptibility to stimulation or blockade by agonists and antagonists, may differ in the synapses that serve inner and outer hair cells.

Underlying Principles Involved in a Study of Cochlear Afferent Transmission

It is appropriate here to discuss briefly the underlying principles involved in a study of the effects of drugs on auditory afferent synaptic transmission. The CAP is obtained by recording the response of the afferent fibers to a click stimulus. A click stimulus will evoke simultaneous firing of a large number of fibers at one time. This summed response is recorded extracellularly as a volume-conducted potential by a gross electrode. Because the response recorded is a measure of the number of fibers firing synchronously, any drug that will block a percentage of the afferent synapses will reduce the amplitude of this potential. However, any drug (i.e., any viable afferent transmitter candidate) that will increase the firing rate of single fibers in the VIII nerve will also reduce the amplitude of the CAP by decreasing the probability that most of the fibers will fire simultaneously in response to the stimulus or by depolarization of some of the afferent terminals. Consequently one cannot discover whether an agent is an agonist or an antagonist simply by determining its effect on the CAP.

The CM is considered to be the response of the hair cells (primarily the outer hair cells) to stimulation and may be a reflection of the receptor potential. Consequently it is generally assumed that an agent acting specifically on the postsynaptic receptors of the hair cell–receptoneural synapse will not significantly affect the CM. The possibility that the afferent transmitter may have presynaptic actions that could affect the nature of the receptor potential should be kept in mind. The afferent transmitter might cause presynaptic as well as postsynaptic depolarizations and the presynaptic depolarization could lead to a decrease in CM. The reasoning here is the converse of that applied to explain the increase in CM induced by the olivo-cochlear bundle's supposed hyperpolarization of the hair cells. If a drug reduces the CAP and the CM, then the possibility that this action is associated with a diminution of the EP must also be considered. Such an effect should not be interpreted as an interference of transmission at the afferent synapse.

It is also important to ascertain that the ability of an agent to decrease the CAP is not due to stimulation or mimicking of the efferent, presumably cholinergic, system. If an agent decreases the CAP, then its effects on single-unit activity should be determined. This is especially applicable to putative transmitters, which should increase the firing rate of single-unit fibers at appropriate concentrations.

Cochlear Afferent Transmitter Candidates

The criteria that must be met before a particular substance may be accepted as the afferent transmitter have not been satisfied for any chemical substance at the present time. On the contrary, most substances have been eliminated as likely transmitter candidates at this synapse. The evidence favoring or eliminating transmitter candidates at the afferent synapse follows.

γ-AMINOBUTYRIC ACID

Flock and Lam[57] suggested that γ-aminobutyric acid (GABA) may be the neurotransmitter at the afferent synapse after finding that the bullfrog (*Rana catesbeiana*) basilar papilla (which has no efferent innervation[22,58]), the lateral line canal organ of a teleost fish, the toadfish (*Opsanus tau*), and the crista ampullaris of the semicircular canal in the skate (*Rana ocellata*) were capable of synthesizing ^{3}H-GABA *in vitro* when incubated with 1-^{3}H-glutamic acid. The possibility that the synthesis of ^{3}H-GABA was associated with the efferent system was diminished by the fact that the frog basilar papilla, which contains no efferent innervation, also synthesized ^{3}H-GABA. They also found that glutamate decarboxylase activity was present in the bullfrog basilar papilla and the lateral line canal organ of the toadfish. In preliminary experiments, picrotoxin, an agent capable of blocking the action of GABA at some synapses,[59,60] blocked both spontaneous and evoked activity in the nerve fibers of the crista ampullaris of the skate.

Their proposal has not been substantiated by further investigation. Fex and Wenthold[61] studied the quantitative distribution of glutamic acid decarboxylase (GAD) in the cochlea and various regions of the brain in the guinea pig. GAD activity, although present, was low in the inner and outer hair cell regions of the cochlea. Flock and Lam[57] demonstrated the presence of GAD in the frog basilar papilla and in the skate crista ampullaris. Because their results were not quantitative, it was difficult to compare them with those of Fex and Wenthold,[61] who suggest that the low specific activity of GAD in the guinea pig cochlea makes it unlikely that GABA is the afferent transmitter in the organ of Corti. Godfrey et al.[62] suggest that synthesis of ^{3}H-GABA from 1-^{3}H-glutamic acid, as reported by Flock and Lam,[57] may be explained by the presence of small quantities of GAD in all neural tissue such that the ability of a specific tissue to synthesize GABA from administered glutamate may not necessarily be related to the role of GABA as a transmitter in that tissue. This suggestion is supported by R. A. Thornhill's unpublished observation that the nonsensory portions of the inner ear of the frog (*Rana temporaria*) had as much ability to synthesize GABA as the sensory portions.[16] Although the predominant pathway for the formation of GABA in neural tissue is the single step α-decarboxylation of 1-glutamate by GAD, alternate pathways of synthesis have been demonstrated[63]; therefore the lack of high GAD activity in the organ of Corti does not necessarily imply that the hair cells are not capable of synthesizing GABA as a neurotransmitter.

Various researchers have been able to detect little or no GABA in the inner ear. Tachibana and Kuriyama[64] were unable to detect the presence of GABA in the hair-cell region of the guinea pig organ of Corti. Thalmann et al.[65] refer to an unpublished study in which they were able to detect only low levels of GABA in the guinea pig organ of Corti (0.2 to 0.3 m*M*/kg). Godfrey et al.[62] found low concentrations of GABA in all regions of the cochlea, including the inner and outer hair-cell region of the guinea pig organ of Corti. R. A. Thornhill, in an unpublished study, found low levels of GABA in the inner ear of *Rana temporaria*. All these authors suggest that the low levels of GABA demonstrated make it unlikely that GABA is the afferent transmitter.

The effect of GABA and its antagonists on the VIII nerve CAP and CM has been studied by several investigators. In the cat[66] intra-arterial injection of GABA in high concentrations produced a decrease in the CAP and CM, but the effect was assumed to be structurally nonspecific because equimolar concentrations of dextrose, sodium chloride, glycine, and α-amino-butyric acid produced the same effect. In the same study intracochlear infusion (into the perilymph of the scala tympani) of 10 m*M* GABA in the guinea pig decreased the amplitude of the CAT, but again the effect was mimicked by infusion of 10 m*M* α-aminobutyric acid and was thus considered to be a nonspecific effect. In another study[67] intracochlear administration of 10 m*M* GABA was without effect on the CAP or CM of the guinea pig, whereas 100 m*M* GABA and 100 m*M* dextrose decreased the CAP. Intracochlear infusion of 10 m*M* GABA in the cat did not affect the CAP or CM.[68] These results are not consistent with the hypothesis that GABA is the afferent transmitter released by the hair cells. Because the CAP may be a reflection of activity at the inner hair cells, the possibility exists that the outer hair cells of the cat cochlea, and perhaps the synapses of the guinea pig hair cells which do not possess the synaptic body, may release GABA, although in light of the neurochemical data this hypothesis becomes tenuous.

Pharmacological evidence also opposes the hypothesis that the transmitter is GABA. Picrotoxin is an agent known to block the action of GABA at some synapses.[59,60] Picrotoxin administered intramuscularly at doses of 100 mg/kg failed to block spontaneous or evoked activity in the lateral line organ of the mudpuppy (*Necturus maculosa*).[44] Intravenous administration of picrotoxin in convulsive doses in the cat did not alter the CAP or the CM.[66] Intracochlear administration of as much as $10^{-3}M$ picrotoxin in the guinea pig[69] or as much as $10^{-2}M$ picrotoxin in the cat[70] did not affect the CAP or the CM.

Bicuculline is another agent that has as one of its actions the ability to block GABA at some synapses.[60] Intracochlear instillation of bicuculline in the guinea pig at concentrations in the range of $10^{-3}M$ did not affect the CAP or the CM.[69] Similarly, intracochlear instillation of bicuculline at its limit of solubility and bicuculline methachloride at $10^{-3}M$ failed to alter the CAP or the CM in the cat.[70] Intracochlear administration of $10^{-2}M$ bicuculline methiodide in the guinea pig greatly reduced the amplitude of the CAP without significantly altering the CM,[67] but the authors attribute the effect to an action independent of blockade of GABA in light of the failure of similar concentrations of GABA to produce an effect. Sand et al.[44] administered bicuculline intramuscularly at 3 mg/kg in the mudpuppy and failed to block spontaneous or evoked activity in the nerve fibers of the lateral line organ.

Aminooxyacetic acid (AOAA) is a drug that inhibits GABA-aminotransferase[71] and consequently the termination of action of GABA. AOAA decreased the amplitude of the CAP and CM[72] but also produced a reduction in the EP.[73] Thus its action to reduce the CAP cannot be specifically attributed to an interference with GABA metabolism at the afferent synapse. Pretreatment of the African clawed toad (*Xenopus laevis*) with AOAA caused no significant alterations in the ultrastructure of the afferent synapse in lateral line sensory cells.[16]

Thiosemicarbazide, an agent capable of inhibiting glutamic acid decarboxylase,[74] thus GABA synthesis, was without effect on the CAP at doses up to 40 mg/kg when administered intravenously in the cat.[66] This study confirmed the results of Desmedt and Monaco.[75a] 3-Mercaptopropionic acid, which inhibits glutamate decarboxylase, had no significant effect on the ultrastructure of the lateral line hair cells when administered to the African clawed toad.[16]

Felix and Ehrenberger[75b] demonstrated the ability of iontophoresed GABA to increase the firing rate in VIII nerve fibers that innervate the saccular macula of the cat, an action which was blocked along with spontaneous discharge by the iontophoresis of bicuculline HCl. These observations indicate that GABA could play a role in vestibular afferent synaptic transmission. Further study of this phenomenon is warranted before conclusions can be drawn about the specificity of action of GABA or bicuculline in this preparation.

When all the evidence is weighed it is apparent that GABA is probably not the afferent transmitter. The most direct evidence is the inability of exogenously applied GABA to affect the CAP in a structurally specific manner (i.e., α-aminobutyric acid was as potent as GABA). The argument can be made, however, that this only proves that GABA is not the afferent transmitter at the inner hair cells because the CAP reflects activity at the afferent synapse of the inner hair cells. The low levels of GABA again contribute to the evidence that GABA is not the afferent transmitter, although anatomical evidence points out the paucity of vesicles at the synapse and suggests that the afferent transmitter may not be stored in appreciable quantities. Although the low-specific activity of GAD tends to rule out the possibility that GABA is the transmitter, the possibility also exists that GABA is synthesized by an alternate pathway, which might also explain the inability of thiosemicarbazide and 3-mercaptopropionic acid to affect the CAP or the ultrastructure of the afferent synapse. Although it is difficult to rule out completely the possibility that GABA is the afferent transmitter, neither is there reason to accept that possibility.

CATECHOLAMINES

The suggestion that a catecholamine may be the afferent transmitter[16,25,27] is based on the ability of drugs known to alter storage of catecholamines to affect the ultrastructural characteristics of the afferent synapse. Pretreatment of frogs (*Rana temporaria*) with reserpine produced a reduction in the density and diameter of the synaptic bars of the vestibular epithelium. The "halo" of vesicles surrounding the bar was depleted. Pretreatment with nialamide, a monoamine oxidase (MAO) inhibitor, produced a decrease in size but an increase in the electron density of the synaptic bars. If nialamide were given with 5-hydroxytryptophan, an indoleamine precursor, the appearance of the bars would be similar to that seen with nialamide treatment alone; but pretreatment with nialamide and 3,4-dihydroxyphenylalanine resulted in a marked increase in synaptic bar size and a corresponding increase in electron density. Thornhill[27] interpreted his results to indicate that the afferent transmitter is a monoamine and probably a catecholamine. His interpretation is based on the fact that reserpine depletes stores of monoamines,[76] an action made evident by a decrease in the number and density of dense-cored vesicles in norepinephrine-containing neurons.[77,78] Using the Falk-Hillarp histofluorescence technique, Fuxe[79] observed that treatment with an MAO inhibitor and 3,4-dihydroxyphenylalanine increased the fluorescence in cells known to contain catecholamines. Because pretreatment with nialamide and 3,4-dihydroxyphenylalanine increased the size and density of the synaptic bar but pretreatment with nialamide and 5-

hydroxytryptophan did not, he postulated that the transmitter is a monoamine and that it is more likely to be a catecholamine or its precursor rather than an indoleamine. The hypothesis was tested further by Osborne and Thornhill[25] in *Rana catesbeiana*. Pretreatment with reserpine and guanethidine resulted in a decrease in the electron density of the synaptic bars. Pretreatment with *p*-chloroamphetamine, an agent presumed to inhibit the storage of serotonin selectively,[80,81] did not alter the appearance of the synaptic bars. The authors conclude, on the basis of the present knowledge of the drugs used, that serotonin is not the afferent transmitter but that a catecholamine is the afferent transmitter. Monaghan[16] has tested the hypothesis by pretreating the African clawed toad (*Xenopus laevis*) with drugs known to alter catecholamine storage and observed their effects on the ultrastructural characteristics of the afferent synapse in hair cells of the lateral line organ. Pretreatment with reserpine produced a mean decrease in synaptic bar diameter and in the number of synaptic vesicles surrounding the synaptic bar. Pretreatment with FLA-63, a dopamine β-hydroxylase inhibitor,[82] decreased the electron density of the synaptic bar and the number of vesicles surrounding the bar. On the basis of these observations, the author proposes that the afferent transmitter is a catecholamine or a similar chemical such as octopamine.

It is hard to reconcile the suggestion that the afferent transmitter is a catecholamine-like substance with the observations that others have made. Using a histofluorescence technique, Fex et al.[83] did not observe monoamine-containing cells in the sensory structures of the organ of Corti of the cat. Similarly, using the Falk-Hillarp histofluorescence technique for the detection of catecholamines, Densert[84] could not demonstrate catecholamine-containing cell bodies in the organ of Corti in the rabbit. Borg et al.[5] studied the effects of various drugs known to interfere with catecholamine storage and found that these drugs had little effect on the ultrastructural characteristics of the rabbit's afferent synapse. Pretreatment with reserpine did not alter the electron density of the synaptic bodies. Pretreatment with 5-hydroxydopamine, a false transmitter in adrenergic systems,[85] increased the electron density in vesicles of the sympathetic nerves of the organ of Corti but did not affect the appearance of vesicles or the synaptic body at the afferent synapse. In addition, 6-hydroxydopamine, which is generally assumed to produce depletion of adrenergic vesicles,[86] did not alter the appearance of the afferent synapse. The authors conclude that it is unlikely that a catecholamine is the afferent transmitter.

The apparent discrepancy between the results in the rabbit and those in the amphibian may be bridged by postulating an explanation based on the existence of a blood-cochlea barrier. Bobbin and Guth[66] suggested that the reason *d*-tubocurarine blocked the efferent synapse when administered intracochlearly but did not affect transmission when applied intraarterially is that a blood-cochlea barrier, similar in nature to the blood-brain barrier, prevented access of systemically applied substances to the hair-cell synapses. Although the existence of a blood-brain barrier in mammals is well established,[87–90] it is possible that in amphibians the blood-brain barrier is not so well developed and it is conceivable that the "blood-cochlea" barrier is also not well developed. In light of the ability of drugs to alter the structure of the sympathetic nerve endings, it must be postulated that the sympathetic nerves lie outside the blood-cochlea barrier. If these arguments are accepted, then we may postulate that the dosage regimen of the drugs used in the study of rabbit cochlea did not produce the effects noted in the amphibian studies because the concentration of drugs at the hair cells was not so high in the rabbit.

In addition, Osborne and Thornhill[25] and Thornhill[27] used considerably higher doses of reserpine for longer periods, which may also account for their ability to observe effects that were not demonstrable in the rabbit cochlea. This argument does not imply that Borg's conclusion, that a catecholamine is not the afferent transmitter, is based on faulty evidence. On the contrary, perhaps it is an indication that extreme doses of reserpine are necessary to produce depletion of the afferent terminal vesicles and that the depletion observed in the amphibian hair cells may be due to an action of reserpine *other than* a specific ability to inhibit storage of catecholamines or indolamines. It should be pointed out that the transmitter might be a monoamine that cannot be made to fluoresce by the standard histochemical methods but might still be depleted by reserpine. Tyramine might be used as an example. Also, reserpine may inhibit the vesicular transmitter "pump" of the unknown afferent transmitter as it does for monoamines at high concentration.

Other neurochemical and pharmacological evidence is not supportive of the hypothesis that a catecholamine is the afferent transmitter. Flock and Lam[57] incubated the frog basilar papilla, the skate crista ampullaris, and the toadfish lateral line canal organ with various radiolabeled precursors, including 1-3,5-^{3}H-tyrosine (a catecholamine precursor), and were unable to detect an increase in the synthesis of tritiated norepinephine (noradrenaline) or dopamine. Klinke and Evans[91a] tested the effect of adrenaline, noradrenaline, and several α- and β-adrenergic blocking agents on the CAP and on single-unit activity in the VIII nerve of the cat. Cochlear instillation of adrenaline and noradrenaline, at $5 \times 10^{-5}M$, had no effect on the single-unit firing rate. Practolol, a β-adrenergic blocking agent, did not affect the CAP or the CM at $10^{-4}M$. Propranolol, also a β-blocking agent, produced a small (15–30%) decrease in the CAP but the effect was attributed to the drug's local anesthetic properties. Phenoxybenzamine, an α-adrenergic blocking agent, did not affect the CAP or the CM at $10^{-4}M$. Phentolamine, another α-adrenergic blocking agent, irreversibly reduced the CAP and CM at $1.4 \times 10^{-4}M$, but its effects were attributed to its ability to depress the EP. The observations of Klinke and Evans[91a] have been substantiated by Comis and Leng,[91b] who found that intracochlear infusion of noradrenaline bitartrate at concentrations between 30 and 300 μM produced no change or a reversible depression in spontaneous or evoked single-fiber discharge in the VIII nerve of the guinea pig. In addition, Bobbin and Thompson[67] administered norepinephrine, epinephrine, and dopamine at 10 m*M* intracochlearly in the guinea pig and observed no change in the CAP or CM.

Thus it would seem that a catecholamine is not the afferent transmitter. The inability of the catecholamines to affect the CAP when administered in high concentrations and the lack of tyrosine hydroxylase activity[61] are strong indications that the afferent transmitter is not a catecholamine. The possibility that the afferent transmitter is a "catecholaminelike" compound cannot be eliminated and the observation that drugs known to interfere with catecholamine storage affect the ultrastructural characteristics of the afferent synapse in amphibians, when administered in high concentrations, suggest that the storage mechanism of the afferent transmitter may be similar to that of the catecholamines.

SEROTONIN (5-HYDROXYTRYPTAMINE)

Much of the evidence which demonstrates that a catecholamine is not the afferent transmitter also indicates that serotonin is not the afferent transmitter.[5,25,27,83,84] Flock and Lam[57] incubated the crista ampullaris of the skate with 1-methylene-^{14}C-tryptophan and could detect no synthesis of serotonin. Intracochlear instillation of serotonin at concentrations up to 10 m*M* in the cat did not affect the CAP or the CM.[92] On the other hand, infusion of serotonin in the guinea pig cochlea produced a 50% decrease in the CAP at 10 m*M* and a smaller decrease at 1 m*M* without affecting the CM.[67] Methysergide is an agent that antagonizes the action of a number of drugs, including serotonin.[93] When instilled intracochlearly in the guinea pig it reduced the CAP and CM but its action was attributed to a nonspecific effect.[67] Cyproheptadine is an antagonist of serotonin peripherally[94] and in the central nervous system.[95] When instilled intracochlearly in the cat it failed to alter the CAP or the CM.[92] In the same study instillation of lysergic acid diethylamide (LSD), a potent inhibitor of serotonergic transmission,[96] failed to alter the CAP or CM at 10^{-6} and $10^{-5}M$ concentrations. Slight decreases in the amplitude of the CAP were obtained with infusion of LSD at 10^{-4} and $3 \times 10^{-4}M$ concentrations, but the effects were attributed to LSD's demonstrated local anesthetic action.[97]

Serotonin appears to be a poor candidate for the afferent transmitter substance. The neurochemical and histological evidence indicates that the afferent transmitter is not serotonin. The pharmacological evidence is generally inconclusive. Some drugs that have the ability to block serotonin elsewhere also to block cochlear transmission. These drugs, however, cannot be expected to have, as their sole action, the ability to block serotonin. The effect of serotonin to depress the CAP in the guinea pig might be taken as evidence that it is the transmitter, but in light of the histological and neurochemical data it would seem that serotonin is probably not the afferent transmitter released by the hair cell.

ACETYLCHOLINE

Although there is much evidence that acetylcholine (Ach) is the neurotransmitter associated with the efferent innervation of the hair cell[98–100] (see also Chapter 6), there is little experimental support for the suggestion[101–103] that Ach also mediates afferent transmission. Gisselsson's[101] suggestion in 1950 that Ach is the afferent transmitter was unfortunately based on several assumptions that have since been proved false and, because of incomplete knowledge at the time of the pharmacology of the efferent innervation of the organ of Corti, also unfortunately based on the assumption that any observations noted might apply to the afferent transmitter processes. It is enlightening to review the circumstances leading to this hypothesis. Derbyshire and Davis [104,105] had postulated that VIII nerve excitation by the hair cell was mediated by a chemical transmitter. Evidence that Ach was the chemical mediator at a large number of synapses was rapidly accumulating.[106] Gray[107] demonstrated that Ach was capable of generating action potentials in cutaneous and mesenteric nerves. With these observations in mind Gisselsson[101] felt that Ach was the logical candidate to be the afferent transmitter and that, if this were so, the demonstration of cholinesterase activity in the cochlear fluid would be strong evidence in support of his hypothesis. He made several unfortunate assumptions that produced his incorrect conclusion. First, he assumed that the nerve endings of the hair cells are in contact with the endolymph rather than the perilymph. Although the assumption appeared to be logical at the time, later investigation has demonstrated that the nerve endings are probably in diffusional contact with the perilymph.[100] Second, the tacit assumption was made that acetylcholinesterase (AchE) was present only in regions in which Ach acts as a neurotransmitter. It is now evident that AchE is an almost ubiquitous enzyme.[108] Martini[109] had demonstrated the presence of a choline esterase in the perilymph of the pigeon, but Gisselsson[101] felt that the observation was irrelevant to the role of Ach in VIII nerve excitation because he believed that the hair cells' nerve endings were not in contact with the perilymph. Gisselsson[101] did confirm Martini's[109] observation by demonstrating that perilymph of the pigeon, guinea pig, and cat is capable of breaking down Ach. He also demonstrated that the endolymph of the cod, cat, and guinea pig contained a substance capable of breaking down Ach and that in the cat the ability of the endolymph to do so was greater than that of the perilymph. In the same study physostigmine produced an increased latency in the generation of the cochlear potentials (CM). In light of these observations Gisselsson proposed a complex role for Ach in the cochlea; that is, that Ach was synthesized in the tectorial membrane and released with mechanical stimulation of the cochlea to stimulate the hair cells [producing the cochlear (microphonic) potential]. At that point Ach diffused to, or was generated at, the nerve endings to produce excitation of the VIII nerve. The tremendous advancement in knowledge of cochlear anatomy and physiology has reduced Gisselsson's[101] idea to an imaginative, but no longer sound, hypothesis, but the example serves to demonstrate that extreme caution should be used in interpreting evidence that purports to show that a given substance may be the afferent transmitter.

The requirements that must be fulfilled before accepting Ach as the transmitter at the efferent synapse have, for the most part, been fulfilled.[100] In contrast, most evidence indicates that it is not involved in afferent transmission.

At synapses in which Ach mediates synaptic transmission its action is terminated by AchE-induced hydrolysis. It has been demonstrated that AchE is associated with the presynaptic endings of the olivocochlear fibers (reviewed by Iurato et al.[110]). In addition, Jasser and Guth[111a] showed that cholineacetyltransferase (the enzyme associated with synthesis of Ach) is present in the cochlea of the cat and that with section of the crossed and uncrossed olivocochlear bundles the activity was greatly reduced or abolished. This observation may be taken as evidence that Ach synthesis is associated with efferent innervation rather than at the afferent synapse. Godfrey et al.[111b] also measured cholineacetyltransferase and AchE activities in the organ of Corti and other cochlear tissues. These authors found the highest enzyme activity was associated with the inner hair cell regions, followed by outer hair cell regions, and little or no enzyme activity in Reissner's membrane, stria vascularis, basilar membrane, or spiral ganglion. Their results were also declared compatible with the suggestion that the cholinergic innervation of the organ of Corti is by means of the olivocochlear (efferent) fibers. Fex and Wenthold[61] measured cholineacetyltransferase activity in several turns in the organ of Corti of the guinea pig and noted that the activity was graded from apex to base (highest in the basal turns). Because the density of efferent (presumably cholinergic) innervation is also graded from apex to base and in light of other evidence (below), the authors conclude that it is likely that the cholineacetyltransferase activity in the cochlea is associated with the cochlear efferents. Flock and Lam[57] incubated the bullfrog basilar papilla, the crista ampullaris of the skate, and the toadfish lateral line organ with methyl-^{3}H-choline chloride and noted that whereas the crista ampullaris of the skate and the toadfish lateral line organ were capable of synthesizing radiolabeled Ach the frog basilar papilla, which has no efferent innervation,[22,58] was not. The presence of cholineacetyltransferase in the lateral line organ, but not in the basilar papilla, led the authors to suggest that the efferent rather than the afferent fibers are cholinergic.

Pharmacological evidence also supports the hypothesis that the efferent rather than the afferent synapse is cholinergically mediated. Bobbin and

Konishi[112] demonstrated that intracochlear infusion of Ach and eserine (a cholinesterase inhibitor) mimicked the effects of crossed olivocochlear bundle stimulation but that increasing the dose would not abolish the CAP. [This agrees with the observation that COCB stimulation has only a limited effect on the CAP (see Chapter 2).] Robertson and Johnstone [113a] showed that the intracochlear infusion of Ach plus eserine mimics the effect of olivocochlear bundle stimulation on VIII nerve, single-fiber discharge rates in the cochlea. Fex[113b] found that *d*-tubocurarine, which has the ability to block the action of Ach when applied intracochlearly, blocked the efferent stimulation-induced slow intracochlear potential. Bobbin and Konishi[112] found that several cholinomimetics, nicotine (1 m*M*), arecoline (1m*M*), and carbachol (50 m*M*), did not affect the CM or CAP when administered intracochlearly in the guinea pig. Galley et al.[114a] demonstrated that intracochlearly applied hexamethonium, gallamine, curare, and atropine (all cholinergic blocking agents) in the cat abolished the crossed olivocochlear bundle effect on CAP and CM, thus confirming the findings of Konishi.[114b] In addition, hemicholinium-3, an agent that interferes with the uptake of choline by cholinergic neurons and eventually blocks Ach synthesis, inhibited the effects of crossed olivocochlear bundle stimulation after long periods of stimulation but did not block the CAP in response to sound stimulation.[114a,115] The addition of 5 m*M* *d*-tubocurarine, 2 m*M* atropine, and 2 m*M* acetylcholine to the bathing solution of an *in vitro* preparation of medium phasic electroreceptors (''bald'' hair cells) of the mormyrid fish also produced negligible changes in the synaptically evoked response (reflected in single-unit, nerve-action potentials).[116] Thus there is strong evidence, both neurochemical and pharmacological, that Ach is not the afferent transmitter released by the hair cells. One observation that is inconsistent with those discussed, however, forms the basis for Vinnikov's[103] suggestion that Ach is the afferent transmitter. He reports that brief stimulation of the cochlea with sound results in an increase in concentration of Ach in the cochlear fluid (endolymph or perilymph) and that after cutting the olivocochlear bundle the Ach content of the cochlear fluid still rises (but only by half as much). He presumes that the efferent and the afferent synapses are cholinergically mediated. Although release of Ach during sound stimulation in the pigeon has been reported by Martini,[109] others have been unable to repeat this observation in this[101] and other animals, including the guinea pig.[101,117]

With all the evidence at hand it seems that Ach can be ruled out as a possible transmitter candidate at the hair cell–VIII nerve afferent junction.

AMINO ACIDS

Aspartate and Glutamate. Steinbach and Bennett[116] proposed that a chemical similar to 1-glutamate may be the afferent transmitter in hair cells of the medium phasic electroreceptors in the mormyrid fish (*Gnathonemus petersii*). These modified hair cells respond to the onset or termination of a rectangular electrical pulse applied to the outer surface of the skin. They are innervated by the lateral line nerves and have a synaptic morphology similar to most other hair cells in that a synaptic body and vesicles are present in the hair cell adjacent to afferent nerve endings. Steinbach and Bennett[116] bathed the inner surface of the *in vitro* electroreceptor–lateral-line nerve preparation with various drug-containing solutions while stimulating the receptors with a rectangular electrical pulse (termed the synaptically evoked response because it evokes synaptic transmission) and while stimulating the lateral line nerve at a point near the receptor (termed the electrically evoked response which is independent of synaptic transmission). Single-unit nerve responses were obtained from the lateral-line nerves by gross electrodes. Ten (10) m*M* 1-glutamate and 10 m*M* 1-aspartate, but not 10 m*M* d-glutamate, 10m*M* propionate, or 10 m*M* acetate, first depressed and then eliminated synaptically evoked responses. At lower doses 0.5 m*M* 1-glutamate transiently enhanced the synaptically evoked response and lowered the threshold for stimulation. During a constant application of 1-glutamate the electrically evoked response showed an increase in threshold and often failed completely but returned within 10 min, whereas the depression of the synaptically evoked response was reversible only after washing with saline. The effects of 1-glutamate were consistent with, and attributed to, postsynaptic depolarization and subsequent desensitization. Unfortunately the effects of lower doses of 1-aspartate were not studied. The inactivity of propionate, *d*-glutamate, and acetate indicate that the responses to 1-glutamate and 1-aspartate are not due simply to the presence of the carboxyl group on the molecule. The inactivity of *d*-glutamate suggests that the effect is structure-dependent. Steinbach and Bennett[116] proposed that 1-glutamate was acting in a manner similar to the endogenous transmitter; therefore a chemical similar to 1-glutamate may be the afferent transmitter at this receptor.

Steinbach and Bennett's[116] observations have been substantiated to a degree in the mammalian organ of Corti. Intracochlear instillation of 10 m*M* 1-glutamate or 10 m*M* 1-aspartate in the cat[68] produced a 50% decrease in the amplitude of the CAP without affecting the CM. The decrease in the CAP was interpreted to mean that 1-glutamate and 1-aspartate were affecting transmission at the afferent synapse either by blocking the action of the transmitter postsynaptically or increasing the spontaneous firing rate. Similar responses to intracochlear administration of 10 m*M* 1-aspartate and 10 m*M* 1-glutamate were obtained in the guinea pig[67] in which 85 and 84% reductions, respectively, were seen in the CAP. Because 1-glutamate and 1-aspartate have the ability to complex calcium,[60] citrate, which is a more powerful calcium complexing agent than glutamate or aspartate,[118] was infused into the guinea pig cochlea.[67] Ten (10) m*M* citrate reduced the CAP only by 65%. It was suggested, therefore, that the effects of glutamate and aspartate were not simply due to their ability to chelate calcium ions. That these effects were not the result of the presence of the carboxylic acid grouping was confirmed by the infusion of 10 m*M* acetate, which had no effect on the CAP.

The hypothesis that glutamate was decreasing the amplitude of the CAP by inducing a synchronous firing in VIII nerve fibers was verified by applying l-glutamate intracochlearly at 50 m*M* while monitoring the activity of single-nerve fibers.[91b,119,120a,b] The infusion of l-glutamate produced a significant rise in the spontaneous firing rate of the units monitored. Infusions of 50 m*M* l-aspartate were less effective.

Fex and Martin[120c] applied DL-α-amino adipate locally to the cat cochlea and found that it had no effect on the amplitude, latency or shape of auditory nerve compound action potentials. This agent was tested because it antagonizes the actions of excitatory amino acids at a receptor called the N-methyl-D-aspartate, aspartate-preferring receptor. These results suggest that if glutamate or aspartate were the primary afferent transmitter, its receptor on the primary afferent dendrite is not of the type tested. Bobbin et al[120d] tested N-methyl-D-aspartate itself on cochlear electrical activity and found it to be without activity.

Godfrey et al.[62] found high concentrations of glutamate in the hair cell region of the guinea pig organ of Corti (60 to 70 m*M*/kg dry weight), but the concentration of glutamate in nonsensory tissues of the organ of Corti was also high. The basilar membrane contained 50 m*M*/kg dry weight, the stria vascularis, 25 m*M*/kg dry weight, and other tissues, 5 to 15 m*M*/kg dry weight. Aspartate concentrations were also high and were graded in the cochlear hair cells from apex to base. The concentrations of aspartate in nonsensory tissues presented a pattern similar to that described for glutamate.

It would seem that although there is little reason to reject the hypothesis that glutamate or aspartate is the afferent transmitter,[67,68,116,119] there is also little reason to accept it. Steinbach and Bennett[116] and Bobbin and Thompson[119,120a] have suggested that glutamate rather than aspartate may play a role in transmission at the afferent synapse. These suggestions are apparently based on the slightly higher potency of l-glutamate in affecting afferent transmission.

The suggestions that glutamate is the afferent transmitter imply that glutamate is acting to produce its effect by combining with "glutamatergic" postsynaptic receptors. Little direct evidence shows that glutamate is actually acting in such a manner. The fact that relatively large concentrations of glutamate are necessary to produce effects on the firing rate detracts from the argument that glutamate is the afferent transmitter. Several alternate hypotheses for the mechanism of action of glutamate at this synapse must be tested before any conclusions can be reached. The first is that glutamate may be acting presynaptically to induce transmitter release. This hypothesis is compatible with the observations of Steinbach and Bennett[116] that apparent glutamate desensitization was accompanied by apparent desensitization to the afferent transmitter if those observations are interpreted differently. If glutamate were causing transmitter release, the firing rate in lateral-line nerve fibers would most certainly increase, and if that release were followed by depletion of transmitter stores the synaptically evoked response after 10 min would, of course, be ineffective. This would present a picture of apparent desensitization. This hypothesis could be tested by subjecting a hair cell preparation to large concentrations of 1-glutamate and then examining the ultrastructural characteristics of the afferent synapse to determine whether depletion had actually occurred. A second hypothesis is that glutamate may be acting to inhibit reuptake of the transmitter or some precursor to the transmitter. Third, glutamate may actually interact with the receptor, when administered in relatively high concentrations, to produce excitation. It may then remain on the receptor to present a picture consistent with desensitization (this mechanism would be similar to that of the depolarizing ganglionic or neuromuscular blocking agents).

The apparent similarity between the effects of 1-glutamate and 1-aspartate suggests that, whatever the mechanism, some fundamental physicochemical property is shared by these compounds. If they are acting at the postsynaptic receptor, then it might be postulated that they also share some fundamental physicochemical property with the afferent transmitter.

Although the concentrations of glutamate and aspartate are somewhat higher in the hair cell regions than in other regions of the cochlea, both amino acids are fundamental metabolic substrates closely associated with the tricarboxylic acid cycle. Both are capable of contributing NH_3 moieties by the action of a transaminase (and entering the tricarboxylic acid cycle) and of accepting NH_3 to form glutamine or asparagine. A conservative explanation for their higher concentrations may be that they are involved in energy production in the hair cells, that in some way they contribute NH_3 moieties to the transmitter substance, or that they are structurally modified to produce the afferent transmitter.

The suggestion that glutamate is the afferent transmitter[67,68,116,119] seems to be based predominantly on the observation that glutamate will produce depolarization of the VIII nerve dendrites. In almost all regions of the brain in which it has been tested,[121] 1-glutamate has been excitatory, and it is suggested that the effects may, in many cases, be unrelated to synaptic function. Because of the widespread sensitivity of neural tissue to depolarization by relatively high concentrations of applied glutamate, any interpretation of these data in the inner ear must be made with extreme caution.

A necessary criterion for the proof that any substance serves as a neurotransmitter is the demonstration of its release during presynaptic stimulation. Sewell et al.[122] have demonstrated the release of an auditory-nerve-activating substance (ANAS) into the perilymph of frogs and guinea pigs during acoustic stimulation. Aspartate and glutamate levels are not increased in perilymph that contains this substance compared with levels in perilymph collected during silence. Thus, if ANAS is, or contains, the afferent transmitter, then glutamate and/or aspartate cannot serve that role.

The results of experimental data concerning the action of glutamate on the hair cell VIII nerve synapse are interesting, but much more investigation is necessary before glutamate can be considered a serious candidate for the role of afferent transmitter. In light of the similarity of the effect of 1-aspartate on the hair cell–VIII nerve synapse the role of 1-aspartate in synaptic transmission at this synapse should be investigated as thoroughly as that of 1-glutamate.

Glycine. The available evidence indicates that glycine is not the afferent transmitter in the cochlea. Godfrey et al.[62] found that levels of glycine in the cochlea of guinea pigs were as high as those found in the cat spinal cord gray matter, where glycine is purported to be an inhibitory transmitter,[123] but similarly high levels of glycine were present in nonsensory portions of the cochlea. The intra-arterial administration of glycine in the cat was equipotent, on a molar basis, to dextrose and sodium chloride, which indicates that the effect was probably due to the high osmolality of the injection fluid.[66] Klinke and Oertel[68] found that intracochlear instillation of glycine at concentrations up to 30 m*M* did not affect the CAP or CM. Perfusion of glycine in the guinea pig cochlea had no effect on the CAP or CM at 10 m*M*. Infusion of 100 m*M* glycine decreased the amplitude of the CAP, an effect that was duplicated by the infusion of 100 m*M* dextrose.[67] Furthermore, strychnine, an agent known to block the action of glycine elsewhere,[124] does not block at the afferent synapse.

Thus it would seem that there is little reason to believe that glycine is the afferent transmitter.

MISCELLANEOUS TRANSMITTER CANDIDATES (HISTAMINE, TAURINE, SUBSTANCE P, ATP, PROSTAGLANDINS, OCTOPAMINE, TYRAMINE)

Histamine was not detected in the organ of Corti by a fluorescent histochemical technique.[125a] Intracochlear infusion of histamine in the guinea pig at 10 m*M* produced only a slight decrease (19%) in the CAP.[67] It would appear, then, that histamine is probably not a candidate for the afferent transmitter substance. Taurine, when instilled intracochlearly in the guinea pig[67] did not affect the CAP or CM at 10 m*M*. Substance P did not affect the CAP or CM when administered intracochlearly in the guinea pig.[69] Although adenosine triphosphate (ATP) reduced the CAP 38 and 95% when administered intracochlearly at concentrations of 1 and 10 m*M*, respectively, the effects were attributed to ATP's ability to chelate calcium.[67]

Intra-arterial injection of prostaglandin E_1 (PGE_1) in the cat was found to produce an increase in the amplitude of the CAP, as well as a blockade of efferent stimulation effects.[125b] Administered intracochlearly in the guinea pig[67] PGE_1, PGA_1, PGE_2, PGF_2, and PGF_{2a}, all produced depression of the CAP when infused at 1 m*M* concentrations. Because salicylate, a prostaglandin synthesis inhibitor, also reduces the CAP when applied intracochlearly, Bobbin and Thompson[67] suggested that the prostaglandins may play a regulatory role in afferent synaptic transmission.

Although octopamine was without effect during intracochlear infusion of 10 m*M* in the guinea pig, tyramine produced, at 1 and 10 m*M* concentrations, 2 and 94% reductions, respectively, in the CAP.[67] The authors suggest that the data indicate that tyramine may be a transmitter candidate in the cochlea.

TRANSMITTERLIKE ACTIVITY (TLA) OR AUDITORY NERVE ACTIVATING SUBSTANCE (ANAS)

Among ourselves we call it "the transmitter." When strangers are present, we call it, with a wink, "transmitterlike activity" (TLA). In print it is called "auditory nerve activating substance" (ANAS).[122] ANAS is detectable by bioassay in the bullfrog (*R. catesbeiana*). It appears in the perilymph of guinea pigs or bullfrogs during sound stimulation of these animals and causes an increase in the firing rate of single units in the frog auditory nerve.[122] The perilymph of animals maintained in quiet has no detectable ANAS. It appears to be stable in the frozen state over several days. So far it has eluded detection by standard physical means, probably because of its low concentration in perilymph. Our approach to this problem is to attempt the separation of ANAS from the other constituents of perilymph by a means as simple as possible. At the moment we are using thin layer and high pressure liquid chromatography and apparently have found a component that appears on chromatograms of perilymph collected during sound stimulation but not on chromatograms of perilymph collected in quiet. The success of these separations will be monitored by the bioassay.

SUMMARY

Much of the evidence indicates that the afferent transmitter substance is a chemical compound not yet included in the list of putative transmitters. It is reasonable to suggest that the afferent transmitter is probably not acetylcholine, one of the catecholamines, γ-aminobutyric acid, serotonin, histamine, or glycine. Based on a limited amount of evidence, taurine, substance P, ATP, and octopamine seem to be eliminated as possible candidates. Although glutamate and aspartate cannot be eliminated as possible transmitter candidates, considerably more investigation is necessary before a role for these amino acids in synaptic transmission can be postulated with any certainty. The ability of tyramine to reduce the amplitude of the CAP in the guinea pig is interesting. However, a putative transmitter should produce its effect at concentrations near those achieved in synaptic transmission. The high concentration required for tyramine's effect argues against its role as a transmitter at the hair cell VIII nerve junction.

It must be restated that these conclusions are based on these assumptions:

1. The transmitter released by the hair cell is identical from species to species and is present in all hair cells, regardless of their sensory function.
2. A single transmitter substance is released and functions in afferent synaptic transmission.

5.3 TRANSMITTERS OF THE COCHLEAR NUCLEUS

The problem of correlating specific transmitters with specific cell types or aggregates in a structure as complicated as the cochlear nucleus is difficult but not impossible with today's techniques. Only in the last few years have scientists interested in transmission turned their attention to this challenging task in this important auditory structure. The purpose of this subchapter is to inform the interested reader of the studies that have attempted to describe the distribution of transmitters in the cochlear nucleus. The only attempts in this review to correlate the complicated anatomy, physiology, and transmitter distributions are *en passant* and are not meant to be comprehensive.

5.3.1 α-Amino Acids

The leading candidates for the role of secondary auditory transmitter (i.e., the transmitter released by VIII nerve endings in the cochlear nucleus) are glutamate and aspartate.[125c,126] Following cochlear ablation in the guinea pig, the concentrations of both amino acids decreased in the ventral cochlear nucleus (an area that receives VIII nerve endings) but not in the superficial dorsal cochlear nucleus (an area that receives few VIII nerve endings). The decrease in concentration of aspartate followed the degeneration of VIII nerve endings with greater fidelity than the decrease in the concentration of glutamate. Alanine dropped less than glutamate or aspartate and then not in parallel with the degeneration of nerve endings. Although all auditory nerve terminals were degenerating one day after the lesion, glutamic acid showed no decrease at this time. Glutamic acid decreased two days after cochlear ablation and continued to decrease for 28 days after ablation, a puzzling finding, because within three days postablation virtually all VIII nerve endings were gone. The close relation between the time course of decrease of aspartic acid in the cochlear nucleus and the morphological degeneration of the VIII nerve terminals after cochlear ablation suggests that aspartic acid may be concentrated in the terminals of the auditory nerve. The time course of the decrease in glutamic acid and the continued slow decrease that occurred after most primary terminals had degenerated suggests a secondary effect.

In an extension of this work Wenthold[126] subdivided the cochlear nucleus into seven anatomical regions and repeated the procedures of amino acid determinations in these regions after cochlear ablation. In this study aspartic acid distribution fits that of a putative transmitter better than the distribution of glutamic acid. Glutamic acid concentration was relatively uniform throughout the areas sampled. This finding confirms the results of Godfrey et al.[127-129] According to Wenthold[126] and Godfrey et al.[129] aspartate showed a less uniform distribution among cochlear nucleus subdividisions. As a further test of the suggestion that glutamate is the transmitter released by VIII nerve endings in the cochlear nucleus Bird et al.[130] injected kainic acid into the brainstem roughly equidistant from the anteroventral, posteroventral, and dorsal cochlear nuclei. Kainic acid destroys glutamatoceptive neurons somewhat specifically. The rate and extent of degeneration correlated with the distribution of VIII nerve terminals, which supports the hypothesis that glutamate may be the transmitter of these sites. As pharmacologists, however, we may be permitted to comment that kainic acid is only relatively specific, such specificity depending on its concentration.

Wenthold and Gulley[130a] also studied the content of glutamate and aspartate in the cochlear nucleus of waltzing guinea pigs which become deaf after 30 to 90 days of life. This deafness is caused by the degeneration of the spiral ganglion and primary auditory afferents. In these animals the cochlear nucleus content of glutamate and aspartate decreases after 90 days of life.

Two enzymes associated with glutamate and aspartate (glutaminase and aspartate amino-transferase) were found by Wenthold[130b] to be two to five times higher in auditory nerves than in other nerves tested. The activities of both enzymes decreased in the ventral cochlear nucleus after auditory nerve lesion.

The transport of radiolabeled glutamate, aspartate, and leucine from cochlea to cochlear nucleus was studied by Kane.[130c] The label from glutamate was transported to all the major subdivisions of the cochlear nucleus as was the label of leucine. The heaviest labeling was seen where the primary afferents were densest. The label from aspartate was transported primarily to the ventral cochlear nucleus. The author tilts cautiously in favor of aspartate over glutamate as the transmitter released by the auditory nerve endings, based on the relatively lower grain counts in cochlear nucleus after aspartate administration, compared with glutamate administration. These relatively lower grain counts suggest greater release and therefore loss of the aspartate label from auditory nerves.

Release of labeled glutamate and aspartate from cochlear nucleus on acoustic stimulation was found[130d] in superfusates of cochlear nucleus. There was no increase in labeled valine release occasioned by acoustic stimulation. Similarly, Wenthold[130e] and Canzek and Reubi[130f] demonstrated a calcium-dependent, potassium-stimulated release of both glutamate and aspartate from slices of cochlear nucleus. When the auditory nerve was allowed to degenerate the release of these amino acids from the slices decreased. The calcium dependency of the release was clearer with glutamate than with aspartate, thus causing these authors to lean in favor of glutamate.

Both Caspary and Havey[130g] and Martin and Adams[130h] found excitation of cochlear nucleus units by glutamate and aspartate. In addition, Martin and Adams[130h] found excitation by kainic acid and *N*-methyl D-aspartate. The amino acid antagonist DL-α-amino adipate was able to block sound-evoked activity in some cochlear nucleus units but not in others. The units that were activated by glutamate and aspartate were those whose sound-evoked excitation was inhibited by DL-α-amino-adipate.

The distributions of other amino acids and their associated enzymes have been examined in the cochlear nucleus. Glycine levels in the cochlear nucleus are similar to those reported for spinal cord gray matter in which it is presumed to be a transmitter. Godfrey et al.[129] suggest that part of the glycine is associated with small cells that may be interneurons. Caspary and Havey[131] applied glycine iontophoretically to various areas of the cochlear nucleus and found a generalized depression or a striking inhibition of activity with little reduction in driven neuronal firing.

5.3.2 γ-Aminobutyric Acid

The distributions of γ-aminobutyric acid (GABA) and associated enzymes also suggest a neurotransmitter role for this amino acid in the cochlear nucleus. First, is a striking range of values for GABA, with the highest levels in the granular regions and dorsal cochlear nucleus[128]; the posteroventral cochlear nucleus has about 1/6 to 1/8 as much. GABA was also found in high concentration in the dorsal cochlear nucleus and low in the ventral cochlear nucleus by Tachibana and Kuriyama.[132] These authors suggest that the dorsal cochlear nucleus receives GABA-ergic neurons.

They also studied the distribution of GABA transaminase (GABA-T) by histochemical means.[132] The enzyme, considered an important means of terminating GABA's action, was localized more in the dorsal cochlear nucleus than in the ventral cochlear nucleus, thus correlating with GABA's distribution.

In contrast, Davies[133] found that most of the GABA-T-containing cells were in the anterior ventral cochlear nucleus, although cells throughout the cochlear nucleus stained for this enzyme. He concluded that GABA might be the transmitter for pathways intrinsic as well as extrinsic to the cochlear nucleus. That GABA might function as an inhibitory transmitter in the cochlear nucleus was supported by the observation of Whitefield and Comis[134] that GABA produces a strong depression of firing rate when applied locally.

The enzyme that synthesizes GABA, glutamic acid decarboxylase (GAD), was found in the cochlear nucleus[135,136] and auditory nerve.[135] In his most recent publication on the subject Davies[136] has shown that both GAD and GABA seem to concentrate in the dorsal cochlear nucleus in rats, cats, and guinea pigs. Davies[136] also showed that sectioning the dorsal acoustic stria led to a significant (but less than total) decrease in GAD and GABA-T, whereas decochleation did not produce a lasting fall in enzyme activity. He concluded that aboug 30% of the GAD in the cochlear nucleus can be attributed to centrifugal fibers coursing through the dorsal acoustic stria and terminating in the dorsal cochlear nucleus. The remainder of GAD activity exists in nerve endings of intrinsic nerve fibers. The auditory nerve had low GAD activity which did not change after cochlear lesions[135]; this suggests that GABA is not the transmitter released by the auditory nerve.

5.3.3 Acetylcholine

Likewise, Ach apparently is not the transmitter released by auditory nerve endings in the cochlear nucleus.[135,137] Within the cochlear nucleus, however, the strikingly uneven distribution of AchE[138] could be taken as evidence for a neurotransmitter role for Ach. AchE is known to be a less reliable indicator of the location of cholinergic neurons than cholineacetyltransferase. Godfrey et al.[139] therefore examined the cochlear nucleus for the distribution of both enzymes. Conclusions concerning specific distributions of cholinergic pathways are not to be had from the current literature, but it does appear that Ach may be a transmitter released from cells intrinsic as well as extrinsic to the cochlear nucleus. The major extrinsic cholinergic pathways seem to be collaterals of the crossed olivocochlear bundle and a separate excitatory pathway from the superior olivary complex which ends in the ipsilateral anteroventral cochlear nucleus.[137] Using hemicholinium-3 because of its known ability to inhibit Ach synthesis, Comis and Davies[137] determined the effect of this agent on the Ach content of the cochlear nucleus after ipsilateral superior olivary stimulation. They found a marked reduction in Ach content of cochlear nucleus under these conditions and concluded that this pathway represented a major extrinsic source of cholinergic neurons. Furthermore, these authors[137] demonstrated a reduction in the Ach content of the cochlear nucleus by sound stimulation in the presence of hemicholinium-3. This decrease occurred only with the superior olive intact. This finding provides evidence that the cholinergic innervation is centrifugal, not centripetal.

The findings of Godfrey et al.[139] of high AchE and cholineacetyltransferase activities in the granular layer superficial to the anteroventral cochlear nucleus agree with Rasmussen's[140] report that most crossed olivocochlear collaterals enter and terminate in this region. The especially high cholineacetyltransferase activity in the ventrolateral area of the granular layer superficial to the anteroventral cochlear nucleus is supported by the findings of Osen and Roth[138] that AchE-positive fibers, presumably of the olivocochlear bundle, travel through this part of the cochlear nucleus and may end in the superficial layer of the dorsal cochlear nucleus.[140] The release of Ach from the dorsal cochlear nucleus on olivocochlear bundle stimulation[141] is evidence of this projected path. Comis and Whitfield[142a] have demonstrated by single unit studies that when Ach applied locally has an effect it is invariably excitatory. This suggests that the olivocochlear endings exert opposite effects in the cochlea and cochlear nucleus. The olivocochlear collaterals (if true collaterals) to the cochlear nucleus would then be producing excitation, whereas cochlear units would be simultaneously inhibited, an interesting arrangement, perhaps suited to shaping information.

In an interesting and circumspectly written paper Hunt and Schmidt[142b] reported on the binding patterns of radioiodinated α-bungarotoxin in the rat central nervous system. These authors studied the distribution of the toxin radioautographically. It was presumed that α-bungarotoxin exhibited a certain specific affinity for cholinoceptive sites in the central nervous system. This concept has been questioned[142c] and Hunt and Schmidt go to great lengths to present a balanced view of their results. All these caveats notwithstanding, they[142b] found high concentrations of silver grains over the cochlear nucleus, particularly the ventral cochlear nucleus. The source of the prejunctional (presumed) cholinergic nerves that serve the toxin binding site can only be guessed at. It is parsimonious, however, to assume that these nerves might be intrinsic as well as crossed and uncrossed olivocochlear cholinergic inputs to the cochlear nucleus.

Pickles and Comis[143] and Pickles[144] have studied the influence of atropine applied to the dorsal surface of the cochlear nucleus on behavorial responses to sound stimuli. They found that the ability to detect an auditory signal in noise following the application of atropine is impaired, whereas the absolute threshold is much less affected. Pickles[144] points out that atropine increases the width of the critical band and plumps for the homolateral rather than the contralateral olivocochlear bundle or an intrinsic cholinergic synapse as the site of atropine's action.

5.3.4 Norepinephrine and Serotonin

The cochlear nucleus also receives a significant projection of noradrenergic neurons.[145,146] The norepinephrine-containing fibers reach the cochlear nucleus by two distinct pathways. One enters through the dorsal region of the anteroventral cochlear nucleus and the second enters the dorsal and posteroventral cochlear nucleus via the dorsal acoustic stria. At least some of these fibers originate from the locus coeruleus. The local application of norepinephrine to the cochlear nucleus[147] leads to inhibition of single unit activity. Pickles[148a] in a companion piece to his earlier work with atropine applied norepinephrine directly to the surface of the cochlear nucleus. In this study norepinephrine increased the absolute and masked thresholds significantly, affecting both to the same extent. The influence of wideband noise masking was greater than that of the narrowband after norepinephrine application, which led Pickles[148a] to suggest that, as with atropine, norepinephrine had increased the width of the critical band. Fuxe[148b] has reported the presence of serotonergic nerve endings in the dorsal cochlear nucleus.

5.3.5 Polypeptides

Two polypeptides with presumed transmitter roles have been found in the cochlear nucleus, substance P, and somatostatin.

Substance P is an undecapeptide which has been nominated as the transmitter of primary afferent transmission in the spinal cord.[149] In an extensive investigation of the distribution of substance P-like immunoreactivity in the central nervous system of the rat Ljungdahl et al.[150] found substance P positive-cell bodies and nerve terminals in many areas of the rat central nervous system. A few substance P-like immunoreactive cell bodies were found in the dorsal cochlear nucleus but none in the ventral cochlear nucleus.

Somatostatin has also been found in the cochlear nucleus by radioimmunoassay.[151]

5.3.6 Summary

Any attempts at summarizing these data can only lay the author open to charges of oversimplification. Nonetheless, by way of attempting some sorely needed clarification, here is a summary of transmission in the cochlear nucleus:

1 The transmitter released by the auditory nerve in the cochlear nucleus is unlikely to be Ach, GABA, glycine, or a catecholamine. It may be glutamate or aspartate, with aspartate receiving somewhat stronger evidential support for this role.

2 GABA seems to be involved as an extrinsic and intrinsic transmitter.

3 Cholinergic neurons investing the cochlear nucleus derive from the contralateral and homolateral olivocochlear bundle. There may be intrinsic cholinergic neurons but there seem to be few, if any, cholinergic neurons projecting from the cochlear nucleus.[139]

4 Noradrenergic neurons investing the cochlear nucleus arrive in two bundles. At least some of the noradrenergic fibers derive from the locus coeruleus.

5 The function of most of these transmitters is unknown. Ach, however, seems generally excitatory, whereas norepinephrine, GABA, and glycine are generally inhibitory.

6 An atropine-sensitive (cholinergic) pathway and a noradrenergic pathway appear to be important for the detection of signals in noise.

REFERENCES

1. C. A. Smith and F. Sjostrand, *J. Ultrastruct. Res.*, **5,** 184 (1961a).
2. C. A. Smith and F. Sjostrand, *J. Ultrastruct. Res.*, **5,** 523 (1961b).

3. K. Kikuchi and D. Hilding, *Acta Oto Laryngol.*, **60,** 207 (1965).
4. H. Engstrom and H. W. Ades, in E. Friedman, Ed., *The Ultrastructure of the Sensory Organs*, Elsevier, New York, 1973.
5. E. Borg, O. Densert, and A. Flock, *Acta Oto Laryngol.*, **87,** 321 (1974).
6. R. A. Dunn and D. K. Morest, *Proc. Nat. Acad. Sci. USA*, **72,** 3599 (1975).
7. H. Spoendlin, in L. Ruedi, Ed., *Advances in Oto-Rhino-Laryngology*, Vol. 13, S. Karger, Basel, Switzerland, 1966, pp. 227.
8. E. L. Rodriguez-Echandia, *Z. Zellforsch. Microsk. Anat.*, **78,** 30 (1967).
9. C. A. Smith, in S. Iruato, Ed., *Submicroscopic Structure in the Inner Ear*, Pergamon, New York, 1967, pp. 107–131.
10. R. L. Gulley and T. S. Reese, *J. Comp. Neurol.*, **171,** 517 (1977).
11. K. Hama, *J. Cell Biol.,* **24,** 193 (1965).
12. A. Flock, *Cold Spring Harbor Symp. Quant. Biol.*, **30,** 133 (1965).
13. S. S. Jande, *J. Ultrastruct. Res.*, **15,** 496 (1966).
14. Y. Yamanda, *J. Ultrastruct Res.*, **43,** 1017 (1973).
15. A. Flock and J. M. Jorgensen, *Cell Tissue Res.*, **152,** 283 (1974).
16. P. Monaghan, *Cell Tissue Res.*, **163,** 239 (1975).
17. J. M. Jorgensen and A. Flock, *J. Neurocytol.*, **5,** 33 (1976).
18. A. M. Mullinger, *Proc. R. Soc. London*, **160,** 345 (1964).
19. K. Hama, *Z. Zellforsch. Microsk. Anat.*, **94,** 155 (1969).
20. A. Mullinger and J. J. B. Smith, *Tissue Cell,* **1,** 403 (1969).
21. T. Takasaka and C. A. Smith, *J. Ultrastruct. Res.*, **35,** 20 (1971).
22. L. Frishkopf and A. Flock, *Acta Oto Laryngol.*, **77,** 176 (1974).
23. D. Bagger-Sjoback, *Cell Tissue Res.*, **165,** 141 (1976).
24. D. W. Hamilton, *J. Ultrastruct. Res.*, **23,** 98 (1968).
25. M. P. Osborne, and R. A. Thornhill, *Z. Zellforsch. Microsk. Anat.*, **127**, 347 (1972).
26. R. A. Thornhill, *Proc. R. Soc. London*, **181,** 175 (1972a).
27. R. A. Thornilll, *Comp. Gen. Pharmacol.* , **3,** 85 (1972b).
28. F. S. Sjostrand, *J. Ultrastruct. Res.*, **2,** 122 (1958).
29. R. J. Wurtman, J. Axelrod, and D. Kelly, in *The Pineal*, Academic, New York, 1968.
30. P. H. Jepson, *Acta Oto Laryngol.,* **55,** 1 (1969).
31. E. G. Gray, and H. L. Pease, *Brain Res.*, **35,** 1 (1970).
32. K. Hama and K. Saito, *Gunma Symp. Endocrinol.*, **11,** 15 (1974).
33. M. Tachibana and H. Morioka, *J. Electron. Microsc.*, **25,** 95 (1976).
34. S. Iurato, K. Franke, L. Luciano, G. Wermbter, E. Pannese, and E. Realle, *Acta Oto Laryngol.*, **82,** 57 (1976).
35. (a) R. L. Gulley and T. S. Reese, *Anat. Rec.*, **189,** 109 (1977); (b) D. Bodian, *Proc. Nat. Acad. Sci. USA*, **75,** 4582 (1978).
36. H. Davis, *Physiol. Rev.*, **41,** 391 (1961).
37. E. G. Wever and C. Bray, *Proc. Nat. Acad. Sci. USA*, **16,** 344 (1930).
38. H. Davis, *Cold Spring Harbor Symp. Quant. Biol.*, **30,** 181 (1965).
39. H. Davis, in S. S. Stevens and H. Davis, Eds., *Hearing*, Wiley, New York, 1938.
40. G. Harris, L. Frishkopf, and A. Flock, *Science*, **167,** 76 (1970).
41. M. J. Mulroy, D. W. Altmann, T. F. Weiss, and W. T. Peake, *Nature*, **249,** 482 (1974).
42. H. Davis, *Physiol. Rev.*, **37,** 1 (1957).
43. P. Dallos, in *The Auditory Periphery*, Academic, New York, 1973.

44. O. Sand, S. Ozawa, and S. Hagiwara, *J. Comp. Physiol.*, **102,** 13 (1975).

45. I. J. Russell and P. M. Sellick, *Nature*, **267,** 859 (1977).

46. A. Flock, J. M. Jorgensen, and I. Russell, *Acta Oto Laryngol.*, **76,** 190 (1973).

47. (a) T. F. Weiss, M. J. Mulroy, and D. W. Altmann, *J. Acoust. Soc. Am.*, **55,** 606 (1974); (b) A. Flock and I. Russell, *Nature London New Biol.*, **243,** 85 (1973); (c) I. J. Russell and P. M. Sellick, *J. Physiol.*, **284,** 261 (1978); (d) A. J. Hudspeth and D. P. Corey, *Proc. Nat. Acad. Sci. USA*, **74,** 2407 (1977).

48. T. Furukawa, Y. Ishii, and S. Matsuura, *Jpn. J. Physiol.*, **22,** 617 (1972).

49. T. Furukawa and Y. Ishii, *J. Neurophysiol.*, **30,** 1377 (1968).

50. Y. Ishii, S. Matsuura, and T. Furukawa, *Jpn. J. Physiol.*, **21,** 79 (1971b).

51. A. R. Martin, *Physiol. Rev.*, **46,** 51 (1965).

52. B. Katz, in *Nerve Muscle and Synapse*, McGraw-Hill, New York, 1966.

53. Y. Ishii, S. Matsuura, and T. Furukawa, *Jpn. J. Physiol.* **21,** 91 (1971a).

54. R. Glenn, *J. Acoust. Soc. Am.*, **64,** Suppl. S-2 (1978).

55. H. Spoendlin, *Acta Oto Laryngol.*, **73,** 235 (1972).

56. D. Morrison, R. A. Schindler, and J. Wersall, *Acta Oto Laryngol.*, **79,** 11 (1975).

57. A. Flock, and D. M. K. Lam, *Nature*, **249,** 142 (1974).

58. R. G. Robbins, R. S. Bauknight, and V. Honrubia, *Acta Oto Laryngol.*, **64,** 436 (1967).

59. E. A. Kravitz, in G. C. Quarton, T. Melnechuk, and F. O. Schmitt, Eds., *The Neurosciences*, Rockefeller University Press, New York, 1967, p. 433.

60. K. Krnjevic, *Physiol. Rev.*, **54,** 418 (1974).

61. J. Fex and R. Wenthold, *Brain Res.*, **109,** 575 (1976).

62. D. A. Godfrey, J. A. Carter, S. J. Berger, and F. M. Matschinsky, *J. Histochem. Cytochem.*, **24,** 468 (1976).

63. N. Seiler, and M. J. Al-Therib, *Biochem. J.*, **144,** 29 (1974).

64. M. Tachibana and K. Kuriyama, *Brain Res.*, **69,** 370 (1974).

65. R. Thalmann, T. Miyoshi, J. Kusasari, and I. Ise, *The Otolaryngol. Clinics of N. Am.*, **8,** 313 (1975).

66. R. P. Bobbin and P. S. Guth, *Neuropharmacology*, **9,** 567 (1970).

67. R. P. Bobbin and M. H. Thompson, *Ann. Otol. Rhinol. Laryngol.*, **87,** 185 (1978a).

68. R. Klinke and W. Oertel, *Exp. Brain Res.*, **30,** 145 (1977).

69. C. H. Norris, P. S. Guth, and R. C. Hastings, *Fed. Proc. Fed. Am. Soc. Exp. Biol.*, **35,** 621 (1976).

70. R. Klinke and W. Oertel, *Exp. Brain Res.*, **28,** 311 (1977).

71. P. D. Roa, J. K. Tews, and W. E. Stone, *Biochem. Pharmacol.*, **13,** 477 (1964).

72. R. P. Bobbin, G. Gonzalez, and P. S. Guth, *Nature London*, **223,** 70 (1969).

73. R. P. Bobbin and M. Gondra, *Neuropharmacology*, **12,** 1005 (1973).

74. K. F. Killam and J. A. Bain, *J. Pharmacol. Exp. Ther.*, **119,** 255 (1957).

75a. J. F. Desmedt and P. Monaco, *Proc. 1st Int. Congr. Pharmacol.*, **8,** 183 (1962).

75b. D. Felix and K. Ehrensberger, in *Inner Ear Biology*, Vol. 68, M. Portmann and J. M. Aran, Eds., Editions of the National Institute of Health and Medical Research, Paris, 1977, pp. 147–154.

76. A. N. Bertler, N. A. Hillarp, and B. Rosengren, *Acta Physiol. Scand.* **52,** 44 (1962).

77. A. Pellegrino de Iraldi and E. De Robertis, *Experientia*, **17,** 122 (1961).

78. D. J. Curtis and G. A. Kerkut, *Comp. Gen. Pharmacol.*, **30,** 835 (1969).

79. K. Fuxe, *Z. Zellforsch Microsk. Anat.*, **65,** 573 (1965).

80. A. Pletscher, M. DaPrada, W. P. Burchand, A. Bartholini, F. A. Steimer, H. Bruderen, and F. Bifler, *J. Pharmacol. Exp. Ther.*, **154,** 64 (1966).

81. H. H. Frey and M. P. Magnusson, *Biochem. Pharmacol.*, **17,** 1299 (1968).

82. M. Corrodi, H. Fuxe, B. Hamberger, and A. Ljungdahl, *Ear: J. Pharmacol,* **12,** 145 (1970).

83. J. Fex, K. Fuxe, and G. Lennerstrand, *Acta Physiol. Scand.,* **64,** 259 (1965).

84. O. Densert, *Acta Oto Laryngol.*, **78,** 345 (1974).

85. J. P. Tranzer and H. Thoenen, *Experientia Basel*, **23,** 743 (1967).

86. R. M. Kostrzewa and D. M. Jacobowitz, *Pharmacol. Rev.,* **26,** 199 (1974).

87. D. P. Rall and C. G. Zubrod, *Ann. Rev. Pharmacol.*, **2,** 109 (1962).

88. L. S. Schanker in G. L. Hobby, Ed., *Antimicrob. Agents Chemother.,* Amer. Soc. Microbiol., Ann Arbor, 1965

89. C. F. Barlow and A. V. Lorenzo, in Y. Cohen, Ed., *Radionuclides in Pharmacology*, Pergamon, New York, 1971.

90. W. H. Oldendorf, *Ann. Rev. Pharmacol.*, **14,** 239 (1974).

91a. R. Klinke and E. F. Evans, *Exp. Brain Res.*, **28,** 315 (1977).

91b. S. D. Comis and G. Leng, *Exp. Brain Res.*, in press (1979).

92. R. Klinke and W. Oertel, *Exp. Brain Res.*, **30,** 141 (1977b).

93. W. W. Douglas, in L. F. Goodman and L. Gilman, Eds., *The Pharmacological Basis of Therapeutics*, Macmillan, New York, 1975.

94. S. A. Stone, H. C. Wenger, J. M. Ludden, J. M. Staverski, and C. A. Rossi, *J. Pharmacol. Exp. Ther.*, **131,** 13 (1961).

95. H. J. Haigler and G. K. Aghajanian, *J. Neural. Transm.*, **35,** 257 (1974).

96. G. K. Aghajanian, *Neuropharmacology*, **15,** 521 (1976).

97. V. diCarlo, *Arch. Ital. Sci. Farmacol.*, **11,** 3 (1961).

98. J. Fex, in *Basic Mechanics of Hearing*, A. Moller, Ed., Academic, New York, 1973, pp. 377–420.

99. R. Klinke and N. Galley, *Physiol. Rev.*, **51,** 316 (1974).

100. P. S. Guth, C. H. Norris, and R. P. Bobbin, *Pharmacol. Rev.*, **28,** 95 (1976).

101. L. Gisselsson, *Acta Oto Laryngol. Suppl.* **82,** 3 (1950).

102. Ya. A. Vinnikov, and L. K. Titova, *The Organ of Corti*, Consultants Bureau, New York (1964).

103. Ya. A. Vinnikov, in *Sensory Reception, Cytology, Molecular Mechanisms and Evolution*, Springer Verlag, Heidelberg, 1974.

104. A. J. Derbyshire and H. Davis, *Am. J. Physiol.*, **113,** 476 (1935a).

105. A. J. Derbyshire and H. Davis, *Am. J. Physiol.*, **113,** 35 (1935b).

106. J. F. Fulton, in *Physiology of the Nervous System*, Oxford, 1943.

107. J. P. Gray, *J. Physiol.*, **106,** 1 (1947).

108. D. Jacobowitz, *Life Sci.,* **4,** 297 (1965).

109. V. Martini, *Arch. Sci. Biol.*, **27,** 94, 1941.

110. S. Iurato, L. Luciano, E. Pannese, and E. Reale, *Acta Oto Laryngol. Suppl.* **279** (1971).

111a. A. Jasser and P. S. Guth, *J. Neurochem.*, **20,** 45 (1973).

111b. P. A. Godfrey, J. J. Krzanowski, and F. M. Matschinsky, *J. Histochem. Cytochem.*, **24,** 470 (1976).

112. R. P. Bobbin and T. Konishi, *Acta Oto Laryngol.*, **77,** 56 (1974).

113a. D. Robertson and B. M. Johnstone, *Hear. Res.,* **1,** 31 (1978).

113b. J. Fex, in A. S. DeReuck and J. Knight, Eds., *Hearing Mechanism in Vertebrates*, Little, Brown, Boston, 1968.

114a. N. Galley, R. Klinke, W. Oertel, M. Pause, and W. H. Storch, *Brain Res.*, **64,** 55 (1973).

114b. T. Konishi, *Acta Oto Laryngol.*, **74,** 252 (1972).

115. P. S. Guth and J. Amaro, *Neuropharmacology*, **8,** 49 (1969).

116. A. B. Steinbach and M. V. L. Bennett, *J. Gen. Physiol.*, **58,** 580 (1971).

117. C. H. Norris and P. S. Guth, *Acta Oto Laryngol.*, **77,** 318 (1974).

118. D. R. Curtis, D. D. Perrin, and J. C. Watkins, *J. Neurochem.*, **6,** 1 (1960).

119. R. P. Bobbin and M. H. Thompson, *Fed. Proc. Fed. Am. Soc. Exp. Biol.*, **37,** 2111 (1978b).

120a R. P. Bobbin and M. H. Thompson, *Ann. Otol. Rhinol. Laryngol.*, **87,** 1 (1978).

120b. R. P. Bobbin, *Exp. Brain Res.*, **34,** 389 (1979).

120c. J. Fex and M. R. Martin, *Neuropharmacology,* **19,** 809 (1980).

120d. R. P. Bobbin, S. C. Bledsoe, and D. M. Chihal, *Assoc. Res. Otolaryngol. Abstr.,* 4th Midwinter Meeting, p. 27 (1981).

121. P. N. R. Usherwood, in C. N. Hockman and D. Biegler, Eds., *Chemical Transmission in the Mammalian Central Nervous System*, University Park Press, Baltimore, 1976.

122. W. J. Sewell, C. H. Norris, M. Tachibana, and P. S. Guth, *Science*, **202,** 910 (1978).

123. L. F. Graham, R. P. Shank, R. Werman, and M. H. Aprison, *J. Neurochem.*, **14,** 465 (1967).

124. D. R. Curtis, Q. W. Duggan, and G. A. K. Johnston, *Exp. Brain Res.*, **12,** 547 (1971).

125a. H. Spoendlin and W. Lichtensteiger, *Acta Oto Laryngol.*, **61,** 423 (1966).

125b. R. D. Brown, *Arch. Int. Pharmacodyn. Ther.*, **198,** 372 (1972).

125c. R. J. Wenthold and R. L. Gulley, *Brain Res.*, **138,** 111 (1977).

126. R. J. Wenthold, *Brain Res.*, **143,** 544 (1978).

127. D. A. Godfrey, J. A. Carter, S. J. Berger, and F. M. Matschinsky, *J. Histochem. Cytochem.*, **26,** 468 (1976).

128. D. A. Godfrey, J. A. Carter, S. J. Berger, O. H. Lowry, and F. M. Matschinsky, *J. Histochem. Cytochem.*, **25,** 417 (1977).

129. D. A. Godfrey, J. A. Carter, O. H. Lowry, and F. M. Matschinsky, *J. Histochem. Cytochem.*, **26**(2), 118 (1978).

130. S. J. Bird, R. L. Gulley, R. J. Wenthold, and J. Fex, *Science*, **202,** 1037 (1978).

130a. R. J. Wenthold and R. L. Gulley, *Brain Res.*, **158,** 295 (1978).

130b. R. J. Wenthold, *Brain Res.*, **190,** 293 (1980).

130c. E. S. Kane, *Neuroscience*, **4,** 729 (1979).

130d. E. Hansson, J. Jarlstedt, and A. Sellstrom, *Experientia*, **36,** 576 (1980).

130e. R. J. Wenthold, *Brain Res.*, **162,** 338 (1979).

130f. V. Canzek and J. C. Reubi, *Exp. Brain Res.*, **38,** 437 (1980).

130g. D. M. Caspary and D. C. Havey, *Soc. Neuroscience Abstr.,* **9,**17 (1979).

130h. M. R. Martin and J. C. Adams, *Neuroscience*, **4,** 1097 (1979).

131. D. M. Caspary and D. C. Havey, Abstract Society for Neuroscience III, **4** (1977).

132. M. Tachibana and K. Kuriyama, *Brain Res.*, **69,** 370 (1974).

133. W. E. Davies, *Brain Res.*, **83,** 27 (1975).

134. I. C. Whitfield and S. D. Comis, Part II, AF EOAR, **63** (1966).

135. J. Fex and R. J. Wenthold, *Brain Res.*, **109,** 575 (1976).

136. W. E. Davies, in *Inner Ear Biology*, Vol. 68, M. Portmann and J. M. Aran, Eds., Editions of the National Institute of Health and Medical Research, Paris, p. 155 (1977).

137. S. D. Comis and W. E. Davies, *J. Neurochem.*, **16,** 423 (1969).

138. K. K. Osen and K. Roth, *Brain Res.*, **16,** 165 (1969).

139. D. A. Godfrey, A. D. Williams, and F. M. Matschinsky, *J. Histochem. Cytochem.*, **25,** 397 (1977).

140. G. L. Rasmussen, in *Neurological Aspects of Auditory and Vestibular Disorders*, W. S. Fields and B. R. Alford, Eds., Thomas, Springfield, Ill., 1964, pp. 5–19.

141. S. D. Comis and P. S. Guth, *Neuropharmacology*, **13,** 633 (1974).

142a. S. D. Comis and I. C. Whitfield, *J. Physiol.*, **183,** 22 (1965).

142b. S. Hunt and J. Schmidt, *Brain Res.*, **157,** 213 (1978).

142c. S. W. Jones, R. T. Galasso, and R. D. O'Brien, *J. Neurochem.*, **29,** 803 (1977).

143. J. O. Pickles and S. D. Comis, *J. Neurophysiol.*, **36**(6), 1131 (1976).

144. J. O. Pickles, *J. Neurophysiol.*, **39,** 394 (1976).

145. L. F. Kromer and R. Y. Moore, *Brain Res.*, **118,** 531 (1976).

146. L. W. Swanson and B. K. Hartman, *J. Comp. Neurol.*, **163,** 467 (1975).

147. S. D. Comis and I. C. Whitfield, *J. Neurophysiol.*, **31,** 62 (1968).

148a. J. O. Pickles, *Brain Res.*, **105,** 591 (1976).

148b. K. Fuxe, *Acta Physiol. Scand.*, **64,** Suppl. 247, 40 (1965).

149. S. E. Leeman and E. D. Mroz, *Life Sci.*, **15,** 2033 (1974).

150. A. Ljungdal, T. Hokfelt, and G. Nilsson, *Neuroscience*, **3,** 861 (1978).

151. M. Tachibana, J. M. Rothman, and P. S. Guth, *Hear. Res.*, **1,** 369 (1979).

CHAPTER 6

Pharmacology of the Cochlear Efferents

ERNEST A. DAIGNEAULT, Ph.D.

Professor and Head
Department of Pharmacology
East Tennessee State University
College of Medicine, Johnson City

CONTENTS

6.1 INTRODUCTION

As pointed out in earlier chapters, the specific function of the efferent innervation of the cochlea is not definitively established, despite intensive investigation. Electrical stimulation of the contralateral or homolateral olivocochlear bundles[1] (COCB and HOCB, respectively) produces inhibition of auditory afferent activity, as reflected by the suppression of the cochlear action potential (CAP) and the activity of individual auditory afferent fibers. In addition, COCB stimulation augments cochlear microphonics (CM), reduces the positive endocochlear dc potential (EP), and causes a positive shift in the summating potential.[1] The functional significance of these findings is obscure, however. The maximal attenuation of the CAP obtained by COCB stimulation is only 20 to 30 dB[1-4] and HOCB stimulation is even less effective because it produces 4 to 6 dB attenuation.[3,5-8] Furthermore, in an elegant series of experiments Igarashi et al.[9-13] found that transection of the COCB had little effect on the behavioral auditory function of the cat. Thus the auditory efferent system may be influenced primarily by higher levels of the CNS and its function may not be critical for auditory tasks such as pitch discrimination. Perhaps, as Klinke and Galley[1] suggest, these efferents act as a feed-forward system to inhibit auditory input during such acts as vocalization.

In contrast to our vague understanding of the function of the auditory efferents, a significant body of evidence supports the concept that cochlear efferent synapses are chemically mediated and that the neurotransmitter is acetylcholine (Ach). The primary purpose of this chapter is to present this evidence and place it in perspective with that related to other possible mediators.

6.2 CHEMICAL VERSUS ELECTRICAL MEDIATION AT SYNAPSES

An important criterion for the identification of chemically transmitting synapses is the presence of presynaptic vesicles[14]; electrically mediated synapses (electrotonic junctions) have none. The cochlear efferent nerve terminals do contain great numbers of spherical, electron-transparent presynaptic vesicles that are 300 to 400 Å in diameter and congregated close to the synaptic membrane.[15] In addition, the synaptic cleft of a chemically transmitting synapse is about 200 Å in width, whereas that of an electrotonic junction (i.e., a "gap" junction) is 20 to 40 Å wide.[14] The cochlear efferent synapse does have a cleft that is fairly regular and 200 Å wide.[15]

Functionally speaking, a synaptic delay is characteristic of a chemically mediated synapse, whereas electrotonic synapses have no delay. Instead they allow for a passive spread of current from cell to cell (i.e., electrical coupling). The delay in the chemically mediated synapse is due to the time required for the neurotransmitter to be released, diffuse to the postsynaptic membrane, and exert its effect. Accordingly, 12 to 40 msec elapse between stimulation of the COCB and the resultant EP alteration.[16] Even though this is a gross evaluation of synaptic activity and not a discrete measure of the synaptic delay, it is consistent with the presence of a synaptic delay. Another consequence of presynaptic stimulation of a chemically mediated synapse is that there is a prolonged time course; the effects which last for a time after the stimulation ceases are due to the time required for the action of the mediator to be terminated by reuptake into the presynaptic terminal, by enzymatic degradation of the mediator, and/or by diffusion of the mediator away from the postsynaptic membrane. The changes induced by cochlear efferent stimulation have a prolonged time course that outlasts the stimulation by 100 to 150 msec.[1]

Furthermore, it has been demonstrated that calcium plays an essential role in the release of neurotransmitters and hormones.[17] The cochlear efferent synapse is also affected by changes in the calcium concentration of perilymph.[18]

6.3 CRITERIA USED TO ESTABLISH A NEUROTRANSMITTER

The evidence indicates that the cochlear efferent synapse is chemically mediated; therefore we examine next the criteria used to establish the presence of a neurotransmitter originally set forth by Dale,[19] but modified somewhat over the years (e.g., Werman[20]). The essence of the proofs required, however, are the same. The set of criteria is as follows:

1 The putative neurotransmitter and a storage mechanism must be present in the presynaptic terminal.
2 The presynaptic neuron must contain a mechanism for the synthesis of the transmitter candidate.
3 A mechanism must be present to terminate the action of the potential neurotransmitter.
4 The postsynaptic receptor must respond quantitatively to the putative transmitter and related agents (agonists), all of which should mimic the effects produced by the presynaptic stimulation.
5 Drugs that alter presynaptic stimulation effects at synapses known to be mediated by the candidate for neurotransmitter should have predictable effects on presynaptic stimulation at the synapse under examination.
6 The putative transmitter must be released by presynaptic stimulation.

In addition to these six criteria, we could stipulate that presynaptic denervation should induce a hypersensitivity or supersensitivity of the postsynaptic membrane to the exogenously applied transmitter candidate.

The role of Ach and other substances as the neurotransmitter at the cochlear efferent terminals is now evaluated. The foregoing criteria are used to establish a logical framework for the discussion.

6.4 ACETYLCHOLINE AS MEDIATOR

6.4.1 Criterion 1. Presence and Storage in the Presynaptic Terminal

No direct evidence indicates that the Ach contained in the cochlea is actually present in the presynaptic terminals of the cochlear efferents. Electronmicroscopic studies demonstrate, however, that cochlear efferent terminals have synaptic vesicles of size, shape, and morphological appearance[15] similar to cholinergic vesicles identified in the neuromuscular junction.[14]

6.4.2 Criterion 2. Synthesis of Transmitter

Acetylcholine is synthesized in cholinergic presynaptic terminals from choline and acetate by the action of the cholineacetyltransferase enzyme. Therefore this enzyme must be present in cholinergic presynaptic terminals. Jasser and Guth[21] first demonstrated that cholineacetyltransferase is indeed present in the cochlea of the cat and that efferent denervation greatly reduces or abolishes its activity. Other investigators have since obtained similar results in other species (see Chapter 5) and observed that synthesis of Ach is dependent on the presence of efferent nerve fibers.

6.4.3 Criterion 3. Termination of Transmitter Action

The postsynaptic action of Ach is terminated by enzymatic hydrolysis via acetylcholinesterase (AchE). This enzyme, therefore, should be present in the area of cholinergic synapses. In 1956 Churchill and Schuknecht[22] demonstrated that AchE is associated with the presynaptic terminals of the cochlear efferents. By examining normal and deefferentized cat cochleas these investigators[22-24] concluded that most of the AchE activity in the cochlea depended on the integrity of the olivocochlear bundles. If the efferents were cut, most of the AchE activity in the cochlea would disappear after a period of a few days. Hilding and Wersall,[25] who used normal guinea pig cochleas, found a close correlation between the staining reaction for AchE and the localization of the efferent nerve endings. Vinnikov and Titova,[26] with normal guinea pig, cat, and rabbit cochleas, found that AchE was diffusely distributed throughout the space bounded by the base of the hair cells and the nerve fibers and endings situated beneath the hair cells. They also found AchE activity in the intraganglionic spiral bundles and little in the spiral ganglia or their fibers, which again indicates the AchE is more involved with the efferents than afferents. Recent studies (reviewed in the preceding chapter and by Iurato et al.[27]) have extended and confirmed these earlier investigations. Thus AchE appears to be present in sufficient quantities to terminate the action of Ach.

The presence of AchE is certainly necessary at any cholinergic synapse to terminate the postsynaptic action of Ach. As pointed out in Chapter 5, however, AchE is a rather ubiquitous enzyme found in such places as along axons of nerves which are not cholinergic.[28] Thus the fulfillment of this criterion is not sufficient, by itself, to make a strong case for Ach as the efferent mediator.

6.4.4 Criterion 4. Mimicking the Postsynaptic Action of the Transmitter by Exogenously Applied Cholinergic Agonists and Anticholinesterases

Background

The cochlear effects of exogenously applied cholinergic drugs have not been easy to evaluate, predominantly because of the difficulty of delivering a sufficient quantity of drug into the cochlea proper. Early investigators gave the drugs intravenously, which led to the production of systemic effects such as depression of blood pressure. This route of administration yielded few conclusive results because a high enough concentration of the drug was not being delivered to the cochlea. Other investigators have applied drugs to the round window membrane, also for the most part with inconclusive results.

The intra-arterial route of administration has enjoyed more success, however. This route was chosen by Brown,[29] who studied the arterial supply to the cochlea in different species. Because the literature stated that the internal carotid arteries of cats were not patent and that the arterial supply to the inner ear was a branch of the basilar artery, he inserted his cannula in the left subclavian artery so that retrograde injections could be made into the left vertebral artery (the right subclavian artery was not used because it is part of the innominate artery and it was feared that some of the drug solution would escape into the common carotid artery as a consequence). This route of administration made it possible to establish, in cats, that Ach could produce depression of the CAP in a dose-related manner.[30] Discrepancies were still apparent in the actions of cholinergic drugs that were due, in part, to the blood–cochlea barrier (see Chapter 1). Pretreatment with a detergent[29–30] did render the cochlea more sensitive to the intra-arterially administered drugs that had affected it. This experimental manipulation, however, did not render the cochlea sensitive to drugs that were not effective before detergent pretreatment. It was not until Bobbin and Konishi[31–32] perfused the perilymphatic space of the guinea pig cochlea with cholinergic drugs that most of the discrepancies were resolved.

Finally, a few experiments have been performed with iontophoresis to deliver drugs into specific areas of the cochlea. The results obtained with this technique can be misinterpreted because of the localized delivery of a high concentration of drug and the unknown extent of drug diffusion away from the site. Furthermore, this technique does not appear to have any advantage over delivery of the drug by intracochlear perfusion.

It must be pointed out here that a considerable number of experiments dealing with the administration of cholinergic drugs have yielded negative or conflicting results, most of which are due to methodological difficulties. For the sake of brevity only the critical studies are cited in this chapter. The reader is referred to the reviews of Guth et al.[18] and Klinke and Galley[1] for a comprehensive treatment of this specific literature.

Cochlear Effects of Cholinergic Agonists and Anticholinesterases

As already mentioned, electrical stimulation of the COCB or HOCB will produce suppression of the CAP. Intra-arterial (vertebral artery) administration of Ach[30,33–34] does produce suppression of the CAP in doses that do not effect cochlear blood flow adversely.[35] On the other hand, intracochlear perfusion of Ach alone[31–32] produces no significant changes in cochlear potentials, probably because this agent is rapidly hydrolyzed by cochlear AchE. In this regard, when Ach is perfused in combination with the cholinesterase inhibitor eserine (physostigmine) to protect it from degradation, this route of administration also produces suppression of the CAP. An additional characteristic of COCB stimulation is that it augments CM; intra-arterial Ach does not.[30,33–34] However, intracochlear perfusion of the combination of Ach and eserine does. It has also been found that COCB stimulation produces a reduction of the EP and a positive shift in the summating potential. Bobbin and Konishi[32] were unable to detect any effect of the intracochlear perfusion of the combination of Ach and eserine on the EP. They did obtain an increase in EP when the artificial perilymph was perfused alone and they felt that this increase could have masked any effect on the EP that may have been produced when Ach and eserine were perfused in the artificial perilymph. The effects of exogenously applied Ach on the summating potential have not been reported.

Because of the proved relationships between chemical structure and pharmacological activity we would expect that the administration of choline or choline esters other than Ach would also mimic some of the effects of cochlear efferent stimulation. This is apparently the case, although the results are not so conclusive as with Ach itself. Intra-arterial administration of methacholine does produce consistent suppression of the CAP and on occasion augments CM.[29] In addition, intra-arterial administration of choline has suppressed the CAP in the hands of one group of investigators[34] but not in those of others.[36–37]

It might also be expected that administration of other cholinomimetics such as the cholinesterase inhibitors and anticholinesterase insecticides would enhance the effects of intra-arterial Ach by preventing its degradation by AchE and could even exert cholinergic effects themselves, for if Ach were being released at the cochlear efferent synapse a block of AchE would prevent its degradation and allow its accumulation in the region of those synapses. One group of investigators[33] did find that intra-arterial eserine produced suppression of the CAP, although another group[29,34] obtained inconsistent results. In addition, Daigneault[38] found that prolonged exposure of animals to anticholinesterase insecticides caused some suppression of the CAP and also enhanced the cochlear effects of intra-arterial Ach.

Intracochlear perfusion with various cholinergic agonists or eserine alone had no effect on the CAP or CM.[32] This was attributed to the limited range of concentrations tested.

6.4.5 Criterion 5. Effects of Drugs on Presynaptic Stimulation of Cochlear Efferents

Cholinergic Blockers

The effect of intra-arterial Ach on the CAP was blocked[30,34] by intra-arterial atropine and methyl atropine, drugs that are competitive antagonists of Ach at postganglionic parasympathetic nerve terminals (i.e., "muscarinic" blockers). In contrast, such blockade did not occur in response to intra-arterial administration of gallamine (Flaxedil®) or mecamylamine (Inversine®), drugs that block Ach at the neuromuscular junction and the autonomic ganglia, respectively (i.e., "nicotinic" blockers). None of these drugs has any measurable effect on COCB stimulation effects when given intra-arterially. These and other cholinergic blockers, however, are quite active in blocking COCB effects when given by intracochlear perfusion or instillation. The list of effective cholinergic blockers[18] includes *d*-tubocurarine, atropine, methyl atropine, decamethonium, hexamethonium, gallamine, succinylcholine, muscarone, and mecamylamine. Thus intracochlear application of these drugs appears to bypass the blood–cochlea barrier.

Bobbin and Konishi[32] also found that intracochlear perfusion of a high concentration of eserine (800 μM) produces a block of COCB effects, although perfusion of the lower concentration (20 μM) used in combination with Ach does not. They believed that the block with high doses of eserine was due to a curarelike action of the drug because this action has been documented at other cholinergic synapses.[39-40] Furthermore, Galley et al.[41] found that intracochlear instillation of eserine enhanced the COCB stimulation effects, which would be expected if the drug caused an excess of Ach to cumulate at the efferent terminals.

Aminoglycoside Antibiotics

The aminoglycoside antibiotics produce a block of the neuromuscular junction that appears to be due in part to a postsynaptic block of Ach.[42] One or more of these antibiotics have been demonstrated (1) to block the CAP depression produced by intra-arterial Ach when administered acutely[43]; (2) to act as weak agonists themselves and cause CAP depression and/or augmentation of CM when given acutely[44-46]; and (3) to enhance, then block COCB stimulation effects when given chronically.[47-48] Because of these findings and the correlation between aminoglycoside-induced hair-cell damage and the efferent innervation pattern of the cochlea, it has been postulated that the ototoxicity of these antibiotics may, at least in part, be due to their interference with Ach's role as mediator of the cochlear efferents (see Chapter 7 for further evaluation of this postulate).

Cholinergic Agonists

When given alone by intracochlear perfusion, Ach, carbachol, nicotine, and choline have been demonstrated to block COCB stimulation effects partially without mimicking those effects.[32] The blockade of cholinergic synapses by cholinergic agonists is not surprising because these drugs classically demonstrate dose-dependent blocking at cholinergic sites.[49-50]

Strychnine, Brucine, Coniine, and Tetanus Toxin

Intravenous strychnine blocks the mimicking effects of intra-arterial Ach[34] and both COCB and HOCB stimulation effects.[4,51-53] In addition, it has been demonstrated that intravenous brucine and coniine[4,53-54] block COCB stimulation effects. Whether they block intra-arterial Ach or HOCB stimulation effects is not known.

Strychnine is not normally regarded as an anticholinergic; rather, it is usually considered an antagonist of glycine. It has also produced a postsynaptic blockade of peripheral cholinergic sites[55-57] and a presynaptic cholinergic blockade in the superior cervical ganglion.[58] When applied intracochlearly, strychnine and gallamine are roughly equipotent in their blockade of COCB stimulation effects.[37] Coniine, like strychnine, has both neuromuscular and ganglionic blocking activities[57] and blockade of these junctions by both drugs is partially reversed by the cholinesterase inhibitors physostigmine and neostigmine.[59] Brucine's structural relationship to strychnine and its similar pharmacological actions leads us to believe that it is also acting on the cochlear efferents via an anticholinergic effect. These findings prompted Guth et al.[18] to suggest that these alkaloids are antagonists at cochlear *cholinergic* sites.

Tetanus toxin resembles strychnine in its ability to block spinal inhibition and is also generally considered a glycine antagonist. As Guth et al.[18] pointed out, however, it also inhibits cholinergic transmission (e.g., in the iris[60]). When Klinke et al.[61] instilled this drug into the cochlea they obtained a complete block of the effects of COCB stimulation. The mechanism of this action was believed to be due to presynaptic interference with release of the efferent transmitter.

Hemicholinium-3 (HC-3)

HC-3 blocks synthesis of Ach by interfering with the acetylation of choline.[62-63] Therefore, if HC-3 is administered and a cholinergic nerve is stimulated presynaptically to force it to continue to release Ach, depletion of Ach occurs and blockade of presynaptic stimulation effects results. At doses higher than those necessary to produce the presynaptic depletion of Ach, HC-3 also has a curarelike effect.[64-65]

Intra-arterial administration of HC-3[34,36] produces a partial block of COCB stimulation effects when concomitant COCB stimulation is used. Intracochlear instillation of HC-3,[37] even more effective, produces a complete block of COCB stimulation effects. These results are what would be expected if Ach were the mediator at the cochlear efferent terminals. Furthermore, when higher concentrations of HC-3 than those necessary to produce presynaptic depletion of Ach are instilled in the cochlea, COCB stimulation effects are blocked with or without concomitant presynaptic stimulation.[37] The latter effect could be logically attributed to the curarelike action of HC-3.

Appropriate doses of choline can overcome the effect of HC-3 on Ach synthesis.[63] Guth and Amaro[36] demonstrated that intra-arterial administration of choline produced a reversal of the HC-3 effect on COCB stimulation. Although Brown et al.[34] did not observe a reversal after intra-arterial administration of choline, the doses they used were higher than those used by Guth and Amaro and the depression of the CAP obtained due to the direct effect of choline probably obscured any underlying reversal of the presynaptic depletion of Ach. Galley et al.[37] were also unable to reverse the HC-3 effect by intracochlear application of choline but they speculated that it may have been due to their not using a high enough concentration of choline.

6.4.6 Criterion 6. Release of Ach by COCB Stimulation

The technical difficulties surrounding the experiments required to satisfy this criterion are substantial. In the first place it is not possible to perfuse selectively the cochlear compartment that contains cortilymph, the organ of Corti, and the afferent and efferent terminals. Therefore it is necessary to perfuse the perilymphatic compartment and hope that a high enough concentration of mediator can be obtained to be detected after its diffusion from the organ of Corti and its dilution by perilymph. Second, the presence of large amounts of cochlear AchE in the region of the efferent synapse makes it mandatory that adequate anticholinesterase concentrations also be present to minimize the metabolism of Ach.

A number of investigators have reported preliminary positive or negative results but the credit for the in-depth evaluation of this criterion must go to Norris and Guth.[66] These investigators[66-68] calculated the Ach content of normal guinea pig perilymph to be on the order of 10^{-11} mole/ml of perilymphatic perfusate in the presence of cholinesterase inhibition, a concentration that was just detectable by their improved bioassay technique. Furthermore, they found some baseline Ach in the perilymph of guinea pigs perfused in silence and a more than twofold increase when COCB stimulation was performed during perfusion.

6.4.7 Denervation Supersensitivity

Daigneault and Brown[69] found that if the cochlear efferents are sectioned and allowed to degenerate before administering Ach intra-arterially the depression of the CAP by Ach is enhanced. The exact mechanism of the phenomenon of denervation supersensitivity is not clearly understood; at the neuromuscular junction it seems to be due to a spread of Ach receptor sites over the entire surface (in the innervated junction Ach acts only in the end-plate region). Daigneault and Brown[69] postulated that the denervation supersensitivity of the CAP to Ach is due to a similar increase in Ach receptors. On the other hand, Guth et al.[18] suggested that this supersensitivity is the result of the disappearance of most of the cochlear AchE when the cochlear efferent endings degenerate; hence Ach is allowed prolonged access to receptors. Either interpretation, however, is predicated on the logical conclusion obtained from the experiment of Daigneault and Brown; *that Ach is acting on receptors associated with the cochlear efferent synapse.* This finding, in itself, lends support to and strengthens the cholinergic hypothesis of cochlear efferent transmission.

6.5 OTHER SUBSTANCES AS POTENTIAL EFFERENT NEUROTRANSMITTERS

6.5.1 Glycine

A reasonable amount of evidence exists to support the role of glycine as neurotransmitter of the postsynaptic inhibitory sites between α-motoneurons and interneurons in the spinal cord. Iontophoretic application of glycine produces an immediate hyperpolarization of motoneurons, an effect that is rapidly reversible.[70-72] In contrast, Daigneault and Brown[73] were unable to obtain depression of the CAP with intra-arterially administered glycine. Bobbin and Guth[74] and Bobbin and Thompson[75] did find that intra-arterial administration and intracochlear perfusion, respectively, of glycine produced CAP depression but only at concentrations sufficient to produce an osmotic imbalance (equimolar concentrations of dextrose and NaCl also produced depression of the CAP). Furthermore, Klinke and Oertel[76] determined that intracochlear instillation of glycine at concentrations up to $3 \times 10^{-2} M$ caused no change in the CM or the CAP. Thus exogenous application of glycine does not appear to mimic the cochlear changes induced by COCB stimulation.

In addition, glycine is apparently present in higher concentrations in spinal interneurons than in the other neural elements of the spinal cord.[77] Godfrey et al.[78] examined the cochlear distribution of glycine and found that it was present in the region of the inner and outer hair cells at levels similar to those reported in the spinal cord,[79] but they also found similar high concentrations in Reissner's membrane and the stria vascularis and stated that these other high cochlear levels "raise some doubts about a specific synaptic role of glycine in the cochlea." It is worth pointing out that if glycine were the efferent mediator there should have been higher concentrations of this amino acid in the OHC preparations than in the IHC preparations because of the distribution of the efferent nerve terminals; these investigators found no difference, however.

Strychnine blocks the glycine-induced hyperpolarization of the α-motoneuron, the inhibitory hyperpolarizations of motoneurons produced by volleys in appropriate afferent fibers, and the glycine-induced depression of the spontaneous or amino acid-induced firing of spinal interneurons and Renshaw cells.[71] In addition, local tetanus rigidity is associated with significant loss of glycine in spinal gray matter on the side of the local tetanus,[80] thus indicating that tetanus toxin blocks spinal inhibitory transmission by decreasing the glycine content of interneurons. These drug effects, coupled with the demonstration that strychnine will block the effects of COCB stimulation, caused earlier auditory researchers to postulate that glycine is the cochlear efferent transmitter substance. Nevertheless, the presence of substantial negative evidence and the lack of definitive positive results make it unlikely that glycine is the cochlear efferent transmitter. As pointed out earlier, strychnine and tetanus toxin also have anticholinergic activity. It is reasonable to assume that the previously discussed explanations of Guth et al.[18] related to the effects of these drugs on cochlear efferent stimulation are correct.

6.5.2 Other Amino Acids

As stated in Chapter 5, γ-aminobutyric acid (GABA) is unlikely to be the afferent or efferent neurotransmitter in the cochlea because (1) the levels of GABA in the organ of Corti are low; (2) intra-arterial administration and intracochlear perfusion of GABA does not produce a specific effect on the CAP or CM; (3) neither picrotoxin nor bicuculline, agents that are known to block the action of GABA at some synapses, have any effect on the CAP or CM; and (4) thiosemicarbazide, an inhibitor of glutamic acid decarboxylase, is without influence on the CAP and COCB effect.

In addition, neither aspartate nor glutamate appear to be the efferent mediator because, as discussed in Chapter 5, both amino acids produce a selective depression of the CAP after intracochlear instillation in the cat or intracochlear perfusion in the guinea pig; they cause no change in CM. Finally, it does not seem probable that L-alanine, β-alanine, or taurine can be taken seriously as candidates for efferent transmitter because they are inactive after intracochlear perfusion.[75]

6.5.3 Monoamines

Nerve terminals that contain the monoamines epinephrine, norepinephrine, dopamine, or 5-hydroxytryptamine (serotonin) possess dense-cored (electron opaque) synaptic vesicles.[14] "The demonstration of catecholamines and serotonin with the semiquantitative method of fluorescence histochemistry has shown that neurons and their processes that contain these transmitters can be readily identified."[14] As pointed out earlier in this chapter, the synaptic vesicles of the cochlear efferent terminals are transparent, not opaque. Furthermore, histofluorescence studies of the organ of Corti in the cat[81] and rabbit[82] have not been able to demonstrate monoamine-containing cells in the organ of Corti. Moreover, intracochlear applications of epinephrine, norepinephrine, and dopamine in the cat and/or guinea pig have no effect on the CAP or CM (see Chapter 5). Furthermore, intracochlear administration of serotonin does not produce cochlear potential changes in the cat, although it does produce selective depression of the CAP in the guinea pig. Therefore, the preponderance of electronmicroscopic, histochemical, and pharmacological evidence does not support a monoaminergic role in cochlear efferent transmission.

6.6 CONCLUSION

Ach is in all probability the transmitter at the terminals of the cochlear efferents. All criteria used to establish a neural mediator have been satisfactorily fulfilled.

REFERENCES

1. R. Klinke and N. Galley, *Physiol. Rev.*, **54,** 316 (1974).
2. J. Fex, *Acta Oto Laryngol.*, **50,** 540 (1959).
3. J. Fex, *Acta Physiol. Scand. Suppl.*, **55,** 189 (1962).
4. J. E. Desmedt and P. Monaco, *Nature*, **192,** 1263 (1961).
5. J. Fex, *Acta Physiol. Scand. Suppl.*, **59,** 213 (1963).
6. J. Fex, *Acta Physiol. Scand.*, **64,** 43 (1965).
7. J. M. Goldberg and P. B. Brown, *J. Neurophysiol.*, **31,** 639 (1968).
8. A. L. Rupert, G. Moushegian, and M. A. Whitcomb, *Exp. Neurol.*, **20,** 575 (1968).
9. M. Igarashi, B. R. Alford, Y. Nakai, and W. P. Gordon, *Acta Oto Laryngol.*, **73,** 455 (1972).
10. M. Igarashi, B. R. Alford, W. P. Gordon, and Y. Nakai, *Acta Oto Laryngol.*, **77,** 311 (1974).

11. M. Igarashi, J. L. Cranford, Y. Nakai, and B. R. Alford, *Acta Oto Laryngol.*, **83,** 410 (1977).
12. M. Igarashi, J. L. Cranford, Y. Nakai, and B. R. Alford, *Acta Oto Laryngol.*, **87,** 79 (1978).
13. M. Igarashi, J. L. Cranford, E. A. Allen, and B. R. Alford, *Acta Oto Laryngol.*, **87,** 429 (1979).
14. G. D. Pappas, in E. L. Eagles, Ed., *The Nervous System*, Vol. 3, Raven, New York, 1975, pp. 19–30.
15. H. Spoendlin, in L. Ruedi, Ed., *Advances in Oto-Rhino-Laryngology*, Vol. 13, S. Karger, Basel, 1966, pp. 227.
16. J. Fex, in A.V.S. de Reuck and J. Knight, Eds., *CIBA Foundation Symposium on Hearing Mechanisms in Vertebrates*, Churchill, London, 1968, pp. 169–181.
17. R. P. Rubin, *Pharmacol. Rev.*, **22,** 389 (1970).
18. P. S. Guth, C. H. Norris, and R. P. Bobbin, *Pharmacol. Rev.*, **28,** 95 (1976).
19. H. H. Dale, *Pharmacol. Rev.*, **6,** 7 (1954).
20. R. Werman, *Comp. Biochem. Physiol.*, **18,** 745 (1966).
21. A. Jasser and P. S. Guth, *J. Neurochem.*, **20,** 45 (1973).
22. J. A. Churchill and H. F. Schuknecht, *Laryngoscope*, **66,** 1 (1956).
23. J. A. Churchill and H. F. Schuknecht, *Henry Ford Hosp. Med. Bull.*, **7,** 202 (1959).
24. J. A. Churchill, H. F. Schuknecht, and R. Doran, *Arch. Otolaryngol.*, **69,** 549 (1959).
25. D. Hilding and J. Wersall, *Acta Oto Laryngol.*, **55,** 205 (1962).
26. Y. A. Vinnikov and L. K. Titova, *The Organ of Corti—Its Histopathology and Histochemistry*, Consultants Bureau, New York, 1964, pp. 101–110.
27. S. Iurato, L. Luciano, E. Pannese, and E. Realle, *Acta Oto Laryngol. Suppl.*, 279 (1971).
28. G. B. Koelle, in O. Eichler and A. Farah, Eds., *Handbuch der Experimentellen Pharmakologie*, Vol. 15, Springer-Verlag, Berlin, 1963, pp. 189–298.
29. R. D. Brown, M.S. Thesis, L.S.U. Medical Center, New Orleans, 1966, pp. 51.
30. E. A. Daigneault and R. D. Brown, *Arch. Int. Pharmacodyn. Ther.*, **162,** 20 (1966).
31. R. P. Bobbin and T. Konishi, *Nature*, **231,** 222 (1971).
32. R. P. Bobbin and T. Konishi, *Acta Oto Laryngol.*, **77,** 56 (1974).
33. J. Amaro, P. S. Guth, and L. Wanderlinder, *Brit. J. Pharmacol. Chemother.*, **28,** 207 (1966).
34. R. D. Brown, E. A. Daigneault, and J. R. Pruett, *J. Pharmacol. Exp. Ther.*, **165,** 300 (1969).
35. E. A. Daigneault and C. Devia, *Fed. Proc.*, **35,** Abstr. 2294 (1976).
36. P. S. Guth and J. Amaro, *Neuropharmacology*, **8,** 49 (1969).
37. N. Galley, R. Klinke, W. Oertel, M. Pause, and W. H. Storch, *Brain Res.*, **64,** 55 (1973).
38. E. A. Daigneault, *Toxicol. Appl. Pharmacol.*, **21,** 495 (1972).
39. W. Feldberg and A. Vartiainen, *J. Physiol.*, **83,** 103 (1934).
40. J. C. Eccles and W. V. MacFarlane, *J. Neurophysiol.*, **12,** 59 (1949).
41. N. Galley, R. Klinke, W. Oertel, and K. Gottl, *Arch. Ges. Physiol. Suppl.*, **343,** Abstr. R80 (1973).
42. W. E. Sanders, Jr., and C. C. Sanders, in R. George, R. Okun, and A. K. Cho, Eds., *Annual Review of Pharmacology and Toxicology*, Vol. 19, Annual Reviews, Palo Alto, 1979, pp. 53–83.
43. E. A. Daigneault, J. R. Pruett, and R. D. Brown, *Toxicol. Appl. Pharmacol.*, **17,** 223 (1970).

44. R. D. Brown, Ph.D. Dissertation, L.S.U. Medical Center, New Orleans, 1968, pp. 55.
45. F. B. Simmons, R. Galambos, and J. P. Albrite, *Arch. Otolaryngol.*, **72,** 233 (1960).
46. H. Sohmer and M. Feinmesser, *Arch. Int. Pharmacodyn. Ther.*, **144,** 446 (1963).
47. R. D. Brown, *Acta Oto Laryngol.*, **73,** 335 (1972).
48. R. D. Brown and E. A. Daigneault, *Acta Oto Laryngol.*, **76,** 128 (1973).
49. S. Thesleff, *Acta Physiol. Scand.*, **34,** 218 (1955).
50. R. B. Barlow, *Introduction to Chemical Pharmacology*, 2nd ed., Methuen, London, 1964, pp. 452.
51. J. E. Desmedt and V. Lagrutta, *Nature*, **200,** 472 (1963).
52. J. E. Desmedt and P. Monaco, *Arch. Int. Pharmacodyn. Ther.*, **129,** 244 (1960).
53. J. E. Desmedt and P. Monaco, in W. D. M. Paton, Ed., *Proceedings of the First International Pharmacological Meeting*, Vol. 8, Macmillan, New York, 1962, pp. 183–188.
54. V. Lagrutta and J. E. Desmedt, *Arch. Int. Pharmacodyn. Ther.*, **151,** 289 (1964).
55. B. O. Alving, *Arch. Int. Pharmacodyn. Ther.*, **131,** 123 (1961).
56. A. Lanari and J. V. Luco, *Am. J. Physiol.*, **126,** 277 (1939).
57. S. R. Sampson, D. W. Esplin, and B. Zablocka, *J. Pharmacol. Exp. Ther.*, **152,** 313 (1966).
58. D. N. McKinstry and G. B. Koelle, *Nature*, **213,** 505 (1967).
59. R. K. Ferguson, B. Zablocka-Esplin, and D. W. Esplin, *Arch. Int. Pharmacodyn. Ther.*, **185,** 298 (1970).
60. N. Ambache, R. S. Morgan, and G. Payling Wright, *J. Physiol.*, **107,** 45 (1948).
61. R. Klinke, N. Galley, M. Pause, and W. H. Storch, *Brain Res.*, **49,** 447 (1973).
62. D. Elmquist and D. M. J. Quastel, *J. Physiol.*, **177,** 463 (1965).
63. F. C. MacIntosh, *Fed. Proc.*, **20,** 562 (1961).
64. A. R. Martin and R. K. Orkand, *Fed. Proc.*, **20,** 579 (1961).
65. R. E. Thies and V. B. Brooks, *Fed. Proc.*, **20,** 569 (1961).
66. C. H. Norris and P. S. Guth, *Acta Oto Laryngol.*, **77,** 318 (1974).
67. C. H. Norris, McK. Burton, and P. S. Guth, *Proc. 83rd Meet. Acoust. Soc. Am.*, 50 (1972).
68. C. H. Norris, P. S. Guth and M. Stockwell, *Fed. Proc.*, **31,** 580 (1972).
69. E. A. Daigneault and R. D. Brown, *Arch. Int. Pharmacodyn. Ther.*, **177,** 238 (1969).
70. R. Werman, R. A. Davidoff, and M. H. Aprison, *Physiologist*, **9,** 318 (1966).
71. D. R. Curtis, L. Hosli, G. A. R. Johnston, and I. H. Johnston, *Brain Res.*, **5,** 112 (1967).
72. R. Werman, R. A. Davidoff, and M. H. Aprison, *Nature*, **214,** 681 (1967).
73. E. A. Daigneault and R. D. Brown, *Fed. Proc.*, **28,** Abstr. 2884 (1969).
74. R. P. Bobbin and P. S. Guth, *Neuropharmacology*, **9,** 567 (1970).
75. R. P. Bobbin and M. H. Thompson, *Ann. Otol.*, **87,** 185 (1978).
76. R. Klinke and W. Oertel, *Exp. Brain Res.*, **30,** 145 (1977).
77. R. A. Davidoff, R. P. Shank, L. T. Graham, Jr., M. H. Aprison, and R. Werman, *Nature*, **214,** 680 (1967).
78. D. A. Godfrey, J. A. Carter, S. J. Berger, and F. M. Matschinsky, *J. Histochem. Cytochem.*, **24,** 468 (1976).
79. L. T. Graham, Jr., R. P. Shank, R. Werman, and M. H. Aprison, *J. Neurochem.*, **14,** 465 (1967).
80. T. Semba and M. Kano, *Science*, **164,** 571 (1969).
81. J. Fex, K. Fuxe, and G. Lennerstrand, *Acta Physiol. Scand.*, **64,** 259 (1965).
82. O. Densert, *Acta Oto Laryngol.*, **78,** 345 (1974).

CHAPTER 7

Ototoxicity of Aminoglycoside Antibiotics

JIRI PRAZMA, M.D., Ph.D.

Assistant Professor of Otolaryngology
Department of Surgery
Section of Otolaryngology
University of North Carolina Medical School, Chapel Hill

CONTENTS

7.1 INTRODUCTION

Hearing and equilibrium disturbances due to drugs, aspirin, arsenic preparations, and quinine, in particular, have been recognized for some time. However, more attention to this subject came after the introduction of streptomycin for the treatment of tuberculosis. Thousands of papers have been written about aminoglycoside antibiotics (AmAn) and their adverse reactions. Excellent reviews of this subject have been presented by Kohonen,[1] Guth and Bobbin,[2] Federspil,[3] Hawkins,[4-5] Brown and Feldman,[6] and Sanders and Sanders.[7]

Aminoglycoside antibiotics can be subdivided into several groups according to structure. The first group includes streptomycin (STM) and dihydrostreptomycin (DH–STM). The second group consists of kanamycin (KA), amikacin (AK), and tobramycin (TO). The third group includes gentamicin (GE), sisomicin (SI), and netilmicin (NET). Tobramycin can also be placed in the third group because of its structural relation to the gentamicin aminoglycosides. The fourth and final group consists of neomycin (NEO), paramomycin, lividomycin, and ribostatin. The AmAn can also be divided according to origin; for example, aminoglycosides which are produced by *Streptomyces* are identified as "mycin" and those produced by *Micromonospora* are termed "micin." Recently a new generation of aminoglycoside antibiotics was developed by molecular manipulation from the earliest AmAn. This group includes amikacin and netilmicin.

As a group the AmAn share a number of properties:

1 All are organic bases that consist of "polycations containing amino sugars glycosidically linked to streptidine or deoxystreptamine."[7]
2 Their inorganic acid salts are water soluble, the sulfate salts normally being those used therapeutically (except for amikacin, which is sufficiently water soluble).
3 None is absorbed to a significant degree by the normal intestinal tract.
4 Their serum concentrations usually peak 30 to 90 min after i.m. administration.
5 The elimination half-lives (T 1/2s*) of all are relatively short (1.5–3 hr).
6 Excretion is primarily via glomerular filtration.
7 All have nephrotoxic and ototoxic liability, neuromuscular blocking capability, and allergenicity.
8 They are used primarily in the treatment of disease caused by gram-negative bacteria.

One of the factors limiting broad application of AmAn in the treatment of serious gram-negative bacterial infections is the narrow range between ther-

*T 1/2s in this chapter always refer to T 1/2 β's.

apeutic and toxic serum levels; for example, when the peak serum concentration of GE is maintained below 4 μg/ml, bacteremia caused by *Pseudomonas aeruginosa*, which are resistant to these low levels, results in a high fatality rate.[8] However, if its peak serum level is maintained above 8 μg/ml ototoxicity and nephrotoxicity frequently occur.[9]

7.2 GENERAL DISCUSSION OF AMINOGLYCOSIDE ANTIBIOTICS

7.2.1 Antibacterial Action and Resistance

At present the most widely accepted theory is that the AmAn affect bacteria undergoing protein synthesis. They prevent polymerization of amino acids by adhering to the 30s ribosomal subunit, thus interfering with protein synthesis. However, to act inside bacterial cells they must first be transported there, either actively or passively. It has been found that sensitive microorganisms are capable of concentrating these antibiotics inside their cells—up to 250 times the surrounding concentration. Bryan and Van den Elzen[10] and Price et al.[11] were able to prove that AmAn are actively taken up by sensitive microorganisms but not by the insensitive.

Resistance to AmAn is usually caused by enzymes that can acetylate, adenylate, or phosphorylate the antibiotics and inactivate them. Acquired resistance is carried on extrachromosomal elements (R factors or plasmids) that are transferred by conjunction or transduction. Cross-resistance to similar antibiotics may also occur.[12]

7.2.2 Absorption, Distribution, and Excretion

The antibiotics are only partly absorbed from the gastrointestinal tract after oral administration (about 3% of dose); for the most part they are excreted, unchanged, in the feces. To achieve a therapeutic effect they must be administered parenterally. Some of them which are highly toxic can be absorbed from the skin, gastrointestinal tract, and peritoneal and thoracic cavities in quantities sufficient to cause adverse reactions. This is particularly likely when large portions of skin are abraded or denuded or when the gastrointestinal tract mucosa, the serosa, or the pleura are inflammed because of injury or disease.

Serum concentrations usually peak within 30 to 90 min after i.m. administration. In normal adults the serum elimination half-lives (T 1/2s) of the AmAn are in the range of 1.5 to 3 hr. In newborns 6 to 22 days old, however, they are as long as 6 hr and may extend past 18 in premature infants (whose kidneys are not fully developed). The half-lives of these drugs are even longer in anuric or oliguric patients.

The AmAn are distributed mainly in the extracellular fluids. It must be realized, however, that the presence of therapeutic serum concentrations of these drugs is not an adequate indicator of therapeutic concentrations in the interstitial fluids of various organ systems; for example, Chisolm et al.[13] found, using dogs, that a single i.m. injection of GE (80 mg) and TO (50 mg) produced similar serum concentration/time profiles in which TO produced a slightly higher peak serum level than GE (about 10.5 and 9 μg/ml, respectively). In contrast, tissue fluid levels (obtained by using silastic tissue cages placed under the animal's skin) were much higher for GE than for TO, their peak levels being about 5 and 1 μg/ml, respectively, 3 hr after the injection.

At one extreme the AmAn penetrate slowly and inadequately into the CSF. After 3 hr their peak concentrations reach only 1/5 to 1/10 the serum levels. Their concentrations in the liver correspond closely to their serum levels, and, at the other extreme, the AmAn accumulate in the kidney cortex (probably intracellularly). The *T* 1/2s of GE, TO, and KA in renal cortex homogenate have been observed to be 109, 74, and 60 hr, respectively; the shortest *T* 1/2, 4.6 hr, was for STM.[14]

All AmAn are excreted by glomerular filtration—the protein bound portion, by tubular secretion. If kidney function is not normal at the beginning of treatment or if it deteriorates during therapy, the AmAn will not be excreted at normal rates. Therefore the serum levels of the drugs will rise after each dose and may reach toxic levels. For this reason renal function should be determined before and during treatment with AmAn to avoid or minimize adverse effects. If the serum level exceeds the therapeutic range, the AmAn can be removed by peritoneal dialysis or hemodialysis. Various methods (bioassays, immunoassays) for the determination of AmAn levels have been described by Jackson,[15] and complete radioimmunoassay kits are available from New England Nuclear and others.

7.2.3 Ototoxicity

General Pattern of Cochlear Pathology and Pathophysiology

The hearing loss and the disturbances of equilibrium observed in many patients treated by different AmAn are widely recognized. Their ototoxic properties vary (Table 7.1) and have been reproduced many times in laboratory animals, particularly the guinea pig, the animal most commonly used in ototoxicity studies. Only the cochlear toxicity of these drugs is discussed in this section; their vestibular toxicity is presented as each specific drug is covered in a subsequent section of this chapter. A perspective on vestibulotoxicity is also given in Chapter 11.

The pattern of cochlear destruction produced by the AmAn is well known. The threshold for damage to the outer hair cells (OHC) is lower than that for the inner hair cells (IHC) and supporting cells of the organ of Corti. One of the earliest changes in cochlear architecture is the disarrangement of the hairs on the OHC, particularly those of the first row in the basal turn of the

Table 7.1 Relative Frequency of Toxic Reactions After Systemic Administration of Aminoglycosides

Antibiotic	Cochlea	Vestibular Apparatus	Kidney
Streptomycin	+++	+++	++
Dihydrostreptomycin	++++	++	++
Neomycin	+++++	++	+++
Kanamycin	+++	+	+++
Gentamicin	++	++	++
Tobramycin	+	+	+
Amikacin	+++	+	+++
Netilmicin[a]	+	+	+
Sisomicin[a]	++	++	++

Note. + amount of toxic reaction when used clinically.
[a]Greater neuromuscular blocking activity than Tobramycin (based on animal work).

cochlea.[16] Outer hair cell loss usually starts in the basal turn and progresses toward the apex, as the dosage increases. In the basal turn we can see destruction of supporting cells such as the pillar cells sooner than damage to the IHC (Figure 7.1). The IHC destruction starts in the apex and progresses basalward toward the oval and round windows. In addition to this longitudinal gradient, there is a radial gradient because degeneration starts in the first row of OHC and progresses to the second and third rows (Figure 7.2). In other structures of the cochlea, such as the stria vascularis, morphological changes are usually observed only after larger doses.

The cochlear pathology produced by the AmAn is manifested initially in behavioral experiments as elevation of hearing thresholds for the higher frequencies; lower frequencies become involved as the toxicity worsens. Electrophysiologically, the morphological picture is correlated with a decline in amplitude of cochlear microphonics (CM) and cochlear action potential (CAP), first for high frequencies and later for the lower frequencies. Simmons et al.[17] observed a large reduction of CM at high intensities of acoustic stimulation (above 75 dB SPL) and a relatively small decline at the lower intensities. It has also been documented by single-unit recording in the spiral ganglion of guinea pigs that AmAn poisoning, which causes loss of outer hair cells, leads to the loss of sharp, sensitive tuning, thus causing a shift in the damaged region to lower frequencies in the tuning curves.[18]

This information documents that AmAn ototoxicity is caused by the destruction of the cochlea. In karyometric studies no changes were found in the ventral cochlear nucleus,[19] which indicates that the central auditory pathways are not damaged by direct action of the drugs.

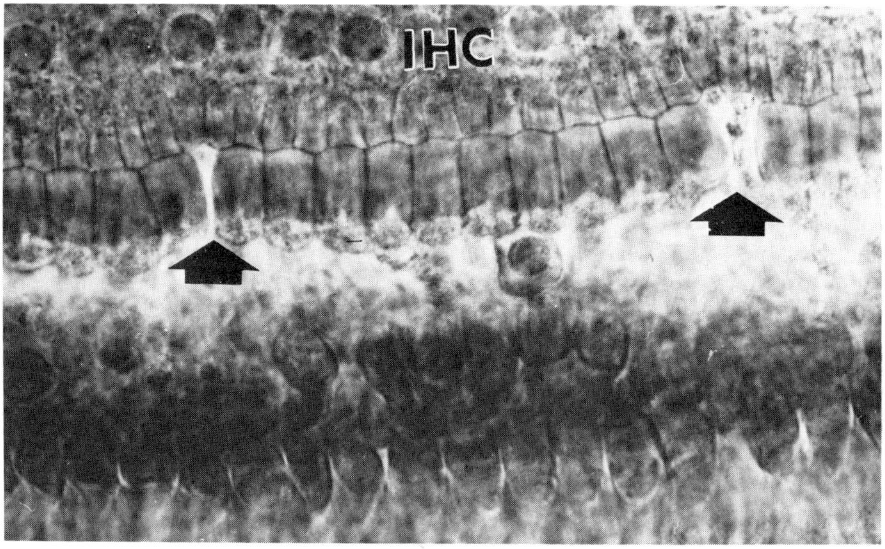

Figure 7.1 Surface preparation of the basal turn from a guinea pig that received 200 mg/kg/day i.m. tobramycin for 14 days. The focus is at the level of the hair-cell nuclei. A large percentage of the OHCs are missing (area between and below arrows). There is also extensive damage to the outer pillar cells (arrows). The IHCs are intact and without observable changes under light microscopy. From Prazma et al.[204] Reprinted by permission of the *Laryngoscope*.

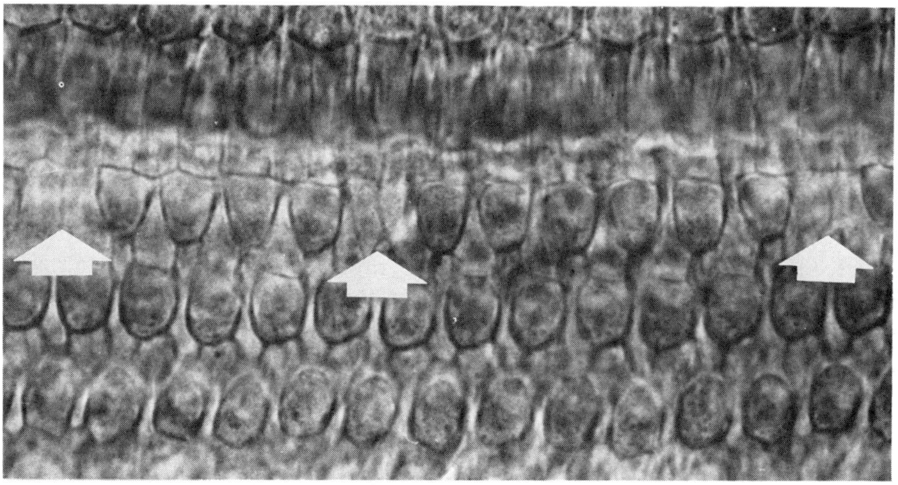

Figure 7.2 Surface preparation from a guinea pig that received 150 mg/kg/day i.m. tobramycin for eight days. Arrows indicate OHC loss in the first row of the second turn. Other structures appear to be normal. From Prazma et al.[204] Reprinted by permission of the *Laryngoscope*.

Relevant Pharmacokinetics

The kinetics of AmAn distribution into the cochlea have been investigated by the use of isotopically labeled AmAn given intraperitoneally,[20] intra-arterially,[21] and intracochlearly.[22] Tritiated DH–STM was observed in the perilymph, but not in the endolymph, 1 hr after its intraperitoneal administration.[20] However, after 2 hr, equivalent concentrations were found in endolymph and perilymph. One hour after intra-arterial administration STM was observed mainly in the supporting structures, particularly in Deiter's cells, but it was also found in Reissner's membrane.[21] After 4 hr it was concentrated mainly in the organ of Corti. The kinetics of GE were also studied by radioimmunoassay technique. After intramuscular drug administration, the serum peak was detected in 15 min and the perilymph peak in 3 hr.[22b] When labeled DH–STM was perfused through the perilymphatic compartment[22a] it was found in both inner and outer hair cells; inside the cells, but not on the surface. This observation of intracellular uptake of the AmAn could be associated with the experiments of Bryan and Van den Elzen[10] and Price et al.,[11] who observed active intracellular uptake of these antibiotics by sensitive microorganisms.

Retention of AmAn in the cochlear fluids of animals is well documented.[23–29] These drugs penetrate rather slowly into the perilymph and endolymph; 2 to 5 hr elapse after subcutaneous administration before peak concentrations are obtained. Although the penetration of AmAn into endolymph is slower than that of perilymph, endolymph and perilymph concentrations are approximately the same 5 hr after administration. They are eliminated from perilymph even more slowly than they gain entrance; for example, after a single subcutaneous or intramuscular administration of STM, AK, TO, GE, KA, or NEO the serum half-lives are 1.5 to 3 hr; however, the perilymph *T* 1/2 ranges from 3.5 to 30 hr (3.5, 10, 11, 12, 15, and 30 hr, respectively). (See Figures 7.3 and 7.4 for illustrations of the serum and perilymph decay profiles of four of these antibiotics.) It is also worth pointing out that these differences in perilymph *T* 1/2s could account for the ototoxic liability being greater with KA and NEO than with GE, TO, or AK. This would be expected if the perilymph were in communication with the fluid surrounding the hair cells (see Chapter 1). Perilymph KA[26] and perilymph NEO[24] concentrations are several times higher after chronic treatment, which indicates that their long perilymph *T* 1/2s do indeed allow cochlear accumulation. On the other hand, the shorter perilymph *T* 1/2s of GE, TO, and AK allow a greater percentage of drugs to be eliminated from perilymph between doses, thus decreasing the likelihood of ototoxicity developing when animals and, presumably, patients are treated chronically with these agents.[27]

Inflammatory processes in the middle ear increase the perilymph concentrations of AmAn when they are administered systemically.[24,27–28a] This may account for the exceptional finding of Wagner et al.,[28a] who observed that

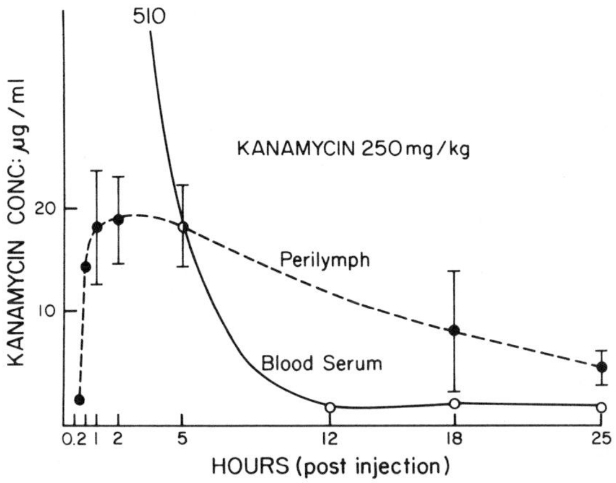

Figure 7.3 Kanamycin concentrations in the perilymph and blood serum of a guinea pig after single i.m. injection of 250 mg/kg. Redrawn from Stupp et al.[26]

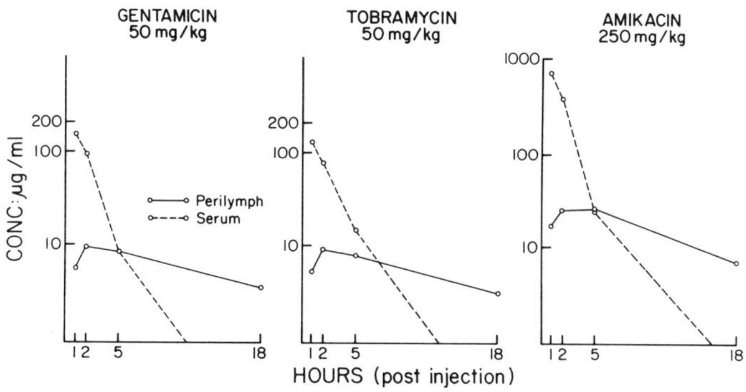

Figure 7.4 Concentration changes in serum and perilymph of guinea pigs after a single s.c. injection of gentamicin, tobramycin, or amikacin. Redrawn from Federspil et al.[27]

unequal concentrations of STM were found between the cochleas in one rabbit. It should also be pointed out that Federspil et al.[27] found other AmAn (GE, TO, and AK) bilaterally distributed into the perilymph of the two cochleas of guinea pigs. Furthermore, inflammation of the middle ear during treatment with TO substantially increased OHC loss in guinea pigs.[18] These observations are probably related to the general inflammatory effect that causes tight junctions to be leaky and thus increases diffusion of AmAn from blood capillaries into the inner ear structures. The important consequences of this finding is that otitis media and other middle and, presumably, inner-ear inflammatory processes may act in an additive (or synergistic) manner with the ototoxic antibiotics.

The increased incidence of ototoxicity observed when AmAn are given to patients with impaired renal function could be due to the perilymph T 1/2s of the AmAn increasing as a consequence of their decreased rate of excretion by the kidney. Federspil et al.[27] found that after a single subcutaneous injection of GE in bilaterally nephrectomized guinea pigs, the perilymph concentration did not fall from the 5-hr peak value for the entire 18-hr observation period, although the serum, CSF, and aqueous humor concentrations did decline slowly.

In an attempt to influence the rate of perilymph production and turnover and thereby arrive at a method of treating the ototoxicity of the AmAn, Federspil et al.[27] studied the effects that cisternal (suboccipital) puncture and diuresis induced by water, osmotic agents, and natriuretics had on perilymph concentrations of GE, TO, and AK. Unfortunately their results indicate that none of these treatment modalities affected the cochlear concentrations of the AmAn.

In our laboratory we are presently investigating the effect of alteration of glomerular filtration and nutrition on the toxicity of AmAn.[28b,c,d] Parts of these experiments were presented at the 1980 ARO meeting in Florida.[28e] In all experiments guinea pigs received i.m. TO or GE once a day. Toxicity decreased in hyperhydrated and increased in dehydrated animals, correlating with the glomerular filtration rate. When the animals were semistarved (restricted to 1/4 of their normal food intake) the ototoxicity of TO more than doubled and increased even more in GE groups in which all the animals died in 6 to 10 days. Other recent studies have shown that semistarvation reduces glomerular filtration and renal plasma flow rate.[28f,g] Therefore the increase in toxicity and ototoxicity in our semistarved groups may have been caused by an alteration of glomerular filtration.

Possible Mechanisms of Ototoxic Action

EFFECT ON RNA METABOLISM

Bactericidal action of AmAn is well established as an interference with ribosomal protein synthesis.[29b] The inhibition of RNA metabolism in the OHC has been considered an initial effect of KA on the inner ear.[30,31] By autoradiography, a decreased incorporation of ^{3}H-uridine in Reissner's membrane after treatment with AmAn was reported by Watanuki et al.[32] In our study,[33] after several days of treatment with high doses of TO, we observed nuclear swelling of the OHC in the apical turns. This swelling disappeared 1 to 2 weeks after terminating treatment. In the lower turns, however, no significant swelling was observed, but a substantial OHC loss showed two weeks after treatment. These cells may have gone through the stage of swelling so fast that they were not noticed in our experiments; possibly, nuclear swelling is a reversible phenomenon and is not necessarily associated with cell death.

INTERACTION OF GLUCOSE TRANSPORT AND ITS METABOLISM

Another ototoxicity mechanism of AmAn involves their effect on carbohydrate metabolism in the organ of Corti. In the past AmAn have been known to suppress different respiratory enzymes in the inner ear[34–36] and cause inhibition of the Embden-Myerhof pathway but not the hexose monophosphate pathway.[37] Interest in the possible interaction between glucose and KA was stimulated by the findings of Owada[38] that 3-aminoglucose, a component of all KA molecules, produced ototoxicity as severe as KA itself.

Some studies of glucose–AmAn interaction may be explained by an increased excretion of AmAn due to osmotic diuresis caused by hyperglycemia. Cronin[39] observed that KA was rapidly eliminated from the plasma when the blood glucose level was elevated by periodic i.v. injections of glucose. The decreased ototoxicity of KA in animals in which hyperglycemia (above 300 mg%) was induced by alloxan[40] may be similarly explained.

Experimental findings however, tend to support the theory of a direct interaction of AmAn with glucose. Interference of aminosugars with glucose transport has been documented in the diaphram[41] and synaptosomes,[42] probably by competing with glucose transport. Glucose transport was also altered in the rat intestine after treatment with NEO.[43] In addition, the glycosuria observed in normoglycemic animals treated with GE and KA implies that the antibiotics are interfering with glucose reabsorption in the proximal tubules.[40,44] Interaction of AmAn with glucose transport was further documented in experiments[47] in which 2-deoxyglucose transport was inhibited by KA in red blood cells and slices of kidney. Furthermore, sodium D-glucuro-1,4-lactone prevents the accumulation of KA in renal tissue and also prevents renal damage if administered before KA.[45,46]

The interactions of AmAn with glucose were also observed in inner-ear experiments. A decrease in the amount of labeled glucose in perilymph and endolymph after KA treatment was observed by Takeda.[48] Thalmann et al.[49] described a higher amount of glycogen in the apex and a lower amount in the basal turn. This has been further documented in histochemical studies by Postma et al.[33] and Falbe-Hansen.[50] We[33] have also investigated the effect of TO on the level of glycogen in the hair cells and found that the damage was largest in the areas of lowest glycogen stores. In areas of highest storage of glycogen (apical turns) the glycogen content increased during treatment. This observation suggests that not only is transport of glucose altered but so is its metabolism. Inhibition of the Embden-Meyerhof pathway in the organ of Corti without altering the hexose monophosphate pathway after KA treatment was reported by Tachibana et al.[37] Interaction of AmAn with glucose in the inner ear was further documented in experiments by Cronin.[39] A large decline in CAP, caused by direct perfusions of scala tympani with KA, was 100% restored only when the scala tympani was perfused by artificial perilymph with $4.4 \times 10^{-1} M$ glucose for 60 min. Artificial perilymph, alone, did not restore the CAP. A decrease in ototoxicity of KA, as mentioned earlier, was also observed in alloxan-induced hyperglycemic animals.[40]

OTOTOXICITY AND EFFERENT NERVE INNERVATION

The distribution of efferent nerve endings has been described by Engstrom[51] and Smith and Sjostrand.[52] These nerve endings are present in all three rows of the OHC in the basal turn, in the first two rows of turn II, and in the first row of turns III and IV. Furthermore, Spoendlin[53] reported that efferent nerve endings are rarely found in contact with thc IHC but rather with the afferent nerve endings or afferent dendrites below the IHC. He has also reported that the great majority of afferent nerves are destined for the IHC rather than the OHC.

Kohonen[1] demonstrated that the pattern of hair-cell degeneration produced by KA and NEO is correlated with the pattern of hair-cell efferent innervation and that the activity of AmAn on the cochlear efferents could be responsible for the damage to the OHC. This idea was extended by experiments by Brown[54] and Brown and Daigneault,[55] who found that several days of treatment with NEO first enhanced, then blocked the contralateral olivocochlear bundle stimulation effect on the CAP. They also stated that the NEO action may be due to its pharmacological effect on the efferent synapses, which occurs before the destruction of hair cells. Aminoglycosides may affect the OHC by a mechanism similar to that which affects the neuromuscular endings[7]; it has been shown that neomycin decreases the number of CA^{2+} binding sites.

An increase in CM and CAP was noted in animals that had received small doses of AmAn.[28a,56,57] This initial rise in the CAP has been considered a result of primary damage to the efferent system.[58]

Capps and Duval[59] observed that the elimination of the crossed olivocochlear bundle in AmAn-treated animals reduced hair cell loss by 50% when investigated 14 days after treatment. Because of preliminary data also cited in their paper, however, they suggest that elimination of the crossed olivocochlear bundle causes retardation of outer hair cell destruction rather than prevention of destructive processes.

EFFECT ON MEMBRANE ENZYMES

Another possible mechanism and, in my opinion, the presently best documented, is the AmAn action on cell membranes and their enzymes that disturbs the transport of ions and nutrients into the cells.

It is currently broadly accepted that polyphosphoinositides control membrane-bound Ca^{2+}, a function that is important to the maintenance of stability and excitability of membranes.[60a,60b] Lodhi et al.[60c] demonstrated that Ca^{2+} is displaced by NEO which is bound to the polyphosphoinositide complex and causes disturbances of the structure of lipid membranes that lead to increased permeability of cells.[60d,60e]

These observations led Schacht[61] to the hypothesis that normally phosphomonoesterase acts on phosphoinositides to cleave the phosphate groups and liberate Ca^{2+}, thus altering the permeability of the membrane to cations. In this model the AmAn compete with Ca^{2+} for exposed phosphate groups. This binding may be reversible in low concentrations of AmAn but is irreversible in high concentrations and thus impairs the membrane permeability and disturbs the transport of ions and nutrients into the cells. This binding has been observed in experiments with synaptozomal membranes, which are considered a good model for excitable membranes (synaptozomes are nerve endings that are separated from axons during homogenization of brain tissue). Incubation of synaptozomal membranes with γ-^{32}P-ATP produced a decrease in formation of phosphatidylinositol diphosphate when $10^{-4}M$ neomycin was present in the medium.[61]

Chronic treatment with NEO inhibits polyphosphoinositide metabolism in the kidney[61a] and in inner-ear tissue.[61b] When the cochlea is perfused with solutions that contain NEO, a correlation is found between the loss of cochlear microphonics and the inhibition of polyphosphoinositides.[60e] Furthermore, polyphosphoinositides were recently isolated from renal and cochlear tissue by affinity chromatography and identified as receptors for NEO.[61c]

These disturbances in membrane structure and function may allow more drug to enter the cochlear cells and further disturb their metabolism.

As presented above, the most favorable theories that explain the mechanism of AmAn action are those that apply to the action of polyphosphoinositides and to AmAn interaction with glucose transport and metabolism.

Onset of Ototoxic Action

Rapid decline of microphonics was observed after topical application of STM to the hair-bearing surface of the hair cells in the lateral line organ.[62] In similar experiments Harada et al.[63] noticed a reversible suppression of spontaneous and evoked discharges from the frog semicircular canal. Later, Matsuura et al.[64] observed that saccular microphonics were rapidly suppressed within 3–4 min of drug administration when STM and KA were administered intraluminally. When administered extraluminally, however, their concentration had to be several times higher to achieve the same effect. Furthermore, Engstrom[65] reported that the earliest morphological sign of antibiotic intoxication is swelling and disarrangement of the hairs of the OHC. These experiments suggest that the primary site of action of the AmAn is the hair-bearing surface of the hair cells and that this effect commences immediately after a high concentration reaches them.

The foregoing observations led us to investigate the acute effect of TO after i.v. administration in the guinea pig.[66] Shortly after administration of 200 mg/kg the EP, CM, and CAP had sharply declined. At an intermediate dose (100 mg/kg) the EP was unaffected for 110 min, but a gradual decline of CM and CAP resulted. When the lowest dose (50 mg/kg) was administered no effect on cochlear potentials was observed. In a few similar experiments Brummett and Brown[67] measured blood pressure and CM. They concluded that changes in cochlear potentials after i.v. administration of TO did not reflect the cochlear effect of this drug but a decline in blood pressure produced by the drug. After our[66] largest dose (200 mg/kg) TO probably did affect the whole body by causing respiratory depression and producing a decline in blood pressure. Thus decline of EP, CM, and CAP in this group may also be the result of a general systemic toxicity. It is our opinion, however, that a direct effect of the aminoglycoside on cochlear potentials was seen, particularly in the group given 100 mg/kg, and it was not a secondary effect due to blood pressure decline. In this group a decline was recorded only in CM and CAP; there was no decline in EP until after 110 min. If these effects were caused by a drop in blood pressure (as Brummett and Brown[67] suggested), then EP, which is more sensitivie to anoxic conditions, would have declined before CM.

Our observations of the rapid onset of AmAn action is also supported by experiments[68] in which the perilymphatic space was perfused by NEO in Ringer's solution. This technique allows the administration of high doses (10^{-4} to $10^{-2}M$) of NEO without significantly affecting the rest of the body; 5 min after perfusion was started the amplitude of CM declined to about 50% of the control value. Similarly, Konishi[69] observed that AmAn suppressed the cochlear potentials more when applied to endolymph than to the perilymph and that the CM were suppressed more than the EP. Furthermore, after i.v. administration of TO to humans[70] a decline in CM and CAP occurred when the serum level exceeded 8 to 10 μg/ml. Within 15 min the cochlear activity declined 50% and stayed at this low level for the next 100 min. All patients recovered after treatment without late auditory or vestibular symptoms. This effect was also documented by Dobbs and Mawer,[71] who observed a 1.3-to-4.2-dB elevation of the hearing threshold at 1 hr after i.v. administration of TO.

In conclusion, these experiments document that the AmAn act in the inner ear immediately when they reach the hair cells in high concentrations. This relatively quick onset of action may be caused by their effect on cell membranes. In addition, hair-cell activity is probably affected independently of the AmAn action on the stria vascularis because CM are affected before the EP is altered. Furthermore, if the inner ear and hair cells are exposed to these antibiotics for only a short time, their effect is apparently reversible.

Cochlear Sequence of Ototoxic Action

The question whether hair-cell destruction is primary or secondary to damage of the stria vascularis has been considered by several authors.[3,72,73–76a]

Kaneka et al.[76b] investigated this problem by direct perfusion of 20% STM through the cochlea to eliminate its systemic effects. They observed that the hair cells of the organ of Corti were damaged first, then the interdental cells and roots of the outer sulcus cells, followed by the destruction of epithelial cells, such as Claudius' and inner sulcus cells. In the final stage, all epithelial cells of the cochlear duct except the stria vascularis and Reissner's membrane were replaced by a single layer of cells. After treatment with AmAn atrophy of the capillary vessels in the stria vascularis or atrophy of the whole stria vascularis is observed in a large number of instances. In some cases atrophy in the basal turn is greater than that seen in the apical turns. Biochemical changes, such as the decline of ATPase activity in the stria vascularis after treatment with KA, have also been reported by Iinuma et al.[34] and Kaku et al.[35] Furthermore, a decrease in $^{42}K^+$ transport from perilymph to endolymph was observed by Rauch et al.[77] after AmAn treatment. Similarly, a decline in K^+ and a rise in Na^+ content in the endolymph was seen after five days of treatment with AmAn.[78]

From these experimental results there is no doubt that the AmAn affect the stria vascularis. It is uncertain however, from these data, whether this action precedes their effects on hair cells. Logan et al.[66] observed a significant decline in CM and CAP without a change in EP. Similar observations were made by Konishi.[69] It is generally known that the EP originates in the stria vascularis and CM, in hair cells. According to the experiments of Logan et al.,[66] hair-cell function was affected earlier than the function of the stria vascularis.

At present it seems that the primary effect of AmAn is on the hair cells and is independent of their effects on the stria vascularis. Hair-cell function further deteriorates when the function of the stria vascularis is affected. This late action of the AmAn on the stria vascularis could, of course, play a role in their clinical ototoxicity.

Intratympanic Administration

Aminoglycoside antibiotics penetrate into the cochlear fluids from the tympanic cavity as well as from the bloodstream. Destruction of the OHC after intratympanic administration of AmAn has been observed by numerous investigators.[79-83] Aminoglycoside antibiotics also cause a decline in cochlear succinic dehydrogenase and DPN diaphorase activity, after intratympanic administration.[84] Topical administration of these antibiotics not only affects the cochlea but also the vestibular system[85]; the greatest damage is observed in the cristae ampullaris, whereas less damage is seen in the macula utriculi, and the least in the macula sacculi.[86] Aminoglycoside antibiotics should therefore be used in the treatment of external otitis only when the tympanic membrane is not perforated and are not to be given intratympanically at all; severe damage to the entire inner ear can result.

Protection and/or Prevention of Aminoglycoside Ototoxicity

Numerous diseases, some serious, are caused by microorganisms sensitive only to the AmAn. Therefore many investigators have done research in an attempt to eliminate their ototoxic properties. The most successful method has been to decrease peak serum concentrations by dividing the total daily dosage, thus avoiding the high serum peak obtained after a single large administration. Some investigators have also tried mixing them with oily solvents, such as the oxidative products of oleum terebinthinae (ozothin),[87] or have linked them to oily substances, such as streptomycin–diacetylpermoat.[88] Another author has suggested the use of adjuvants, such as amino acids (pantothenic acid) and vitamins (ascorbic acid), which allegedly decrease ototoxicity.[89–91] In contrast to the above experiments, however, Hawkins et al.[92] and Kutchinsky et al.[93] found no protective properties in pantothenic acid. Furthermore, the protective effect of the other adjuvants listed above resulted in a reduction in the effectiveness of AmAn.[26–27] The use of 2,3-dimercaptopropanol has also been suggested to decrease AmAn ototoxicity, but Federspil[3] found that this component, itself, was ototoxic.

In conclusion, none of these agents is really effective in decreasing ototoxicity without also altering the effectiveness of these antibiotics. At present, the means of guarding against ototoxicity is to avoid high peak levels with the use of divided doses without compromising the drug's effectiveness. It is hoped that new aminoglycosides less toxic than those now available will be developed.

*Clinical Suggestions Regarding Dosage Regimen**

All AmAn are ototoxic and nephrotoxic. Therefore before prescribing them contributing factors must be considered; for example, an unusually long course of treatment; concomitant treatment with loop diuretics or other nephrotoxic and/or ototoxic drugs; renal impairment as reflected by elevated serum creatinine or reduced creatinine clearance. Additional risk factors include age (premature, elderly), previous treatment with AmAn, preexisting sensorineural deafness, and noise exposure. In patients in whom some of these factors are present vestibular and audiometric examinations and renal function studies should precede treatment.

LOADING DOSE

Therapeutic doses of AmAn are adjusted on the basis of renal function and serum concentration measurements to maintain the minimum inhibitory con-

*The guidelines for dosing given in this section were developed in and are applicable to adults only; they are not applicable to the pediatric population.

centration (MIC) of the antibiotic.[94,95a,95b] All patients, however, regardless of their renal function, should be given a loading dose (Table 7.2) calculated on the basis of lean body weight. Lean body weight (LBW) can be calculated according to the Devine method[95c]:

$$\text{LBW male} = 50 \text{ kg} + 2.3 \text{ kg (each inch} > 5 \text{ ft)}$$

$$\text{LBW female} = 45 \text{ kg} + 2.3 \text{ kg (each inch} > 5 \text{ ft)}$$

It should be noted that these guidelines do not apply to patients with increased muscle mass or cachexia, nor to those who are obese or edematous. In patients with increased muscle mass or cachexia the loading dose should be based on the idealized body weight (IBW) determined from the patient's height and weight according to standardized tables. In obese patients (those

Table 7.2 Dosing Chart of AmAn in Adults

Aminoglycoside Antibiotic	Usual Loading Doses Lean Body Weight[a] (mg/kg)	Expected "Peak" Serum Levels[b] (μg/ml)
Gentamicin and Tobramycin	1.0	2–4
	1.5	4–6
	2.0	6–10
Kanamycin and Amikacin	5.0	15–20
	7.5	20–30

[a] See text for lean body weight equations and discussion of their limitations.
[b] These are estimated levels that would be obtained after the loading dose, based on the following equation:

$$\text{Expected ``peak'' serum level } (\mu\text{g/ml}) = \frac{\text{loading dose (mg/kg)}}{\text{volume of distribution (L/kg)}} = \frac{\text{mg}}{\text{L}} = \frac{\mu\text{g}}{\text{ml}}.$$

This equation allows for the estimation of serum AmAn concentrations immediately following the loading dose, provided the following assumptions are made: (1) the drug is intravenously administered as a "bolus" dose; (2) pharmacokinetically, a one-compartment, open model can be used to describe drug disposition; (3) the volume of distribution for each drug in all patients will fall into the range of those chosen from the literature and used to make these calculations; (4) drug distribution occurs instantaneously after injection; and (5) the "peak" level is obtained simultaneously with the completion of the drug injection. Therefore predictions of "peak" serum levels with this equation may yield results that deviate significantly from those actually obtained if an i.v. infusion or i.m. injection is used for drug administration; or if the drug exhibits disposition characteristics consistent with a 2- or 3-compartment, open pharmacokinetic model (which is usually the case with AmAn in patients with normal renal function). In other words, the expected "peak" serum levels given in this table are to be used only as "ball park" estimates; they are not intended to be taken literally.

who have a body weight $\geqslant$ 30% of their IBW) serum concentrations may be higher than expected because of the limited distribution of the AmAn into adipose tissue. Schwartz et al.[95d] have derived a correction factor for obese patients, based on "normalized" body mass; this factor, however, cannot be used readily because the authors' "normalized" body mass does not equate with the IBW found in standardized tables or with the LBW as defined in this section. In patients with marked edema, serum concentrations may be lower than expected secondary to the expanded distribution space. No reliable correction factor is available for use in this type of patient.

MAINTENANCE DOSE

After calculating the loading dose the initial maintenance dose can be selected according to the patient's (pt's) corrected creatinine clearance [*C*(*c*)*rc*], which is calculated according to the Cockcroft and Gault equations[95e] and adjusted for a LBW of 70 kg or for a body surface area (S.A.) of 1.73 m^2:

$$C(c)rc \text{ male} = \frac{140 - \text{age}}{\text{serum creatinine}} \times \left(\frac{\text{pt's LBW (kg)}}{70} \text{ or } \frac{\text{pt's S.A. in m}^2}{1.73 \text{ m}^2}\right)$$

$$C(c)rc \text{ female} = \frac{140 - \text{age}}{\text{serum creatinine}} \times 0.85 \times \left(\frac{\text{pt's LBW (kg)}}{70} \text{ or } \frac{\text{pt's S.A. in m}^2}{1.73 \text{ m}^2}\right)$$

The measured or endogenous creatinine clearance can be used instead of the *C*(*c*)*rc*; it should also be adjusted to a LBW of 70 kg or a S.A. of 1.73 m^2. With either endogenous creatinine clearance or *C*(*c*)*rc* the initial maintenance dose can then be computed as a percentage of the loading dose and administered 1 to 3 times a day (Table 7.3).

In patients with changing renal function, the *C*(*c*)*rc* or endogenous creatinine clearance must be determined repeatedly and the maintenance dose corrected. These patients require more frequent monitoring of renal function and aminoglycoside serum concentrations. The pharmacokinetics of AmAn are altered in the presence of renal disease, particularly when creatinine clearance is lower than 80 ml/min per 70 kg LBW (or 1.73 m^2). Adjustments of maintenance AmAn doses should therefore be based on indicators of renal function (serum creatinine, [*C*(*c*)*rc*], or endogenous creatinine clearance) and information obtained from serum AmAn levels. In the design of maintenance therapy it is desirable to keep "peak" serum concentrations below 10 μg/ml and "trough" concentrations slightly below 2 μg/ml during the dosing intervals for both GE and TO.[95g] "Peak" concentrations for both AK and KA should not exceed 25 μg/ml and "trough" concentrations should be permitted to fall to approximately 5 μg/ml within a dosing interval.[95g] By designing dosing regimens to provide serum concen-

Table 7.3[a] Maintenance Dose Adjustment for Amikacin, Gentamicin, Kanamycin, and Tobramycin in Adults

$C(c)rc$[b] (ml/min)	Approximate Elimination Half-Life[c] (hr)	Percentage of Loading Dose Required for Dosage Interval Selected		
		8 hr	12 hr	24 hr
90	3.1	84%	—	—
80	3.4	80	91%	—
70	3.9	76	88	—
60	4.5	71	84	—
50	5.3	65	79	—
40	6.5	57	72	92%
30	8.4	48	63	86
25	9.9	43	57	81
20	11.9	37	50	75
17	13.6	33	46	70
15	15.1	31	42	67
12	17.9	27	37	61
10[d]	20.4	24	34	56
7	25.9	19	28	47
5	31.5	16	23	41
2	46.8	11	16	30
0	69.3	8	11	21

Calculate corrected creatinine clearance [$C(c)rc$] as

$$C(c)rc \text{ male} = [140\text{-age/serum creatinine}] \times [\text{patient's LBW (kg)/70}]$$
$$C(c)rc \text{ female} = [0.85 \times C(c)rc \text{ male}] \times [\text{patient's LBW (kg)/70}]$$

[a]Reproduced with permission from Sarrubi and Hull.[95f]
[b]Endogenous creatinine clearance can be substituted for $C(c)rc$.
[c]Alternatively, one-half the chosen loading dose may be given at an interval approximately equal to the estimated half-life.
[d]Dosing for patients with $C(c)rc \leq 10$ ml/min should always be assisted by measured serum levels.

trations above the MIC for the infecting organism for the majority of a dosing interval, yet not exceeding the desired "peak" and "trough" values, both the ototoxicity and nephrotoxicity associated with these agents may be reduced.

The following schedules for monitoring renal function parameters and serum AmAn levels are recommended to assist the clinician in choosing a maintenance dose and a dosing interval that will minimize the chances of drug-associated toxicities. By using the steps outlined in Categories I through III, it is possible to adjust the maintenance dose or dosing interval based on the AmAn *T* 1/2, creatinine clearance, or both. In most cases individually calculated pharmacokinetic parameters (e.g., *T* 1/2) yield the most precise means of forecasting desired maintenance doses. When AmAn levels are not readily available, determination of *C*(*c*)*rc* (or endogenous creatinine clearance) and application to Table 7.3 will usually result in selection of an acceptable AmAn dosing regimen.

Category I. Patients with Normal Renal Function

(a) Select an initial maintenance dose according to established guidelines (i.e., product literature). Determine serum creatinine [calculate *C*(*c*)*rc*] every other day, and determine the endogenous creatinine clearance once a week. Either determination should be standardized to a LBW of 70 kg or an S.A. of 1.73 m^2, as indicated previously.

(b) At steady state (after 5 or more *T* 1/2s; on the second day in these patients*) and on the fifth and tenth day of therapy determine serum AmAn "peak" (if i.v. infusion, 5 min post infusion; if i.m., approximately 1 hr post injection) and "trough" (immediately before the next dose) levels. If the patient's serum creatinine increases or creatinine clearance decreases by more than 15% of normal, or if the patient has trough AmAn concentrations greater than those recommended, this is indicative of unstable renal function and/or drug accumulation. The patient should therefore be monitored as described in Category III. If the peak level is greater than that recommended, the patient is more likely to experience ototoxicity; therefore, in this case the dosage regimen also needs reevaluation.

Category II. Patients Who Have Impaired Kidney Function and Their Renal Function Is Stable

(a) Calculate the endogenous creatinine clearance before initiation of therapy, if possible. Alternatively, determine serum creatinine and calculate *C*(*c*)*rc*. In either case select an appropriate dose and dosing interval using Table 7.3. Creatinine clearance [or *C*(*c*)*rc*] should be monitored every other day and the dosing regimen adjusted accordingly from Table 7.3, if serum AmAn levels cannot be obtained.

(b) Monitor therapy as described in Category I, step b.

Category III. Patients Who Have Unstable Renal Function

(a) Determine the endogenous creatinine clearance [or *C*(*c*)*rc*] and select an initial maintenance dose from Table 7.3. Monitor one of these

**T* 1/2 is approximately 3 hr in patients with normal renal function. Use *C*(*c*)*rc* or endogenous creatinine clearance in conjunction with Table 7.3 for estimating time to steady state in patients with impaired renal function.

parameters every other day during the course of AmAn therapy and use it to adjust dosage, if serum AmAn levels cannot be obtained.

(b) During the first dosing interval determine the AmAn peak serum concentration. In addition, determine the serum level for at least two and preferably three points beyond the 4-hr point post-i.v. infusion or i.m. injection. One of these points should correspond to the trough concentration. Calculate the slope of the least-squares regression line for the resultant natural log (ln) serum concentration (y-axis) versus time (hours, x-axis) plot and calculate the apparent terminal elimination half-life as follows:

$$T\ 1/2\ (\text{hr}) = \frac{\ln 2}{\text{slope}} = \frac{0.693}{\text{slope}}$$

The adjusted maintenance dose for subsequent time intervals can then be estimated from the calculated T 1/2 (see Table 7.3). The new maintenance dose will, of course, begin with the third dosing interval because the time required for AmAn serum level determination will necessitate administration of the initially calculated maintenance dose during the second dosing interval.

(c) In all patients with changing (unstable) renal function serum, AmAn level monitoring should consist of obtaining steady-state peak and trough levels after selection of a new dose or dosing interval. This should be complimented by monitoring of daily trough levels, adjusting the dose (or interval) as needed to maintain desired serum concentrations.

At times the dosage regimen of a particular AmAn *cannot* be designed to be efficacious in a patient with renal compromise, yet provide acceptable therapeutic serum concentrations. In this case, the clinician should consider appropriate alterations of therapy such as switching to an alternate AmAn or discontinuation of AmAn therapy altogether and institution of therapy with an antibiotic of a different class, if possible.

It cannot be overemphasized that the aforementioned guidelines for therapeutic serum level monitoring and dosing of the AmAn are simplified. Many factors have been shown to influence the disposition, hence the serum levels, of these agents in man. Several of the most noteworthy include prematurity, old age, interindividual variation in renal accumulation of the drugs, hematocrit, fever, obesity, hydration and nutrition status, hypoxemia, major burns, and drug interactions (e.g., heparin, carbenicillin, and ticarcillin). Those interested in a more extensive discussion of this topic should consult the Pechere and Dugal review.[95h]

During treatment, patients should also be questioned routinely for signs of auditory and vestibular symptoms, such as fullness and sensation of pressure in the ears, headache, tinnitus, and dizziness. Moreover, in patients with a higher potential for developing ototoxicity (higher than normal doses, impaired renal function, and/or when treatment exceeds 7 to 10 days), audiometric, vestibular, and renal function tests should be done more frequently. In addition to regular audiometry, high-frequency audiometry (9 to 13 kHz) should be used in patients highly suspected of having adverse reactions. In this way hearing changes can be detected many days before they are seen by regular audiometry.[96-97] This high-frequency decline also precedes tinnitus in patients who experience it.

Plasma levels of the AmAn can be determined by the use of HPLC, microbiological assay, or radioimmunoassay methods. Radioimmunoassays are faster (2 hr), give highly reproducible results, and because of their high specificity are not affected by simultaneous administration of other antibiotics.[98a] Complete kits for radioimmunoassays are available from New England Nuclear and others.

It should be mentioned that it is not clear whether the toxicity of AmAn to infants is more or less than to adults. Bernard and Pechere[98b] found GE (20 mg/kg) more ototoxic to kittens treated from birth up to the twentieth day of life than to adult cats treated with the same dose and time exposure. In contrast, clinically significant ototoxicity from GE or KA was not observed during a three-year follow-up of children receiving the drugs during the neonatal period.[98c] It was pointed out, however, that the dosages of GE and KA used were lower than those used now and that "failure to demonstrate ototoxicity with the dosages employed in this investigation does not assure safety of these drugs when used in the currently recommended, higher doses."

7.2.4 Other Adverse Effects

The other common and serious adverse effect of the AmAn is nephrotoxicity. Volumes have been written on this topic. The reader is referred to those treatises (see Sanders and Sanders[7] and Appel and Neu[99] for recent reviews). It should also be pointed out that monitoring AmAn blood levels is an essential part of the prevention of nephrotoxicity. It is quite likely that nephrotoxicity is more related to trough levels of AmAn than to the peak levels. When Dahlgren et al.[100] gave patients GE and used a rise in serum creatinine as the index of nephrotoxicity, they found that "all of the patients who manifested a rise in serum creatinine had a valley (trough) level of gentamicin over 2 μg/ml."

A nondepolarizing blockade of the neuromuscular junction can also be produced by the AmAn when given in large doses. When used concurrently with curare, ether, or after repeated administration of succinylcholine they may cause respiratory depression.[101-107] The blockade is probably biphasic: an initial suppression of acetylcholine release with a secondary reduction in sensitivity of the postjunctional membrane to acetylcholine.[7,107] Competition with Ca^{2+} for common receptor sites seems to be involved. It has also been reported that NEO decreases the number of Ca^{2+} binding sites in vascular smooth muscle.[108] This mechanism produces a decrease in total Ca^{2+} uptake and an increase in Ca^{2+} efflux[7]; consequently the drugs may increase the patient's weakness in myasthenia gravis.[109] This neuromuscular blocking activity can at times be antagonized by Ca^{2+} or neostigmine.[106–107]

In some patients prolonged therapy has also been associated with hypocalcemia, hypomagnesemia, and hypokalemia. Despite the severe hypocalcemia found in these patients, parathormone is not elevated. Thus AmAn may, in some instances, also have a direct toxic effect on the parathyroid, as confirmed by postmortem examination.[110]

Hypersensitivities to AmAn can also occur. They run the gamut from skin rashes, stomatitis, and eosinophilia to fever, exfoliative dermatitis, angioedema, and anaphylactic shock. Fortunately, hypersensitivities to the AmAn do not occur so often as they do to the penicillins.

Finally, when the AmAn are administered intrathecally, radiculitis, arachnoiditis, brain stem irritation, paraplegia, and somnolence may result.

7.3 DISCUSSION OF SPECIFIC AMINOGLYCOSIDE ANTIBIOTICS

7.3.1 Streptomycin

Streptomycin (STM) was isolated from Streptomyces griseus by Schatz et al.[111] It is an organic base made up of three components: streptidine, streptose, and *N*-methyl-1-glucosamine; the streptose moiety is glycosidically linked to each of the other two moities.

Streptomycin is much more potent in an alkaline medium than an acid medium. An increase in acidity, like that in abscessed cavities proximal to damaged tissue, will decrease its activity. Its ototoxicity limits its clinical usefulness to the treatment of tuberculosis and other disease states when less toxic drugs are not available.

Absorption, Distribution, and Excretion

Streptomycin is well absorbed when given parenterally. About 1/3 of it is bound to plasma protein. In people with normal renal function the serum *T* 1/2 is about 2 1/2 hr, but it may increase to 110 hr in anephric patients.[112] It also diffuses through the placenta, as exemplified by the hearing loss that has occurred in children whose mothers received STM during pregnancy.[112–114]

Ototoxicity

The ototoxic effect of STM was first described by Hinshaw and Feldman[115]; the damage to the vestibular system was reported by Berg,[116] Causse,[117] and Prazic and Salaj.[118] In the past, when high doses of 2.0 g/day were used for long periods of time (60 to 120 days), about 75% of the patients had some cochlear or vestibular symptoms. This high incidence decreased to 25% when the daily dose was lowered to 1.0 g/day. The symptoms usually start as headache, nausea, vomiting, and disturbances in equilibrium. Within a few days the person also develops vertigo in the upright position, difficulty sitting and standing with eyes closed, spontaneous nystagmus, and a positive Romberg test. These signs persist for one to two weeks, after which the patient usually has difficulty only when making sudden movements. Within two months, a compensatory mechanism develops, such that the patient has symptoms only with his eyes closed. Hearing loss usually starts after vestibular toxicity has been manifested. The first sign is decreased sensitivity to high frequencies. Substantial variability from this description can occur however; it is caused by differences from patient to patient in the pattern of destruction to the inner ear.

Streptomycin does seem to have a much greater affinity for the vestibular system than the cochlea. Because of this, use of STM was suggested as a mechanism for suppression of the vestibular symptoms of Meniere's disease.[119–120]

Adverse effects of STM on the inner ear have been detailed by Hawkins et al.,[121] who observed only small changes in the stria vascularis but extensive damage to the OHC, particularly in the basal turn of the cochlea.

More severe degeneration was found in the vestibular system. Igarashi[122] observed large-scale destruction of hair cells in the cristae ampullaris and maculae. Wersall and Hawkins[123] described complete destruction of Type I hair cells and less serious degeneration of Type II and supporting cells. The degenerative changes included damage to the stereocilia, pyknosis of the nuclei, swelling of the mitochondria, vacuolization of the cytoplasm, and osmiophilic inclusions in the supranuclear region of the hair cells. Duvall and Wersall[124] suggested that STM also affected cell-membrane permeability. Scanning electron microscopic examination revealed changes in otolithic membranes; otoconia were irregular, shrunken, or fragmented, their calcium content was variably diminished, and it appeared that they were absorbed by dark cells.[125]

OTOTOXICITY OF DIHYDROSTREPTOMYCIN

Dihydrostreptomycin has a greater affinity for the cochlea than for the vestibular system.[126] In fact, it is so cochleotoxic it is no longer used clinically. It is still a useful research tool, however.

In the cat greater damage occurs in the OHC of the basal turn, which corresponds to the decline of high-frequency CM and the CAP reported by Hawkins et al.[127] and Tyberghein.[128] Decrease in mucopolysaccharides in the spiral limbus after DH–STM has been described by Musebeck and Schatzle.[75]

An important observation was recently reported by Hawkins et al.,[129] who noted that the hearing threshold in the monkey, *M. nemestrina,* remained almost unchanged after long treatment (eight months) with 100 mg/kg day of i.m. DH–STM. *M. nemestrina* is native to Indonesian rain forests where water is abundant. *E. patas,* however, a different species of monkey native to arid sub-Saharian Africa and adapted to little use of water, was severely deafened after three months of treatment with the much lower dose of 20 mg/kg day. Unfortunately we do not yet know if this difference in toxicity was caused by changes in excretion of the antibiotic or whether there are basic differences in the enzymatic systems of these two species.

7.3.2 Neomycin

Neomycin was isolated in 1949 by Waksman and Lechevalier[130] from *Streptomyces fradiae*. Although the original neomycin was a complex of three compounds, neomycins A, B, and C, the commercial preparation consists almost entirely of Neomycin B. Neomycin B (NEO) contains neamine and neobiosamine. Because of its extreme degree of ototoxicity, it is presently available only for topical application.

Absorption, Distribution, and Excretion

Similar to the other AmAn, NEO is poorly absorbed from the gastrointestinal tract, demonstrated by the elimination of approximately 97% of the oral dose in the feces. When given parenterally, it is well absorbed; 1.0 g given i.m. to adult humans provides a peak serum level of approximately 20 μg/ml. The serum *T* 1/2 of NEO is about 3 hr.

The perilymph and serum *T* 1/2's of NEO in animals are about 30 and 3 hr, respectively.[24] Therefore, daily administration results in accumulation of NEO in cochlear fluids (Figure 7.5).

Ototoxicity

The ototoxic properties of NEO are well known because it is the most ototoxic of the AmAn; it is more cochleotoxic than vestibulotoxic.[131] Most earlier reports of human ototoxicity were based on parenteral administration. However, recent reports indicate that it can be ototoxic when given by

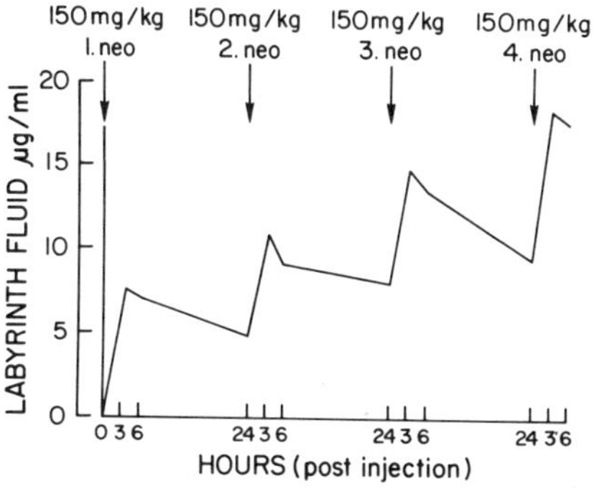

Figure 7.5 Accumulation of neomycin concentration in the perilymph after repeated daily doses of 150 mg/kg. Redrawn from Voldrich.[24]

intrapleural,[132] intraperitoneal,[133] or oral[134] administration. It can also be ototoxic when it is used for colonic or rectal irrigation,[134] after topical application to the ear canal,[79,81,135] and after topical application in burned patients.[136] In other words, it can be ototoxic when applied topically to large surface areas at any time the epithelium to which it is being applied loses its integrity and permits enough of the drug to be absorbed.

7.3.3 Kanamycin

Kanamycin (KAN) is a product of *Streptomyces kanamyceticus* isolated by Umezewa[137] in 1957. The commercial preparation is a mixture of two aminoglycosides, kanamycin A and kanamycin B. Each kanamycin molecule contains two amino sugars in glycoside linkage with 2-deoxystreptamine. The clinical use of KAN is generally restricted to the treatment of infections due to gram-negative organisms which are resistant to the newer, less ototoxic aminoglycosides.

Absorption, Distribution, and Excretion

Kanamycin, like other AmAn, is poorly absorbed from the gastrointestinal tract but well absorbed parenterally. Intramuscular injection of 1.0 g of KA to humans yields a peak serum concentration of 18 to 40 μg/ml at 1 hr. In patients with normally functioning kidneys the serum *T* 1/2 is about 2 hr but is extended to 6 hr in infants 5 to 22 days old and past 18 hr in premature infants. The *T* 1/2 is also extended in patients with renal insufficiency.

Kanamycin penetration into the CSF is slow in that after 3 hr its concentration reaches only about 1/5 to 1/10 that of the serum level. It has been shown to diffuse through the placenta of a pregnant woman, who delivered a deaf child.[138] It, of course, also penetrates into the cochlear fluids, where its perilymph *T* 1/2 is about 15 hr.[26,139]

Kanamycin is not metabolized in the body and is excreted by glomerular filtration; however, some tubular secretion is also hypothesized. About 40 to 80% is excreted during the first 24 hr.[140] Only a small portion is excreted into the intestine; therefore the bacterial flora are not significantly affected after parenteral administration.

The parenteral dose for normal adults and older children is 15 mg/kg/day, given in two or three equally spaced doses. In patients with renal insufficiency, the dose must be reduced according to the serum level of KA. All precautions should be followed as mentioned in the clinical suggestions (see Section 7.2.3). If the serum level exceeds safe margins, it should be removed from the blood by peritoneal dialysis or hemodialysis.[141]

Ototoxicity

The most serious adverse reactions are ototoxicity and nephrotoxicity. Adverse effects are reduced if peak serum concentrations are maintained under

25 μg/ml.[142] (It is worth noting again that nephrotoxicity may be more related to trough than peak levels; studies to confirm this relationship have not been done with any of the AmAn but GE, however.) Shortly after introduction of KA several authors reported its ototoxic effect.[143-147] This damage of the inner ear was enhanced in patients with impaired renal function[145-146] and in patients who had been treated with other AmAn.[148] Clinical studies indicate that KAN is much more cochleotoxic than vestibulotoxic.

Kanamycin ototoxicity has been documented numerous times by different methods in different species of animals. In cats, guinea pigs, and rabbits, chronic treatment produces depression of the CM and CAP, particularly at high frequencies.[84,149-151] Complete suppression of the CM was observed in the guinea pig[152] after 15 to 21 days of treatment with 400 mg/kg/day. Using cats, Simmons et al.[17] observed a substantially larger reduction of CM at high sound intensities, whereas the CM responses to lower sound levels were less affected.

One of the earliest ototoxic changes in cochlear architecture is disarrangement of the stereocilia hairs on the OHC, particularly in the first row of the basal turn of the cochlea.[16] Early ultrastructural changes include swelling of stereocilia, damage to the cuticular plate, and supranuclear clumping of mitochondria and endoplasmic reticulum.[153]

Alteration of enzymatic activity in the basal turn of the cochlea (decreases in succinic dehydrogenase and diphosphopyridine nucleotide diaphorase activities in the OHC and nerve endings) was observed by Kaku et al.[35] and Koide et al.[154] A decrease in ATPase activity in the stria vascularis and spiral ligament after KA treatment was observed by Iinuma et al.[34] and Kaku et al.[35] In addition, decline of acid mucopolysaccharides in the stria vascularis and spiral ligament was observed by Saito and Daly.[155] Microrespirometric studies have shown that the largest oxygen consumption occurs in the basal turn of the cochlea and that KA inhibits cochlear respiration.[156-158]

In addition, Mendelsohn and Katzenberg[78] found a decline in K^+ and a rise in Na^+ in the endolymph after KA treatment for five days. Similarly, Rauch et al.[77] observed that $^{42}K^+$ transport from perilymph to endolymph was reduced in KA-treated animals.

Kanamycin has also affected the efferent nerve endings and nerves. Brown[54] described that chronic treatment with KA blocked contralateral olivocochlear bundle stimulation effects.

7.3.4 Gentamicin

Gentamicin (GE) was first isolated from *Micromonospora purpurea* and described by Weinstein and coworkers[159] in 1963. The commercial preparation consists of a mixture of gentamicins C1, C2, and C1A. Gentamicin's value lies in its activity against a wide variety of gram-negative bacteria; for example, it is specifically effective against *Pseudomonas aeruginosa*, which is inhibited by concentrations of 10 μg/ml or less. Some strains of pseudomonas, however, have developed resistance to GE, which is caused by an adenylating enzyme (GE adenylate synthetase) and is transferred by plasmids.[160] Plasmid transfer is the major cause of the development of antibiotic resistance in gram-negative bacilli.[161]

Absorption, Distribution, and Excretion

Intramuscular injection of a 1.0 mg/kg dose of GE results in a serum concentration of 4 μg/ml in 60 min. It also penetrates into the interstitial fluid better than AK, NET, SI, and TO, the other AmAn with which it is compared in the study.[162] The serum *T* 1/2 in normal adults is about 2 hr. This period is substantially extended when its excretion rate is lowered; for example, in patients with impaired renal function and in newborn or premature infants.[162] Like other AmAn, GE is transported through the placenta and can cause damage to the embryo's inner ear. It also penetrates cochlear fluids; its perilymph *T* 1/2 is about 12 hr (see Figure 7.4).[27] Furthermore, GE is not significantly metabolized. Only a small portion is bound to protein, which is then secreted by the tubules; the rest, in unchanged form, is excreted by glomerular filtration.[163–164]

Gentamicin is usually given by the i.v. route of administration. Dose is established on the basis of weight, renal function, and seriousness of illness. In normal adults 3 mg/kg/day are divided into three doses, given every 8 hr. In life threatening situations, therapy can often be initiated with 5 mg/kg/day given as four divided doses, if supported by individualized pharmacokinetic parameters. This dose should be reduced to the foregoing standard dosage regimen, as soon as possible. In children the recommended dose is 6 to 7.5 mg/kg/day, divided into three doses.

A serum concentration of 10 μg/ml obtained 30 to 60 min after i.m. injection is considered safe,[165] but should not exceed 12 μg/ml.[9,163,166] Determination of serum level should be done frequently and other precautions followed (see Section 7.2.3), particularly when the drug is used in patients with impaired renal function.

Ototoxicity

The predominant ototoxic effect of GE is directed to the vestibular system.[167] In a survey of adverse reactions in 1327 patients treated with GE significant ototoxicity was reported in 31 (2.3%); of these 27 had vestibular impairment and only 12 had high-frequency hearing loss.[165] Similar observation incidences were described by Meyers.[168] When cases of accidental ototoxicity were analyzed several factors that increased the risk of vestibular toxicity were observed. Renal impairment, a long period of treatment, and previous treatment with other ototoxic antibiotics were those most often associated with ototoxic reactions.[168–172] Adverse reactions have been reported not only after parenteral administration of GE but also after its topical use; vestibular toxicity occurred in severely burned patients treated by topically applied GE.[173]

These adverse effects have been reproduced and studied in detail in experimental animals. The high affinity of GE for the vestibular system has been confirmed.[174-177] The largest amount of destruction was observed in the central part of the sensory epithelium of the cristae ampullaris and macula of the utricle, which were more vulnerable to GE than the macula of the saccule. Activity of succinic dehydrogenase was more suppressed in the cristae ampullaris than in the otolithic organs.[177-178] Gentamicin was especially detrimental to the sensory hair cells in the vestibular system.[175] Wersall et al.[178] observed that Type I hair cells were more severely damaged than Type II. Studies of optokinetic nystagmus indicate that the optokinetic neural pathway is not affected and that the damage is localized in the peripheral vestibular system.[175]

Gentamicin's effect on the auditory part of the inner ear in experimental animals was reported by Wersall et al.,[174] Webster et al.,[179] and others. The changes in hearing were manifested by an increase in threshold for frequencies above 3 kHz.[180-181] This hearing loss corresponds to degeneration of the OHC in the basal turn of the cochlea.[180-183] Most of the authors observed a degeneration of the OHC in the basal turn of the cochlea and degeneration of the IHC in the apical turns. Federspil,[183] however, described damage to both OHC and IHC in the basal turn. Ototoxic effects of GE were also observed after its intratympanic administration, as manifested by a decline in CM 24 hr after its application.[184]

7.3.5 Tobramycin

Nebramycin is an aminoglycoside complex isolated from *Streptomyces tenebrarius*.[185-187] Factor Six, now named tobramycin (TO), had the highest specific activity against gram-negative organisms. Although isolated before GE, TO was only recently introduced on the market.

Tobramycin consists of a single aminoglycoside, not a mixture. It is structurally related to kanamycin B and gentamicin C1A. Its uses are similar to those for GE. Some bacteria can inactivate TO by acetylation of amino groups or by adenylation of hydroxyl groups.[188,189] However, it is inert to the phosphorylating enzymes that inactivate some other AmAn.[190]

Absorption, Distribution, and Excretion

After i.m. administration of TO, peak serum concentrations occur in 30 to 60 min. When TO is given by slow i.v. infusion (1 hr) its peak serum concentration is, of course, lower than that following i.m. injection.[191] Serum T 1/2 in normal subjects ranges from 2 to 3 hr and can be extended to 4.5 to 8.7 hr in neonates.[192] In patients with impaired renal function serum T 1/2 ranges from 5.2 to 53 hr, depending on the degree of impairment.[191,193-194] Diffusion of TO into interstitial fluid is poor when compared with GE, SI, and NET.[13,195] Placental transfer of TO was studied by Bernard et al.,[196-197] who found that an i.m. dose of 2 mg/kg given to pregnant women generated a maternal serum level of 5.4 μg/ml and a fetal serum level of 1.2 μg/ml (about 20% of the maternal serum concentration).

Investigation of CSF, perilymph, serum, and aqueous humor levels of TO in animals revealed that only the perilymph showed retention of TO; in the other fluids its concentration declined parallel to serum concentrations.[3] These experiments showed that the perilymph T 1/2 of TO is approximately 11 hr. There is apparently no difference between the concentration of the drug in endolymph and perilymph.[3,198] Penetration of TO into cochlear fluids has also been investigated by the Lilly Toxicology Laboratory. They found that 2 hr after a single i.m. injection of 50, 100, or 150 mg/kg the level of TO in the cochlea was 7,19, and 68 μg/ml, respectively.[192] Long-term treatment did not influence the pharmacodynamics of TO in the perilymph. Increased levels of TO in the perilymph were recorded in uremic animals and in animals with otitis media, although cisternal puncture and diuretics did not change the concentration of this AmAn in the inner ear.[3,198]

Similar to other aminoglycosides, TO is excreted, unchanged, by glomerular filtration. About 75% of TO is excreted during the first 8 hr after injection and about 80 to 90% within 24 hr.[191] If the serum level reaches a toxic value, it can be removed by peritoneal dialysis or hemodialysis.[199]

The usual dose for normal adults and older children is 2 to 3 mg/kg/day, divided into three equal parts, given every 8 hr. In life-threatening infections a dose up to 5 mg/kg/day may be used, but it should be reduced to 3 mg/kg/day as soon as clinically possible. The serum concentration should be monitored when serum concentrations are expected to be high and levels above 12 μg/ml should be avoided. In patients with impaired renal function, doses subsequent to the loading dose should be adjusted according to serum levels. Renal and inner-ear function should be regularly observed when higher doses are used, when renal function is diminished, and when treatment exceeds 7 to 10 days. Tobramycin should be used with caution in prematures, neonates, and infants because of their renal immaturity and the resultant prolongation of the serum T 1/2 of TO.

Ototoxicity

The major side effects of TO are ototoxicity and nephrotoxicity. Clinical experiences with TO have been related by several authors. The largest collection of patients was presented by Neu and Bendush[200] and Bendush et al.[201] In a world-wide collection of 3506 patients treated with TO for various reasons total adverse effects were reported in 3.9%. Certain ototoxicity was observed in 23 cases (0.6%) and ototoxicity of uncertain origin was reported in another 13 (0.4%). In this survey auditory function was impaired far less frequently than vestibular function.

General toxicity was investigated in mice, rats, dogs, and cats.[202] The LD_{50} in mice and rats was 367 and 973 mg/kg, respectively. Toxic signs in dogs and cats that received doses of more than 200 mg/kg included nausea, ataxia, tremor, and respiratory distress.[202]

The acute ototoxicity of TO has been investigated by different methods. Intravenous administration of TO to animals does cause a direct effect on cochlear potentials that is not related to its effect, in higher doses, on blood pressure (see Section 7.2.3).

The effect of chronic treatment with TO was investigated by Postma et al.,[33] Welles et al.,[202] Brummett et al.,[203] and Prazma et al.[204] In cats treated with 50 mg/kg/day of TO administered subcutaneously a reduction of post-rotatory nystagmus was observed after 21 to 32 days. Following treatment with a lower dose of 35 mg/kg/day for the same period of time, reduction of postrotatory nystagmus was observed after 20 to 47 days. Similarly, dogs receiving TO (30 mg/kg/day for two weeks) had a loss of weight and uremia, with severe renal tubular necrosis. When the dose was lowered to 25 mg/kg/day it was noted that no vestibular changes were observed for as long as 65 days of treatment.[202]

Prazma et al.[204] treated guinea pigs with 50, 100, 150, and 200 mg/kg day of s.c. TO and examined their cochleas for degenerative changes, using surface preparation techniques. Administration of TO at a dose of 50 mg/kg day for two weeks caused no significant loss of hair cells. Damage to the OHC appeared after 150 mg/kg/day for eight days or 100 mg/kg/day for two weeks and after 200 mg/kg/day for seven days or longer. The pattern of cochlear damage was similar to that already described (see Section 7.2.3). A comparison of two different dosage schedules (Figure 7.6) in which the total dose in both cases was 1400 mg/kg (100 mg/kg/day for 14 days or 200 mg/kg/day for seven days) showed that high daily doses for shorter periods were more toxic than the lower daily doses spread out over a longer period; the shorter term, higher dose treatment regimen caused twice as much OHC loss. This supports the theory that higher doses of AmAn generate higher blood levels, of which more penetrates into the cochlea and causes larger destruction of hair cells; that is, ototoxicity may be more related to peak serum levels of the AmAn than to their trough levels.

Postma et al.[33] studied the relationship of TO-induced ototoxicity to hair-cell glycogen and found the following:

1. OHC disappearance was not observed earlier than 13 days subsequent to seven days of treatment.
2. Permanent damage of the OHC was most prevalent in areas that normally have the least amount of glycogen. In these areas (particularly in the first turn) glycogen did not increase during treatment and two to three weeks after treatment, it decreased.
3. Swelling of nuclei was observed mostly in the upper turns, not in areas in which the majority of the OHC were later missing. Therefore TO does, at least in animals, interfere with metabolism of glycogen by the hair cells. This could be one of the mechanisms by which the AmAn exert their ototoxicity.

Comparisons of TO and GE show that TO is less ototoxic than GE.[205–206]

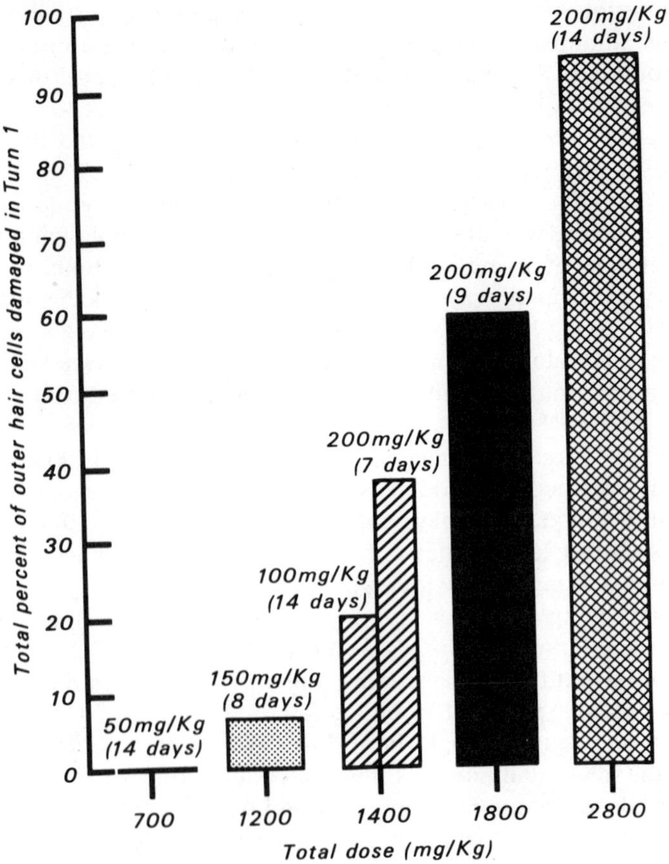

Figure 7.6 Correlation of the ototoxicity produced by tobramycin with dose and duration of treatment. Ototoxicity (total loss of OHC in Turn 1) increases with an increase in total dose, and for the same total dose ototoxicity is increased by a shorter duration of treatment (higher daily dose). From Prazma et al.[204] Reproduced by permission of the *Laryngoscope*.

In addition, the other toxic effects of these two aminoglycosides are similar.[200,207]

7.3.6 Amikacin

Amikacin (AK) is a new semisynthetic AmAn, produced from kanamycin A by acetylation of its 2-deoxystreptamine moiety. The antimicrobial activity of AK is similar to KA[208] but, because it is a poor substrate for *N*-acetylation, O-adenylation, and O-phosphorylation, it has greater effectiveness than KA aginst *P. aeruginosa, E. coli, P. vulgaris, K. pneumoniae, A. aerogenes,* and others. Because it is a poor substrate for many bacterial enzymes, it is particularly useful against resistant microorganisms.[209–211]

Absorption, Distribution, and Excretion

The serum *T* 1/2 of AK is about 2 hr. Intramuscular injections of 3.7, 5, and 7.5 mg/kg to normal adults generate peak serum levels of 12, 16, and 21 μg/ml, respectively.[212] Amikacin does cross the placental and blood-brain barriers. In infants CSF concentration is 10 to 20% of serum concentrations but may reach 50% in patients with meningitis. When it was administered to humans every 6 hr in doses of 150 mg/m^2 the drug had a tendency to accumulate in serum.[213]

During the first 8 hr after administration about 91.9% is excreted, unchanged, in the urine by glomerular filtration, and because 0 to 11% of it is bound to plasma protein, a small percentage is also secreted by the kidney tubule.

The recommended dose of AK in adults and older children with normal kidney function is 15 mg/kg, divided into two to three doses (q. 12 or 8 hr, respectively). If used in patients with impaired renal function, doses should be adjusted according to the creatinine clearance and the plasma level of AK (see Section 7.2.3).

Ototoxicity

Like kanamycin, AK is more toxic to the cochlea than to the vestibular system. In a large group of 1548 patients treated with AK,[165] high-frequency hearing loss was reported in 71 (4.59%), conversational hearing loss in 8 (0.52%), and vestibular symptoms in 10 (0.65%). Analysis of 328 audiograms, before and after treatment, revealed a 15-dB hearing deficit in 3.35% of the subjects.[214] Valdivieso et al.[215] observed hearing loss in 6% of their patients. They also found that toxicity was directly related to serum concentrations and the duration of treatment. A higher incidence of ototoxicity was observed in patients by Black et al.[216] and in leukopenic patients by Lau et al.[217] In 20% of their patients (105 total) they observed unilateral or bilateral perceptive hearing loss greater than 15 dB. Furthermore, Reiffenstein et al.[218a] found that after seven days of treatment the ototoxicity of AK is similar to that of KA. Prosen et al.[218b] found AK somewhat more destructive in the guinea pig cochlea when compared with KA administered at the same doses (100 mg/kg) and time schedule. Amikacin was predominantly cochleotoxic with little effect on the vestibular sense organ when guinea pigs were treated with high doses of 450 mg/kg/day.[218c] Theopold[219] reported that in experiments on guinea pigs AK is more toxic to the cochlea than GE or TO. When he gave AK in a dose 10 times higher than recommended, the damage was greater than that caused by TO and GE given in doses 50 times higher than the recommended.

Amikacin penetration into the cochlear fluid of animals was investigated by Federspil et al.[198] Its perilymph *T* 1/2 is similar to those of GE and TO; about 10 hr. One caution must be observed when interpreting experimental literature on AK as shown in Figure 7.4; it is not given in the same dosages as GE, TO, and SI. For example, when AK, TO, GE, and SI are given in equal doses to guinea pigs,[220] AK and TO are both less ototoxic than GE and SI. However, the recommended human daily dose of AK is 2 to 4 times that of TO and the result is that when given to humans the reported incidence of ototoxicity associated with its use is higher than that for TO or GE.

7.3.7 Netilmicin

Netilmicin (NET, SCH 20569) is an ethyl derivative of dehydrogenated gentamicin C1A. It is highly active against enterobacteriaceae. In addition, it is a poor substrate for some GE inactivating enzymes and therefore is active against many GE-resistant microorganisms. This drug is presently undergoing clinical trials and is not yet on the market. A disadvantage of NET is that it has significant neuromuscular blocking activity.[221,222]

Absorption, Distribution, and Excretion

One hour after parenteral administration of 50 mg/m^2 to volunteers the serum level of NET was about 5.5 μg/ml.[223] After 6 hr about 55% of it was excreted and the serum level was decreased to 1.4 μg/ml.[223] The serum T 1/2 of NET is similar to that of GE (1.3 hr).[224] Interstitial concentration of NET after i.m. injection was initially lower than that obtained after equal doses of GE, but it was the highest of all tested AmAn after 12 hr.[195]

Netilmicin is excreted by glomerular filtration. Renal cortex concentrations are reported to be much higher than medullary concentrations.[221] It is less nephrotoxic than GE or TO, even when the renal cortex concentrations of the drugs are the same.[225–227]

A single subcutaneous injection of 150 mg/kg of NET or GE produces peak serum and perilymph concentrations in 1 and 2 hr, respectively, in experimental animals.[221] The NET levels are lower, however, than the GE levels. In chronic experiments with 50, 100, and 150 mg/kg/day of GE and NET, serum and perilymph concentrations of GE were again higher than those of NET and NET did not accumulate in the perilymph after these daily doses.[221]

A daily dose of 6 to 7.5 mg/kg, divided into three (q. 8 hr), is recommended for normal adults with serious systemic infection.

Ototoxicity

Like GE and TO, NET is considered primarily vestibulotoxic. On a weight basis NET was less ototoxic than GE[222,228–231a] and AK[229] and had about the same ototoxicity as TO[231b] when cochlear and/or vestibular toxicity were examined. In chronic experiments the cochlear damage was smaller after the administration of 200 mg/kg/day of NET than after 50 mg/kg/day of GE.[229]

An interesting feature of NET ototoxicity is that the pattern of cochlear destruction is different from that produced by the other AmAn[198]; NET causes more extensive OHC loss in the upper than in the basal turn.

A low degree of NET ototoxicity to vestibular sensory cells has been demonstrated.[231] Postrotatory vestibular reactions of guinea pigs were not altered when the animals were treated with 100 mg/kg/day for three weeks or 50 mg/kg/day for one month. Development of ataxia and impairment in righting reflex was studied in cats.[222] Gentamicin (40 mg/kg/day) caused ataxia and impairment in righting reflex after 9 to 18 days, whereas the same dose of NET caused this effect only after 92 doses (days). Similarly, NET was less toxic than GE in squirrel monkeys.[230]

7.3.8 Sisomicin

Sisomicin (SI) is produced by *Micromonospora inydensis*. Structurally it is closely related to gentamicin C1A; some cross-resistance exists as a consequence. Its antibacterial activity parallels those of GE and TO.[232] It is not yet on the market.

Absorption, Distribution, and Excretion

Sisomicin is quickly absorbed after parenteral administration. After i.m. administration of 1.0 mg/kg to normal adults it reaches a peak serum value of 4.48 μg/ml within 30 min and its serum *T* 1/2 is about 2.2 hours.[233-234] It does not penetrate into interstitial fluid as well as GE.[195] It is predominantly excreted by glomerular filtration.

Ototoxicity

In animal experiments, SI appears to be the same or slightly more toxic than GE[235,236]; it is considered to be predominantly vestibulotoxic.[207]

ACKNOWLEDGMENTS

I wish to express my appreciation to Gregory L. Kearns, Pharm. D., for his assistance in the formulation of the guidelines for dosage regimens of the AmAn.

REFERENCES

1. A. Kohonen, *Acta Otolaryngol. Suppl.*, **208,** 1 (1965).
2. P. S. Guth and R. P. Bobbin, in *Advances in Pharmacology and Chemotherapy*, Vol. 9, Academic, New York, 1971, pp. 93–130.

3. P. Federspil, *Infection*, **4,** 239 (1976).
4. J. E. Hawkins, in *Handbook of Sensory Physiology*, Vol. 5, Wolf D. Keidel and William D. Neff, Eds., Springer, Berlin, 1976, pp. 707–748.
5. J. E. Hawkins, in *Childhood Deafness*, Fred H. Bess, Ed., Grune & Stratton, New York, 1977, pp. 37–51.
6. R. D. Brown and A. M. Feldman, *Ann. Rev. Pharmacol. Toxicol.*, **18,** 233 (1978).
7. W. E. Sanders, Jr., and C. C. Sanders, *Ann. Rev. Pharmacol. Toxicol.*, **19,** 53 (1979).
8. G. G. Jackson and L. Riff, *J. Infect. Dis.*, (Suppl.)**124,** 185 (1971).
9. G. G. Jackson and G. Archieri, *J. Infect. Dis. Suppl.*, **124,** 130 (1971).
10. L. E. Bryan and H. M. Van den Elzen, *J. Antibiot. Tokyo*, **28,** 696 (1975).
11. K. E. Price, M. D. DeFuria, and T. A. Pursiano, *J. Infect. Dis.*, **134,** 249 (1976).
12. J. Davies and P. Courvalin, *Am. J. Med.*, **62,** 868 (1977).
13. G. D. Chisholm, P. M. Waterworth, J. S. Calnan, and L. P. Garrod, *Br. Med. J.*, **1,** 569 (1973).
14. F. C. Luft and S. A. Kleit, *J. Infect. Dis.*, **130,** 656 (1974).
15. G. G. Jackson, *Clin. Ther.*, **1,** 200 (1977).
16. J. E. Hawkins and H. Engstrom, *Acta Otolaryngol. Suppl.*, **188,** 100 (1964).
17. F. B. Simmons, R. Galambos, and J. P. Albrite, *Arch. Otolaryngol.*, **72,** 233 (1960).
18. D. Robertson and B. M. Johnstone, *J. Acoust. Soc. Am.*, **66,** 466 (1979).
19. I. Galasinska-Pomykol, E. Krochmalska, B. Oldak, and S. Hryszko, *Laryngol. Rhinol. Otol.*, **54,** 418 (1975).
20. K. Balogh, F. Hiraide, and D. Ishii, *Ann. Otol. Rhinol. Laryngol.*, **79,** 641 (1970).
21. M. Portmann, J. Darrouzet, and C. Coste, *Arch. Otolaryngol.*, **100,** 473 (1974).
22a. Ch. von Ilberg, H. Spoendlin, and W. Arnold, *Acta Otolaryngol.*, **71,** 159 (1971).
22b. P. Tran-Ba-Huy, Ch. Manuel, and O. Sterkers, Abstracts of 3rd midwinter research meeting of the Association for Research in Otolaryngology, Florida, 1980, p. 61.
23. V. S. Muraveiskaya, *Antibiotics*, **10,** 245 (1965).
24. L. Voldrich, *Acta Otolaryngol.*, **60,** 243 (1965).
25. D. P. Vrabec, T. H. Cody, and J. A. Ulrich, *Ann. Otol. Rhinol.*, **74,** 688 (1965).
26. H. Stupp, K. Kupper, F. Lagler, H. Sous, and M. Quante, *Audiology*, **12,** 350 (1973).
27. P. Federspil, W. Schatzle, and E. Tiesler, *J. Infect. Dis.*, **134,** 200 (1976).
28a. H. W. Wagner, J. T. Y. Chou, Ch. von Ilberg, R. Ritter, and K. H. Vosteen, *Arzneim Froch* (Drug Res.), **12,** 2006 (1971).
28b. J. Prazma, S. A. Kidwell, A. Drake, J. Fischer, S. D. Ferguson, H. G. Garrison, and L. E. Klingler (submitted to *J. Infect. Dis.*).
28c. J. Prazma, S. D. Ferguson, S. A. Kidwell, H. G. Garrison, A. Drake, and J. Fischer (submitted to *Ann. Otol. Rhinol. Laryngol.*).
28d. J. Prazma, H. G. Garrison, S. A. Kidwell, S. D. Ferguson, J. Fischer, and A. Drake (submitted to *Ann. Otol. Rhinol. Laryngol.*).
28e. J. Prazma, H. G. Garrison, S. A. Kidwell, A. Fischer Drake, J. Fisher, and S. D. Ferguson, Abstracts of 3rd midwinter research meeting of the Association for Research in Otolaryngology, Florida, 1980, p. 61.
28f. G. A. Alleyne, *Pediatrics*, **39,** 400 (1967).
28g. I. Ichikava, M. L. Purkerson, S. Klahr, J. L. Troy, M. Martinez-Maldonado, and B. M. Brenner, *J. Clin. Invest.*, **65,** 982 (1980).
29a. H. Stupp, *Acta Otolaryngol. Suppl.*, **262,** 5 (1970).
29b. S. Pestka, *Ann. Rev. Biochem.*, **40,** 697 (1971).

30. C. Beck, *Arch. Otolaryngol.*, **81,** 548 (1965).
31. G. Stange, E. Holz, Y. Terayama, and Ch. Beck, *Arch. Otorhinolaryngol.*, **186,** 229 (1966).
32. K. Watanuki, H. Kashiwazaki, K. Kawamoto, and S. Katagiri, *Arch. Otorhinolaryngol.*, **192,** 369 (1968).
33. D. S. Postma, J. B. Pecorak, J. Prazma, S. S. Logue, and N. D. Fischer, *Arch. Otolaryngol.*, **102,** 154 (1976).
34. T. Iinuma, O. Mizukoshi, and J. F. Daly, *Laryngoscope*, **77,** 159 (1967).
35. Y. Kaku, J. C. Farmer, and W. R. Hudson, *Arch. Otolaryngol.*, **98,** 282 (1973).
36. Y. Koide, A. Hata, and R. Hando, *Acta Otolaryngol.*, **61,** 332 (1966).
37. M. Tachibana, O. Mizukoshi, and K. Kuriyama, *Biochem. Pharmacol.*, **25,** 2297 (1976).
38. K. Owada, *Chemotherapy*, **5,** 277 (1962) (Tokyo).
39. R. L. Cronin, Masters Thesis, Tulane University Graduate School, July 1978.
40. J. Garcia-Quiroga, C. H. Norris, L. Glade, G. M. Bryant, M. Tachibana, and P. S. Guth, *Res. Comm. Chem. Pathol. Pharmacol.*, **22,** 535 (1978).
41. H. T. Nakada, T. N. Morita, and A. N. Wick, *J. Biol. Chem.*, **215,** 803 (1955).
42. C. H. Tan, N. A. Peterson, and E. Raghupathy, *Biochem. Biophys. Acta*, **464,** 459 (1977).
43. D. Waitzova, K. Kubat, M. Melicharova, and O. Koldovsky, *Physiol. Bohemoslov.*, **20,** 11 (1971).
44. D. S. Ginsburg, A. P. Quintanilla, and M. Levin, *J. Infect. Dis.*, **134,** 119 (1976).
45. K. S. Furuno, K. Matsubara, K. Ando, and S. Suzuki, *J. Antibiot.*, **29,** 950 (1976).
46. K. Furuno, K. Ando, and S. Suzuki, *J. Antibiot.*, **29,** 187 (1976).
47. C. H. Norris, G. Bryant, R. Cronin-Schreiber, and P. S. Guth, *Pharmacologist*, **21,** 3 (1979).
48. T. Takeda, *Pract. Otolaryngol.*, **61,** 991 (1968).
49. R. Thalmann, T. Miyoshi, and I. Thalmann, *Laryngoscope*, **82,** 2249 (1972).
50. J. Falbe-Hansen, *Acta Otolaryngol. Suppl.*, **188,** 108 (1964).
51. H. Engstrom, *Acta Otolaryngol.*, **49,** 109 (1958).
52. C. S. Smith and F. S. Sjostrand, *J. Ultrastruct. Res.*, **5,** 523 (1961).
53. H. Spoendlin, *J. Laryngol. Otol.*, **81,** 717 (1967).
54. R. D. Brown, *Acta Otolaryngol.*, **73,** 335 (1972).
55. R. D. Brown and E. A. Daigneault, *Acta Otolaryngol.*, **76,** 128 (1973).
56. G. Stange, M. Spreng, and U. O. Keidel, *Pfluegers Arch.*, **279,** 99 (1964).
57. E. Krochmalska, *Acta Otolaryngol.*, **77,** 44 (1974).
58. Ch. Beck, *Acta Otolaryngol.*, **71,** 206 (1971).
59. M. J. Capps and A. J. Duvall, *Laryngoscope*, **87,** 1100 (1977).
60a. J. T. Buckley and J. N. Hawthorne, *J. Biol. Chem.*, **247,** 7218 (1972).
60b. M. Kai and J. N. Hawthorne, *Ann. N.Y. Acad. Sci.*, **165,** 761 (1969).
60c. S. Lodhi, N. D. Weiner, and J. Schacht, *Biochem. Biophys. Acta*, **426,** 781 (1976).
60d. J. Schacht, S. Lodhi, and N. D. Weiner, *Membrane Toxicity*, 191–208, Plenum, New York, 1977.
60e. E. Stockhorst and J. Schacht, *Acta Otolaryngol.*, **83,** 401 (1977).
61. J. Schacht, *Ann. Otol. Rhinol. Laryngol.*, **83,** 613 (1974).
61a. A. Schibeci and J. Schacht, *Biochem. Pharmacol.*, **26,** 1769 (1977).
61b. A. Orsulakova, E. Stockhorst, and J. Schacht, *J. Neurochem.*, **26,** 285 (1976).
61c. J. Schacht, *Arch. Otorhinolaryngol.*, **224,** 129 (1979).

62. J. Wersall and A. Flock, *Life Sci.*, **3,** 1151 (1964).
63. Y. Harada, E. Musso, and E. Mira, *Acta Otolaryngol.*, **64,** 327 (1967).
64. S. Matsuura, K. Ikeda, and T. Furukawa, *Jpn. J. Physiol.*, **21,** 590 (1971).
65. H. Engstrom, *Acta Otolaryngol.*, **67,** 254 (1969).
66. T. B. Logan, J. Prazma, W. G. Thomas, and N. D. Fischer, *Arch. Otolaryngol.*, **99,** 190 (1974).
67. R. E. Brummett and R. T. Brown, *Arch. Otolaryngol.*, **101,** 540 (1975).
68. A. L. Nuttall, D. M. Marques, E. Stockhorst, and J. Schacht, *J. Acoust. Soc. Am.*, **57,** S60 (1975).
69. T. Konishi, *Acta Otolaryngol.*, **88,** 41 (1979).
70. P. Wilson and R. T. Ramsden, *Br. Med. J.*, **1,** 259 (1977).
71. S. M. Dobbs and G. E. Mawer, *J. Infect. Dis.*, **134,** S114 (1976).
72. F. Nakamura, *Ann. Otolaryngol. Chir. Cervicofac.*, **66,** 1080 (1957).
73. J. R. Lindsay, L. R. Procter, and W. P. Work, *Laryngoscope*, **70,** 382 (1960).
74. K. Musebeck, *Arch. Otorhinolaryngol.*, **182,** 583 (1963).
75. K. Musebeck and W. Schatzle, *Arch. Otorhinolaryngol.*, **181,** 530 (1964).
76a. L. G. Johnsson and J. E. Hawkins, Jr., *Laryngoscope*, **82,** 1105 (1972).
76b. Y. Kaneko, Y. Terayama, K. Kawamoto, K. Kasajima, and I. Ise, *Acta Otolaryngol.*, **86,** 375 (1978).
77. S. Rauch, N. Kostlin, E. A. Schnieder, and K. Schindler, *Laryngoscope*, **73,** 135 (1963).
78. M. Mendelsohn and I. Katzenberg, *Laryngoscope*, **82,** 397 (1972).
79. A. Kohonen and J. Tarkkanen, *Acta Otolaryngol*, **68,** 90 (1969).
80. H. Davis, B. H. Deatherage, B. Rosenblut, C. Fernandez, R. Kimura, and C. Smith, *Laryngoscope*, **68,** 596 (1958).
81. R. E. Brummett, R. F. Harris, and J. A. Lindgren, *Laryngoscope,* **86,** 1177 (1976).
82. H. F. Schuknecht, *Laryngoscope*, **66,** 859 (1950).
83. G. Stange, C. L. Schmidt, and H. Orthenberger, *Arch. Otorhinolaryngol.*, **217,** 361 (1977).
84. Y. Koide, A. Hata, and R. Hando, *Acta Otolaryngol.*, **61,** 332 (1966).
85. H. Spoendlin, *ORL*, **28,** 305 (1966).
86. H. H. Lindeman, *Acta Otolaryngol.*, **67,** 177 (1968).
87. E. Holz, G. Stange, T. Soda, and C. Beck, *Arch. Otolaryngol.*, **87,** 359 (1968).
88. R. Ritter, J. Chou, Ch. von Ilberg, and W. H. Wagner, *Arch. Otorhinolaryngol.*, **199,** 573 (1971).
89. S. Courvoisier and O. Leau, *Antibiot. Chemother.*, **6,** 411 (1956).
90. B. Prescott and H. J. Stone, *Proc. Soc. Exp. Biol. Med.*, **114,** 433 (1963).
91. B. Prescott and H. J. Stone, *Il Farmaco.*, **21,** 471 (1966).
92. J. E. Hawkins, Jr., H. Wolcott, and W. J. O'Shanny, in *Antibiotics Annual*, New York: Medical Encyclopedia, 1957, p. 554.
93. G. Kutchinsky, H. Lullmann, and W. Pracht, *Dtsch. Med. Wochenschr*, Stuttgart, **84,** 364 (1959).
94. J. V. Bennett, J. L. Brodie, E. J. Benner, and W. M. M. Kirby, *Appl. Environ. Microbiol.*, **14,** 170 (1966).
95a. L. D. Sabath, J. I. Casey, P. A. Ruch, L. L. Stumpf, and M. Findland, *Antimicrob. Agents Chemother.*, **1,** 83 (1970).
95b. S. A. Lerner and G. J. Matz, *Am. J. Otolaryngol.*, **1,** 169 (1980).

95c. B. J. Devine, *Drug Intell. Clin. Pharm.*, **8,** 650 (1974).

95d. S. N. Schwartz, G. J. Pazin, J. A. Lyon, M. Ho, and A. W. Pasculle, *J. Infect. Dis.*, **138,** 499 (1978).

95e. D. W. Cockcroft and M. H. Gault, *Nephron*, **16,** 31 (1976).

95f. F. A. Sarubbi and J. H. Hull, *Ann. Int. Med.*, **89**(1), 612 (1978).

95g. C. V. Sanders, *Syva Monitor*, **6,** 1 (1980).

95h. J. C. Pechere and R. Dugal, *Clin. Pharmacokin.*, **4,** 170 (1979).

96. E. J. Jacobson, M. P. Downs, and J. L. Fletcher, U. S. Army Medical Research Laboratory, Report No. 820, Fort Knox, Kentucky, 1–8 (1969).

97. D. A. Greene, *Rocky Mt. Med. J.*, **74,** 254 (1977).

98a. J. Plantier, A. W. Forrey, M. A. O'Neill, A. D. Blair, T. G. Christopher, and R. E. Cutler, *J. Infect. Dis.*, **134,** 5323 (1976).

98b. R. H. Bernard and J. C. Pechere, Abstracts of 3rd midwinter research meeting of the Association for Research in Otolaryngology, Florida, 1980, p. 59.

98c. T. F. Hieber, G. H. McCracken, R. J. Roeser, D. A. Allen, D. F. Chrane, and J. Morrow, *Pediatrics*, **63,** 443 (1979).

99. G. B. Appel and H. C. Neu, *N. Engl. J. Med.*, **296,** 663 and 784 (1977).

100. J. G. Dahlgren, E. T. Anderson, and W. L. Hewitt, *Antimicrob. Agents Chemother.*, **8,** 58 (1975).

101. O. V. Brazil and A. P. Corrado, *J. Pharmacol. Exp. Ther.*, **120,** 452 (1957).

102. C. B. Pittinger and J. P. Long, *Antibiot. Chemother.*, **8,** 198 (1958).

103. J. C. Timmerman, J. P. Long, and C. B. Pittinger, *Toxicol. Appl. Pharmacol.*, **1,** 299 (1959).

104. R. H. Adamson, R. L. Borgman, J. R. Fouts, and J. P. Long, *Antibiot. Chemother.*, **11,** 429 (1961).

105. G. H. Wagman, E. M. Oden, M. J. Weinstein, and S. Irwin, *Antimicrob. Agents Chemother.*, **6,** 175 (1966).

106. O. V. Brazil and J. Prado-Franceschi, *Arch. Int. Pharmacodyn. Ther.*, **179,** 65 (1969).

107. C. Pittinger and R. Adamson, *Ann. Rev. Pharmacol. Toxicol.*, **12,** 169 (1972).

108. F. R. Goodman, G. B. Weiss, and H. R. Adams, *J. Pharmacol. Exp. Ther.*, **188,** 472 (1974).

109. E. Hokkanen, *Acta Neurol. Scand.*, **40,** 346 (1964).

110. M. J. Keating, M. R. Setho, G. P. Bodey, and N. A. Samaan, *Cancer*, **39,** 1410 (1977).

111. A. Schatz, S. Bugie and S. A. Waksman, *Proc. Soc. Exp. Biol. Med.*, **57,** 244 (1944).

112. G. B. Appel and H. C. Neu, *N. Engl. J. Med.*, **296,** 722 (1977).

113. G. C. Robinson and K. G. Cambon, *N. Engl. J. Med.*, **271,** 949 (1964).

114. E. Varpela and J. Hiertralahti, M. J. T., *Scand. J. Respir. Dis.*, **50,** 101 (1969).

115. H. C. Hinshaw and H. W. Feldman, *Mayo Clin. Proc.*, **20,** 313 (1945).

116. K. Berg, *Ann. Otol. Rhinol. Laryngol.*, **58,** 448 (1949).

117. R. Causse, *Ann. Otolaryngol. Par.*, **66,** 518 (1949).

118. M. Prazic and B. Salaj, *Audiology*, **14,** 173 (1975).

119. H. F. Schuknecht, *Acta Otolaryngol. Suppl.*, **132,** 5 (1957).

120. D. N. F. Fairbanks, H. Shimizu, and D. Warfield, *Arch. Otolaryngol.*, **93,** 590 (1971).

121. J. E. Hawkins, N. J. Rahway, and M. H. Lurie, *Ann. Otol. Rhinol. Laryngol.*, **61,** 789 (1952).

122. M. Igarashi, *Audiology*, **12,** 337 (1973).

123. J. Wersall and J. E. Hawkins, *Acta Otolaryngol.*, **54,** 1 (1962).

124. A. J. Duvall and J. Wersall, *Acta Otolaryngol.*, **57,** 581 (1964).
125. Y. Harada and Y. Sugimoto, *Acta Otolaryngol.*, **84,** 65 (1977).
126. G. E. Shambaugh, E. L. Derlacki, W. H. Harrison, H. House, W. House, V. Hildyard, H. Schuknecht, and J. J. Shea, *J. Am. Med. Assoc.*, **170,** 1657 (1959).
127. J. E. Hawkins, Jr., N. J. Rahway, and M. H. Lurie, *Ann. Otol. Rhinol. Laryngol.*, **62,** 1128 (1953).
128. J. Tyberghein, *Acta Otolaryngol. Suppl.*, **171,** 5 (1962).
129. J. E. Hawkins, Jr., W. C. Stebbins, L. G. Johnsson, D. B. Moody, and A. Muraski, *Acta Otolaryngol.*, **83,** 123 (1977).
130. S. H. Waksman and H. A. Lechevalier, *Science*, **109,** 305 (1949).
131. L. Ruedi, K. Graf, and B. Tschirren, *Schweiz. Med. Wochenschr.*, **83,** 951 (1953).
132. M. Myerson, H. F. Knight, A. J. Gambarini, and T. L. Curran, *Ann. Thorac. Surg.*, **9,** 483 (1970).
133. H. L. Engel and J. S. Denson, *Surgery*, **42,** 862 (1957).
134. R. L. Fields, *Arch. Otolaryngol.*, **79,** 67 (1964).
135. R. N. Khodabnova, T. N. Oberyukhtina, and K. A. Dmitriyeva, *Vestn. Otorinolaringol.*, **33,** 109 (1971).
136. W. C. S. Graham, *Panminerva Med.*, **11,** 44 (1969).
137. H. Umezawa, *J. Antibiot. A. Tokyo*, **10,** 181 (1957).
138. H. C. Jones, *J. Nat. Med. Assoc.*, **65,** 201 (1973).
139. R. Meyer, A. Gottesberge, and H. F. Stupp, *Acta Otolaryngol.*, **67,** 171 (1969).
140. C. M. Kumin, *Ann. N.Y. Acad. Sci.*, **132,** 811 (1966).
141. R. C. Atkins, C. Mion, E. Despaux, N. Van-Hai, J. Christian, and H. Mion, *Kidney Int.*, **3,** 391 (1973).
142. I. Kass, *Ann. N.Y. Acad. Sci.*, **132,** 892 (1966).
143. P. A. Bunn, A. Baltch, and O. Krajnyak, *Ann. N.Y. Acad. Sci.*, **76,** 109 (1958).
144. I. Donomae, *Ann. N.Y. Acad. Sci.*, **76,** 166 (1958).
145. J. O. Frost, J. F. Daly, and J. E. Hawkins, *Antibiotica*, 700 (1958).
146. R. F. Nauton and P. Ward, *Arch. Otolaryngol.*, **69,** 398 (1959).
147. S. M. Finegold, *Ann. N.Y. Acad. Sci.*, **132,** 942 (1966).
148. M. B. Jorgenson and M. R. Schmidt, *Acta Otolaryngol.*, **55,** 537 (1962).
149. J. E. Hawkins, *Ann. Otol. Rhinol. Laryngol.*, **68,** 698 (1959).
150. J. Ouchi and I. Ohtani, *ORL*, **31,** 218 (1969).
151. P. Dallos and C. Y. Wang, *Audiology*, **13,** 277 (1974).
152. R. F. Marseillan, *Acta Physiol. Lat. Am.*, **15,** 300 (1965).
153. J. Farkashidy, R. G. Block, and T. D. R. Briant, *Laryngoscope*, **73,** 713 (1963).
154. Y. Koide, R. Stern, H. K. Roester, and J. F. Daly, *Laryngoscope*, **76,** 1769 (1966).
155. H. Saito and J. F. Daly, *Acta Otolaryngol.*, **71,** 22 (1971).
156. Y. Sato, O. Mizukoshi, and J. F. Daly, *Ann. Otol. Rhinol. Laryngol.*, **78,** 1201 (1969).
157. G. A. Misrahy, J. F. Spradley, S. Dzinovic, and C. J. Brooks, *Ann. Otol. Rhinol. Laryngol.*, **70,** 572 (1961).
158. O. Mizukoshi and J. F. Daly, *Acta Otolaryngol.*, **64,** 45 (1967).
159. M. J. Weinstein, G. M. Luedemann, E. M. Oden, G. H. Wagman, J. P. Rosselot, J. A. Marquez, C. T. Conglio, W. Charney, H. L. Herzog, and J. Black, *J. Med. Chem.*, **6,** 463 (1963).
160. R. Benveniste and J. Davies, *FEBS Lett.*, **14,** 293 (1971).

161. S. A. Kabins, C. R. Nathan, and S. Cohen, *J. Infect. Dis.*, **124,** 65 (1971).

162. G. H. McCracken, D. F. Chrane, and M. L. Thomas, *J. Infect. Dis.*, **124,** S214 (1971).

163. A. M. Gyselynch, A. Forrey, and R. Cutler, *J. Infect. Dis.*, **124,** S70 (1971).

164. R. C. Gordon, C. Regamey, and W. M. M. Kirby, *Antimicrob. Agents Chemother.*, **2,** 214 (1972).

165. G. M. Archieri, F. G. Falco, H. M. Smith, and L. B. Hobson, *Med. J. Acoust. Suppl.*, **1,** 30 (1970).

166. P. T. Frame, J. P. Phair, C. Watanakunakorn, and T. W. Bannister, *J. Infect. Dis.*, **135,** 952 (1977).

167. P. G. Lundquist and J. Wersall, Gentamicin: First International Symposium, Schwabe, Basel, 24–26 (1976).

168. R. M. Meyers, *Arch. Otolaryngol.*, **92,** 160 (1970).

169. G. Banck, S. Belfrage, I. Juhlin, L. Nordstrom, O. Tjernstrom, and N. G. Toremalm, *Acta Pathol. Microbiol. Scand. (B) Suppl.*, **241,** 54 (1973).

170. L. Nordstrom, G. Banck, S. Belfrage, I. Juhlin, O. Tjernstrom, and N. G. Toremalm, *Acta Pathol. Microbiol. Scand. (B)*, **241,** 58 (1973).

171. G. B. Galioto, C. Grassi, G. Manara, and P. Santarelli, *Int. J. Clin. Pharmacol.*, **10,** 95 (1974).

172. J. G. Dahlgren, E. T. Anderson, and W. L. Hewitt, *Antimicrob. Agents Chemother.*, **8,** 58 (1975).

173. V. S. Dayal, E. L. Smith, and W. G. McCain, *Arch. Otolaryngol.*, **100,** 338 (1974).

174. J. Wersall, P. G. Lundquist, and B. Bjorkroth, *J. Infect. Dis.*, **119,** 410 (1969).

175. M. Igarashi, P. G. Lundquist, B. R. Alford, and H. Miyata, *J. Infect. Dis.*, **124,** S114 (1971).

176. J. A. Waitz, E. L. Moss, Jr., and M. J. Weinstein, *J. Infect. Dis.*, **124,** S125 (1971).

177. K. Watanuki, H. F. Stupp, and A. Meyer, Zum Gottesberge, *Laryngoscope*, **82,** 363 (1972).

178. J. Wersall, B. Bjorkroth, A. Flock, and P. G. Lundquist, *Arch. Otorhinolaryngol.*, **200,** 1 (1971).

179. J. C. Webster, R. Carrol, J. T. Benitez, and T. M. McGee, *J. Infect. Dis.* **124,** S138 (1971).

180. J. E. Hawkins, Jr., L. G. Johnsson, and J. M. Aran, *J. Infect. Dis.*, **119,** 417 (1969).

181. J. Ylikoski, J. Wersall, and B. Bjorkroth, *Acta Pathol. Microbiol. Scand. (B)*, **241,** 30 (1973).

182. P. G. Lundquist and J. Wersall, *J. Ultrastruct. Res.*, **18,** 234 (1967).

183. P. Federspil, *Laryngol. Rhinol. Otol. Stuttg.*, **51,** 785 (1972).

184. T. Morizono and B. M. Johnstone, *Med. J. Aust.*, **2,** 634 (1975).

185. W. M. Stark, M. M. Hoehn, and M. J. Knox, *Antimicrob. Agents Chemother.*, **7,** 314 (1967).

186. C. E. Higgins and R. E. Kastner, *Antimicrob. Agents Chemother.*, **7,** 324 (1967).

187. R. Q. Thompson and E. A. Presti, *Antimicrob. Agents Chemother.*, **7,** 332 (1967).

188. R. Benveniste and J. Davies, *Ann. Rev. Biochem.*, **42,** 471 (1973).

189. K. E. Price, T. A. Pursiano, M. D. DeFuria, and G. E. Wright, *Antimicrob. Agents Chemother.*, **5,** 143 (1974).

190. J. Davies, *J. Infect. Dis.*, **124,** S7 (1971).

191. C. Regamey, R. C. Gordon, and W. M. M. Kirby, *Clin. Pharmacol. Ther.*, **14,** 396 (1973).

192. K. S. Israel, J. S. Welles, and H. R. Black, *J. Infect. Dis.*, **134,** S97 (1976).

193. W. R. Lockwood and J. D. Bower, *Antimicrob. Agents Chemother.*, **3,** 125 (1973).

194. K. G. Naber, S. R. Westenfelder, and P. O. Madsen, *Antimicrob. Agents Chemother.*, **3,** 469 (1973).

195. C. Carbon, A. Contrepois, and S. Lamotte-Barrillon, *Antimicrob. Agents Chemother.*, **13,** 368 (1978).

196. B. Bernard, S. J. Garcia, C. A. Ballard, D. Ivler, L. D. Thrupp, A. W. Mathies, and P. F. Wehrle, *Pediatr. Res.*, **7,** 318 (1973).

197. B. Bernard, S. J. Garcia-Caizares, C. A. Ballard, L. D. Thrupp, A. W. Mathies, and P. F. Wehrle, *Antimicrob. Agents Chemother.*, **11,** 688 (1977).

198. P. Federspil, W. Schatzle, and E. Tiesler, *Arch. Otorhinolaryngol.*, **217,** 147 (1977).

199. F. De Rosa, U. Buoncristiani, P. Capitanucci, and R. F. Frongillo, *J. Int. Med. Res.*, **2,** 100 (1974).

200. H. C. Neu and C. L. Bendush, *J. Infect. Dis.*, **134,** S206 (1976).

201. C. L. Bendush, S. L. Senior, and H. O. Wooller, *Med. J. Aust. Suppl.*, **2,** 22 (1977).

202. J. S. Welles, J. L. Emmerson, W. R. Gibson, R. Nickander, N. V. Owen, and R. C. Anderson, *Toxicol. Appl. Pharmacol.*, **25,** 398 (1973).

203. R. E. Brummett, J. A. Vernon, and M. M. Meikle, *Arch. Otolaryngol.*, **94,** 59 (1971).

204. J. Prazma, D. S. Postma, J. B. Pecorak, and N. D. Fischer, *Laryngoscope*, **86,** 259 (1976).

205. R. E. Brummett, D. Himes, B. Saine, and J. Vernon, *Arch. Otolaryngol.*, **96,** 505 (1972).

206. P. Federspil, *Arzneim Forsch.*, **23,** 1739 (1973).

207. P. Federspil and W. Schatzle, in *Inner Ear Biology*, M. Portmann and J. M. Aran, Eds., INSERM, **68,** 319 (1977).

208. B. E. Cabana and J. G. Taggart, *Antimicrob. Agents Chemother.*, **3,** 478 (1973).

209. K. E. Price, D. R. Chisholm, M. Misiek, F. Leitner, and Y. H. Tsai, *J. Antibiot.*, **25,** 709 (1972).

210. J. T. Clark, R. D. Libke, and C. Regamey, *Clin. Pharmacol. Ther.*, **15,** 610 (1974).

211. H. Kawabe, T. Naito, and S. Mitsuhashi, *Antimicrob. Agents Chemother.*, **7,** 50 (1975).

212. J. B. Howard and G. H. McCracken, Jr., *Antimicrob. Agents Chemother.*, **8,** 86 (1975).

213. G. P. Bodey, M. Valdivieso, R. Feld, and V. Rodriguez, *Antimicrob. Agents Chemother.*, **5,** 508 (1974).

214. A. Z. Lane, G. E. Wright, and D. C. Blair, *Am. J. Med.*, **62,** 911 (1977).

215. M. Valdivieso, R. Feld, V. Rodriguez, and G. P. Bodey, *Am. J. Med. Sci.*, **270,** 453 (1975).

216. R. E. Black, W. K. Lau, R. J. Weinstein, L. S. Young, and W. L. Hewitt, *Antimicrob. Agents Chemother.*, **9,** 956 (1976).

217. W. K. Lau, L. S. Young, and R. E. Black, *Am. J. Med.*, **62,** 959 (1977).

218a. J. C. Reiffenstein, S. W. Holmes, G. H. Hottendorf, and M. E. Bierwagen, *J. Antibiot.*, **26,** 94 (1973).

218b. C. A. Prosen, B. D. Moody, W. C. Stebbins, and J. E. Hawkins, Abstracts of 3rd midwinter research meeting of the Association for Research in Otolaryngology, Florida, 1980, p. 36.

218c. Y. Cazals, J. M. Aran, J. P. Erre, A. Guilhaume, and J. E. Hawkins, *Arch. Otorhinolaryngol.*, **224,** 61 (1979).

219. H. M. Theopold, *Acta Otolaryngol.*, **84,** 57 (1977).

220. R. E. Brummett, K. E. Fox, T. W. Bendrick, and D. L. Himes, *J. Antimicrob. Chemother. Suppl. A,* **4,** 73 (1978).

221. Schering-Plough Research Report, Bloomfield, N.J., February 1977.

222. G. H. Miller, G. Arcieri, M. J. Weinstein, and J. A. Waitz, *Antimicrob. Agents Chemother.*, **10,** 827 (1976).

223. B. S. Yap, D. Stewart, and G. P. Bodey, *Antimicrob. Agents Chemother.*, **6,** 717 (1977).

224. L. Riff and G. Moreschi, *Antimicrob. Agents Chemother.*, **11,** 609 (1977).

225. F. C. Luft, M. N. Yum, and S. A. Kleit, *Antimicrob. Agents Chemother.*, **10,** 845 (1976).

226. R. L. Bowman, F. J. Silverblatt, and G. J. Kaloyanides, *Antimicrob. Agents Chemother.*, **12,** 474 (1977).

227. F. C. Luft, R. Block, R. S. Sloan, M. N. Yum, R. Costello, and D. R. Maxwell, *J. Infect. Dis.*, **138,** 541 (1978).

228. R. E. Brummett and K. E. Fox, *Fed. Proc.*, **35,** 621 (1976).

229. P. J. Federspil, *Curr. Chemother.*, **2,** 975 (1978).

230. M. Igarashi, J. K. Levy and J. Jerger, *J. Infect. Dis.*, **137,** 476 (1978).

231a. J. Wersall and B. Bjorkroth, *Curr. Chemother.*, **2,** 976 (1978).

231b. P. A. Bernard, J. C. Pechere and J. C. Jequier, *J. Infect. Dis.*, **139**(4), 418 (1979).

232. L. S. Young and W. L. Hewitt, *Antimicrob. Agents Chemother.*, **4,** 617 (1973).

233. G. Gruenwaldt, A. Doenicke, M. Scheer, and H. Fink, *Infection*, **S4,** 370 (1976).

234. J. C. Pechere, M. M. Pechere, and R. Dugal, *Antimicrob. Agents Chemother.*, **9,** 761 (1976).

235. R. Luthy, *Schweiz. Med. Wochenschr.*, **106,** 450 (1976).

236. A. Arpini, L. Cornacchia, L. Albiero, F. Bamonte, and L. Parravicini, *Arch. Otolaryngol.*, **224,** 137 (1979).

CHAPTER 8

Ototoxicity of Diuretics

JIRI PRAZMA, M.D., Ph.D.

Assistant Professor of Otolaryngology
Department of Surgery
Section of Otolaryngology
University of North Carolina
Medical School, Chapel Hill

CONTENTS

8.1 INTRODUCTION

Diuretics are drugs used to reduce the volume of extracellular fluid by increasing the renal excretion of water and electrolytes. They vary in potency and mechanism of action. Diuretics can generally be divided into six groups: osmotic diuretics, organomercurials, carbonic anhydrase inhibitors, other sulfonamide diuretics, potassium-sparing diuretics, and high ceiling or "loop" diuretics. Hearing impairment has been reported after treatment with "loop" diuretics. This review therefore focuses mainly on that group.

8.2 GENERAL DISCUSSION OF "LOOP" DIURETICS

Loop diuretics (LD), currently the most potent available, include ethacrynic acid (EA), furosemide (FUR), and bumetanide (BUM). In comparison with thiazides, loop diuretics exhibit a shorter duration of action, a steeper dose-response curve, and a greater natriuretic effect. Their action is not additive within the group but they are additive with other classes of diuretic.[1]

Although structural differences exist among the loop diuretics, they are similar in their action. The major site of action is in the medullary and cortical thick ascending limb of Henle's loop, where they inhibit active chloride reabsorption and reduce the positive lumen potential if administered in the lumen.[2] Reports of the action of LD on electrolyte reabsorption in the proximal tubule are conflicting. A decrease in electrolyte reabsorption was found by Clapp et al.,[3] Edwards et al.,[4] and Goldberg,[5] but no effect on transport in the proximal tubules was observed by Berliner et al.[6]

In addition to their effect on NaCl transport in the ascending limb of Henle's loop, loop diuretics redistribute and increase renal blood flow by arteriolar vasodilatation and stimulate renin release. *In vivo,* indomethacin is able to prevent this increase,[7-9] which suggests that prostaglandins (PG) are mediators of this renal vasodilatation.[7] An increased excretion of PGEs and their metabolites in the urine after FUR was observed by Abe et al.[10] Even when the effects of FUR on blood circulation and PG production were repeatedly documented in the kidney neither the production nor the metabolism of PGE_2 was altered by FUR in the uterus. In addition, LD did not increase hemodynamic parameters in the uterus. Therefore the mechanism of LD vasodilatation is probably dependent on the specific PG generated and the presence of receptors for that PG. Before reaching final conclusions about the mechanism of LD-induced renal vasodilatation more studies in this area obviously are necessary.

The molecular mechanism of diuretic action of these drugs is still unresolved. Several basic processes have been suggested: (a) inhibition of Na/K ATPase, (b) inhibition of glycolysis, and (c) inhibition of cAMP formation. The inhibition of Na/K ATPase, as suggested by Duggan and Noll[11] and Hoffman and Kregenow,[12] has been repeatedly disproved by Williamson,[13]

Martinez-Maldonado et al.,[14] and many others. Whatever the mechanism of the LD on NA/K ATPase may be, it is unlikely that this enzyme is directly affected by the loop diuretics. Most authors describe the action of LD on Na/K ATPase as little or none at all.

Similarly, although LD can cause profound inhibition of glycolysis,[15-16] it probably has no direct effect on ion transport but may act nonspecifically because glycolysis inhibition by iodoacetate does not impair Na^+ reabsorption.[17]

Ion transport and membrane permeability may be affected by the interference of the LD with adenylate cyclase. Involvement of cAMP in electrolyte transport has been observed in the toad bladder[18,19] and kidney.[20] The authors cited described a reduction of endogenous cAMP by EA and a displacement of cAMP from its binding sites by FUR, but even this recently described mechanism awaits identification of its role in LD-induced diuresis.

8.2.1 Diuretics and Generation of the Endocochlear Potential

Because of the effect of EA on the generation of the positive endocochlear dc potential (EP), some important observations should be noted. The positive EP in the scala media was discovered by von Bekesy,[21] the ionic composition of endolymph was first established by Smith et al.,[22] and the source of EP generation was localized to the stria vascularis by Tasaki and Spyropoulos.[23] Subsequently a high concentration of Na/K ATPase in the stria vascularis was found by Kuijpers et al.[24] and Matchinsky and Thalmann.[25] The mechanism of EP generation was then studied in anoxia by Konishi et al.[26] and after the application of metabolic poisons (cyanide, tetrodotoxin, and procaine) into the perilymphatic space.[27] Prazma[28] first observed a decline in EP after perfusion of the scala vertibuli with ouabain (*g*-strophanthine) and 2,4-dinitrophenol (2,4-DNP) (Figure 8.1). These observations were confirmed by Konishi and Mendelsohn[29] and Kuijpers and Bonting.[30] These experiments proved that generation of the EP is dependent on an energy source (inhibition by use of 2,4-DNP) and that EP is maintained by a Na/K ATPase-dependent pump (inhibition by ouabain). Because of the high concentration of ATPase found in the stria vascularis, it was postulated[28] that ouabain diffuses from the perilymph of the scala vestibuli through the ligamentum spirale and into the stria, thus inhibiting the enzyme at that site.

Passive endolymph ionic fluxes were studied after inhibition of the ion transport pump. This was accomplished under anoxic conditions by Konishi et al.[26] and later by Johnstone[31] and Bosher and Warren,[32] who studied conductive and ion concentration changes (decrease of K^+, increase of Na^+ by using artificial endolymph). In addition, Prazma[33] studied passive fluxes after inhibition of ion transport by 2,4-DNP. The scala vestibuli was perfused with artificial endolymph and Ringer's solution, both with and without inhibition of active ion transport (Figure 8.2). Perfusion with Ringer's solu-

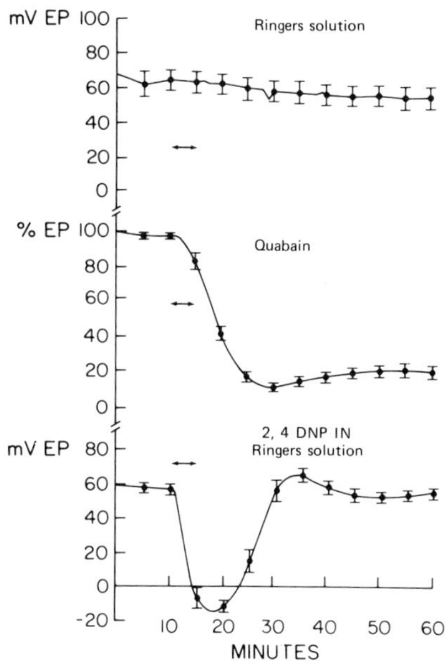

Figure 8.1 Changes in the positive endocochlear d.c. potential (EP) after 5-min perfusion of the scala vestibuli with Ringer's solution, $8.5 \times 10^{-5}M$ ouabain, and $1 \times 10^{-2}M$ 2,4-dinitrophenol in the guinea pig. Vertical bars represent the standard error of mean. Perfusion is indicated by horizontal bar with arrows. (Redrawn from Prazma.[28])

tion resulted in the same EP as that found after perfusion with artificial endolymph (except for a small increase, subsequent decrease, and return to the original level within 10 min after perfusion). Inhibition of active transport by 2,4-DNP in Ringer's solution caused the EP to decline to negative values. In other experiments, however, in which 2,4-DNP was perfused in artificial endolymph, EP declined to 0 mV because both active and passive fluxes were eliminated. Therefore these experiments provided evidence that the positive EP has two portions, a positive potential generated by active transport, and a negative potential which is the result of passive fluxes across the walls of the scala media. A similar conclusion was reached by Kuijpers and Bonting[30] and Johnstone[31] and was later summarized by Sellick and Johnstone.[34a] Bosher's[34b] recent experiments provided further support for this hypothesis which states that the negative portion of the EP is a modified K^+ diffusion potential, largely dependent on K^+ and Na^+ gradients between endolymph and perilymph.

Another explanation of the negative component of the EP was presented by Sitko et al.[38] and Honrubia et al.,[39] who demonstrated that the negative potential in the organ of Corti does not change after EA administration. They postulated that the negative portion of EP is generated in the organ of Corti. Presently most auditory researchers consider the negative component of EP to be the result of the diffusion potential rather than the organ of Corti potential. More experimentation, however, is necessary to resolve this theory's discrepancies.

Because the normal EP in the scala media is large and positive, the func-

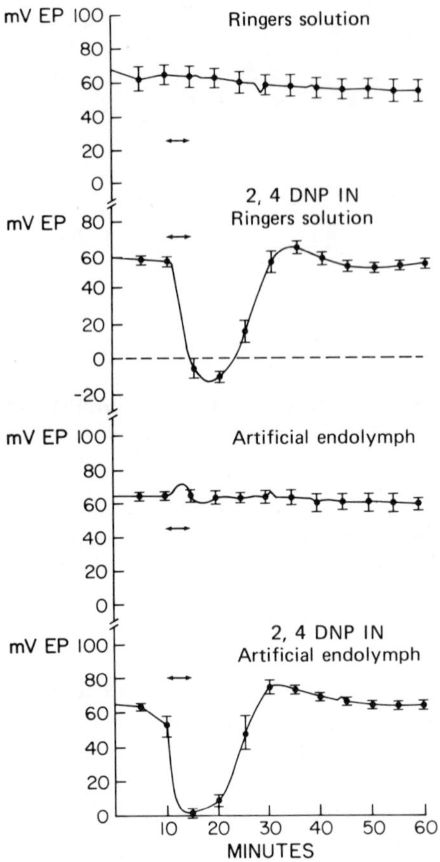

Figure 8.2 Changes in the endocochlear potential (EP) after perfusion of the scala vestibuli with Ringer's solution and $1 \times 10^{-2} M$ 2,4-dinitrophenol in artificial endolymph in the guinea pig. Vertical bars represent the standard error of mean. (Redrawn from Prazma.[33])

tion of Cl^- was also investigated. It has been documented repeatedly that the concentrations of Cl^- are equal in endolymph and perilymph. It has also been suggested that the positive potential in the scala media should cause Cl^- to leak into the endolymph. Konishi and Hamrick[35] found that $^{36}Cl^-$ in the endolymph is higher in concentration after perfusion of the scala vestibuli than of the scala tympani, a finding that indicates that Reissner's membrane is more permeable to Cl^- than other portions of the cochlear duct. This greater permeability appears to be the result of active transport as local application of ouabain and production of anoxia decrease $^{36}Cl^-$ uptake in the endolymph.[35] The greater permeability of Reissner's membrane with other substances has also been reported by several investigators. Ilberg[36] found that thorium dioxide crosses Reissner's membrane in both directions. Hinojosa,[37] however, described the direction of ferritin transport only toward the endolymph. Transport through Reissner's membrane is probably not limited by size of hydrated ions. Smaller, hydrated K^+ ions penetrate from the scala tympani and the scala vestibuli at about the same rate as Cl^-, but Cl^- is transported at a higher rate from the scala vestibuli than from the scala tympani.[35] In addition, Prazma[28] has observed that the EP is not affected by perfusion of the scala vestibuli with Ringer's solution in which Cl^- is replaced by SO_4^{2-}.

Since the discovery of the ototoxic effect of EA by Maher and Schreiner[40] and the later discovery that EA is a dose-dependent inhibitor of the EP by Prazma et al.,[41] numerous studies have been conducted to investigate its other actions. The original hypothesis was that the mode of EA action on the stria vascularis is similar to that of ouabain (inhibition of the Na/K ATPase system); this has not been confirmed, however. *In vitro* experiments have indicated that 50% inhibition of strial Na/K ATPase requires 100 times higher concentrations of EA than those that similarly depress the EP (by 50%) after perilymphatic perfusion.[42] Kuijpers and Wilberts[43] also reported that strial ATPase is inhibited with only high concentrations of EA.

Endolymph ionic composition changes after EA administration have been reported by Bosher et al.,[44] Brusilow and Gordes,[45] and others. With the exception of the experiments in dogs done by Cohn et al.[46] and Brusilow and Gordes,[45] a reversal of the concentrations of K^+ and Na^+ in endolymph has not been produced by EA. Sellick and Johnstone,[47] who used guinea pigs, reported an increase in endolymphatic Na^+ from 1 to 5–8 mM after i.v. injection of EA (25–45 mg/kg) with concomitant small decreases in endolymph K^+. Similarly, small changes of endolymph K^+, but a large decrease in EP, were reported in guinea pigs by Brusilow and Gordes,[45] Prazma[48] (Figure 8.3), and Melichar and Syka.[49] Thus endolymph ionic composition changes produced by EA appear to be dose and species dependent.

Sellick and Johnstone[47] and Thalmann et al.[50] have described the differences in the action of ouabain and EA on the EP of guinea pigs during anoxia. During long-term anoxia after the EP reaches approximately −40 mV it slowly returns to 0 mV. If, however, during maximum EP depression the perilymphatic space was perfused by EA, EP rapidly returned to 0 mV. Conversely, the slow return of EP from −40 to 0 mV was not affected by ouabain.

In conclusion, the effect of EA on EP during anoxia and on ion composition in the endolymph supports the concept that the stria vascularis possesses two pumps that handle sodium, as suggested in the proximal tubule, mammalian gall bladder, and submandibular gland.[51-55] The "first pump" transports Na^+ out of and K^+ into the scala media. This pump is dependent on Na/K ATPase and is inhibited by ouabain. The "second pump" transports Na^+ and Cl^- and is inhibited by EA. This ouabain-insensitive transport is considered by some as an exchange diffusion rather than a second active ion pump.[56,57]

Thus the EP results from active and passive transporting mechanisms. It is hypothesized that the active ion transport has a component inhibited by ouabain and another that is sensitive to EA. This hypothesis, however, needs to be documented more fully in the future.

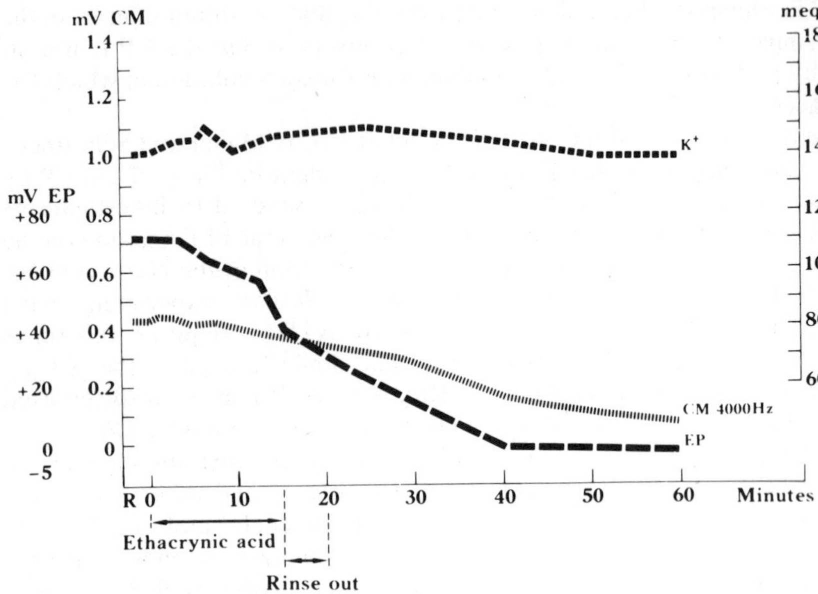

Figure 8.3 The effect of scala tympani perfusion with $1 \times 10^{-3} M$ ethacrynic acid on the endocochlear potential (EP), cochlear microphonics (CM), and K^+ activity in the endolymph of guinea pigs. Potassium activity was measured by ion-specific microelectrodes.

8.2.2 Adverse Reactions

Diuretics may be defined as substances that increase the rate at which urine is formed. They are used to promote loss of salt water from the body and it is not surprising that they sometimes cause unwanted disturbances in electrolyte metabolism. Excessive loss of electrolytes may cause weakness, dizziness, lethargy, leg cramps, anorexia, hypotension, nausea, vomiting, and sometimes mental confusion.

Severe temporary and permanent hearing loss has also been reported in conjunction with the use of these diuretics, particularly EA. The major cochlear damage has been localized to the stria vascularis. Dilation of extracellular spaces and atrophy of intermediate cells has been observed by electron microscopy. Initial reduction in EP and a secondary decline in CM and CAP has been observed after i.v. loop diuretics in many different species. Changes in endolymph ionic composition appear to be a species-dependent effect. Loss of sharpness in tuning of the cochlear nerve fibers and depression of auditory-evoked potentials have also been described. If, as some believe, generalized electrolyte imbalance is responsible for hearing loss reflected by a higher incidence of ototoxic reactions in patients with impaired renal function, the chronic administration of these diuretics should also induce an ototoxic response secondary to potassium depletion. No clinical reports of hearing loss secondary to chronic treatment with LD have been made, however. This suggests that rapid electrolyte changes and/or enzyme alterations in the inner ear are essential in the pathogenesis of the sudden hearing loss caused by loop diuretics. It has also been suggested that the ototoxic effect of EA may be caused by its highly potent metabolite, the cysteine adduct of EA.

Ethacrynic acid and BUM are more potent diuretics than FUR and also more ototoxic. BUM, however, is approximately 40 times more potent as a diuretic when compared with FUR but only 6.5 times more ototoxic.[57b] The ototoxic liability of EA is caused by the narrow range between its therapeutic and toxic doses. The recommended upper limit of EA is 200 mg/day, but ototoxicity has been observed in certain oliguric patients after intravenous administration of only 50 mg.[58] The recommended upper limit of FUR is 600 mg/day; transient hearing loss has been observed after administration of 1000 mg i.v.[59] There is only limited knowledge of BUM ototoxicity in man because of its relatively short history of use, but experimental results are encouraging and early clinical reports suggest that it has a low degree of ototoxicity.

Other adverse reactions that have been found include hyperuricemia, gastrointestinal disturbances, skin rashes, paresthesias, and hepatic dysfunction.[60] Ethacrynic acid and FUR have a moderate effect on lowering the blood pressure, particularly in combination with antihypertensive drugs, and occasionally this combination causes orthostatic hypotension. Therefore coadministration of these two classes of drug may require adjustment of the dosages given. Transient ischemic attacks have also been reported.[61-63] In addition, when LD are administered in high doses they may cause interstitial nephritis.[64] Furthermore, a negative K^+ balance and a fall in serum Cl^- contribute to the development of hypokalemia and hypochloremic alkalosis in patients treated with EA and FUR.[65,66] This effect is particularly severe in patients with K^+ depletion caused by other diseases such as secondary hyperaldosteronism, chronic heart failure, or nephrotic syndrome.[67] From the foregoing it is apparent that urinary loss of Na^+, K^+, H^+ and Cl^- are important factors in the development of extracellular alkalosis. Potassium depletion induced by treatment with these diuretics may also cause digitalis intoxication. Jorgensen and Sorensen[68] reported that under the influence of new potent diuretics, digitalis toxicity increases about 100%. Therefore it is essential that K^+ and Cl^- supplementation be used to avoid electrolyte disturbance.[69-70]

Carbohydrate intolerance and even diabetic coma have been reported after the use of these diuretics. In patients with established diabetes mellitus hyperglycemia is usually exacerbated.[71] A comparison of carbohydrate metabolism in patients treated with chlorothiazide, EA, and FUR showed that the diabetogenic effect of EA and FUR is weaker than that of chlorothiazide.[72-76] Improvement of glucose tolerance and rise of plasma insulin concentration have often been found after withdrawal of these diuretics.[74,77]

8.3 SPECIFIC "LOOP" DIURETICS

8.3.1 Ethacrynic Acid

Chemical Properties

Ethacrynic acid (EA) is an unsaturated ketone derivative of aryloxyacetic acid. Its chemical name is [2,3-dichloro-4-(2-methylenebutyryl)-phenoxy]-acetic acid; its trade name is Edecrin®. The stability of EA and its sodium salt in aqueous solutions is dependent on the pH, temperature, and concentration of the solution. Ethacrynic acid, itself, is slightly soluble in water and highly soluble in organic solvents. Aqueous solutions of the Na^+ salt can be prepared in concentrations as high as 7 to 9%. The stability of EA decreases with increasing pH and temperature.

Absorption, Distribution, and Excretion

Ethacrynic acid is rapidly absorbed from the gastrointestinal tract and diuresis starts within 10 to 30 min after oral administration. In humans the oral dose usually ranges between 50 and 200 mg. If faster onset of action is required, it is administered intravenously with the usual adult dose of 0.5 to 1.0 mg/kg. Its serum elimination half-life (T 1/2) after i.v. administration is less than 1 hr. Approximately 30 to 50% of EA is excreted in the bile and the remainder is excreted in the urine; 30 to 40% of the dose is recovered unchanged, an additional 30% is excreted as the ethylacetate, and 20 to 30% is excreted as the cysteine adduct.

Active transport of EA into cells has not been documented, but its accumulation under aerobic conditions has been observed in cortical slices of the rabbit[78–79] and in rat myometrial cells.[80] The accumulation was depressed by probenecid and 2,4-DNP.[81] Thus there is clear evidence that EA does penetrate intact cells. Accumulation of ^{14}C-EA in the stria vascularis was not seen 30 min after perfusion of perilymphatic space with the drug.[82]

Mechanism and Site of Action

Experimental studies have indicated that EA influences the diluting and concentrating mechanism in the kidney. Its major action is inhibition of Cl^- and Na^+ reabsorption in the ascending limb of the loop of Henle; a less significant effect is exerted on the distal nephron.[40,52,65,69,70,83–88] The diuretic effect is also magnified by additional inhibition of ion reabsorption in the proximal tubule.[40,52,65,87,89]

Some authors have indicated that EA action may be related to its capacity to bind the sulfhydryl groups of renal proteins.[90–93] If EA is a sulfhydryl binding agent, it should be possible to interrupt its action (as in organomercurials) by an injection of dimercaprol (BAL); this antagonism, however, has not been demonstrated.[81]

Another possible mechanism of EA action may be in the inhibition of Mg^{2+} activated Na/K ATPase, suggested by Duggan and Noll,[11] Hoffman and Kregenow,[12] and Bourgoignie et al.[94] Duggan and Noll[11] observed that incubation increased the ability of EA to inhibit isolated renal membrane ATPase by 10 times but did not influence the activity of ouabain and mercurials. The increased activity of EA may be the result of its accumulation, which has been demonstrated in kidney cortex slices.[78-79] Later it was found that the ability of EA to inhibit Na/K ATPase is weaker than that of mercurials and ouabain. The renal cortex membrane ATPase was inhibited 50% by $2 \times 10^{-6}M$ meralluride and $4 \times 10^{-6}M$ ouabain, but to produce similar inhibition a concentration of EA 100 times greater was required. Also, infusion of EA into the renal artery of dogs in sufficient amounts to produce profuse diuresis did not inhibit Na/K ATPase activity.[95] It is therefore doubtful that the concentration of EA in Henle's loop is high enough to inhibit Na/K ATPase, even though accumulation of EA in the renal cortical slices has been documented.[79]

When EA, at a final concentration of $10^{-3}M$, is added 1 min before the addition of glucose in *in vitro* studies of the kidney[16] inhibition of lactic acid production is observed whether or not potassium is present. Maximum inhibition is observed after 20 min exposure to EA; the rate of lactic acid production then decreases to the level seen in the absence of glucose. Although EA (1 m*M*) decreased lactate generation from fructose 1,6-diphosphate by 40%, it did not affect lactate formation from 3-phosphoglyceric acid. The effect of EA in the glycolytic pathway is therefore localized between fructose 1,6-diphosphate and 3-phosphoglyceric acid, but even this mechanism is probably not decisive in EA diuretic action. Bowman et al.[96] demonstrated that inhibition of glycolysis by iodoacetate did not impair Na^+ reabsorption; therefore they postulated that diuresis by EA is not generated by inhibition of glycolysis alone.

Gordon and De Hartog,[15] Jones and Landon,[97] and Gordon[98] have indicated that EA interferes primarily with mitochondrial oxidation and phosphorylation. The blockage of phosphorylation and the prevention of ADP conversion to ATP was reported by Banerjee et al.[99] As these experiments have shown, EA action is extremely complex and the mechanism of its diuresis has not been resolved.

Adverse Reactions

The toxicity of EA is mainly related to its effect on renal extraction of electrolytes. It may cause dehydration, hyponatremia, hypokalemia, hypochloremic alkalosis, hyperuricemia, hypercalcemia, impaired glucose tolerance, and a possible precipitation of latent diabetes. The danger of salt depletion is particularly high in patients who suffer from cirrhosis and its concurrent hypovolemia.

OTOTOXICITY

Sudden temporary and permanent hearing loss has been reported in patients after the use of EA.[40,58,100–108] Temporary hearing loss commences shortly after i.v. injection and returns to normal after 6 to 24 hr. Permanent deafness and vestibular disturbances are primarily associated with renal impairment or concomitant use of other ototoxic drugs.[105–107,109] Sudden ototoxicity is seen mainly after i.v. injection and toxicity after oral administration, even though rare, has been reported.[107,110,111]

Shortly after recognizing that EA caused hearing loss in some patients a search for the mechanism of its ototoxicity began. A decline in CM and CAP was reported after i.v. administration of EA to guinea pigs in doses as low as 10 mg/kg. Greater depressions that lasted for longer times were associated with larger doses. In most of the animals partial or complete recovery occurred after 1 to 2 hr.[102,112–113] Some authors have observed that EA acts in two phases. The rapid first phase occurs shortly after drug administration and the slow second phase begins approximately 20 min later.[112,114] Kohonen et al.[115] and McCurdy et al.[116] reported that hearing was suppressed more in the higher than the lower frequencies after EA administration. A decline in EP and CM after i.v. EA administration was first observed by Prazma et al.[41] Suppression of EP was dose-related and after the highest used dose (50 mg/kg) the EP declined to negative values (Figure 8.4). On the other hand, in

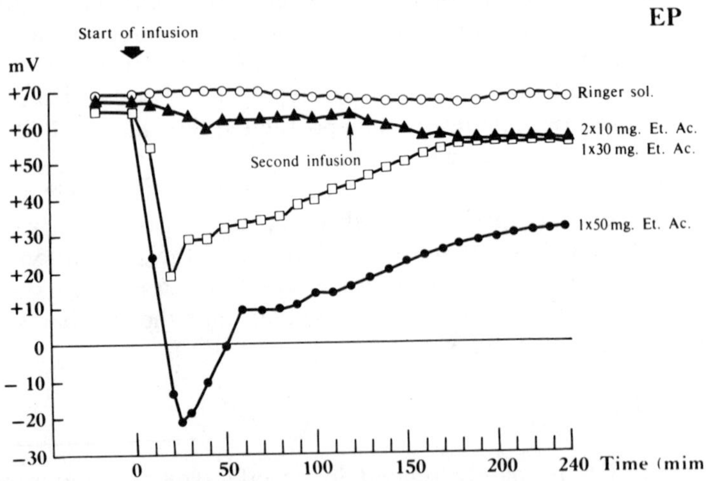

Figure 8.4 Influence of Ringer's solution and ethacrynic acid in concentrations of 2 × 10, 30, and 50 mg/kg on the endocochlear potentials in the guinea pig. Ethacrynic acid and Ringer's solution were administered by i.v. infusion over a 5-min period. The 10 mg/kg infusion of EA was repeated, as indicated, by the arrow and by the 2 × 10 mg note on the figure. From Prazma et al.[41] Reprinted by permission of the American Medical Association.

all tested concentrations EP had a tendency to recover, usually in two phases, first fast, then slow. In contrast, the CM declined at about the same rate as EP but showed no tendency to recover during the subsequent 4 hr (Figure 8.5). This finding suggests that some independent toxic process exists other than that on the stria vascularis or that a reversible effect on the stria produces a less reversible effect elsewhere in the cochlea. Serum *T* 1/2 of EA, as mentioned earlier, is about 1 hr. Another decline in EP, CM, and CAP was observed when a second small dose (10 mg/kg) followed the first dose of 10 mg/kg in a 2-hr period (Figures 8.4 and 8.5). This suggested that an additive adverse effect of EA occurs when another dose is administered before full recovery and may also suggest that the toxic effect of EA on cochlear potentials persists longer than the serum *T* 1/2 of EA because of slower elimination of EA from cochlear tissue. The effect of EA on the EP was later confirmed by Brusilow and Gordes,[45] Dilling et al.,[117] Thalmann et al.,[118] and others.

The role of renal function on EA ototoxicity was studied in a group of nephrectomized guinea pigs.[116] The decline in CM was observed to be larger in this group than in nonnephrectomized animals. The depression of CM was dose-related, appeared in 15 min, and reached a maximum 60 min after EA administration. These experiments suggest that the ototoxicity of EA is dose-related and correlate with the clinical observations that EA is more toxic in patients with poor renal function.

The magnitude of EP decline after EA administration also appears to be

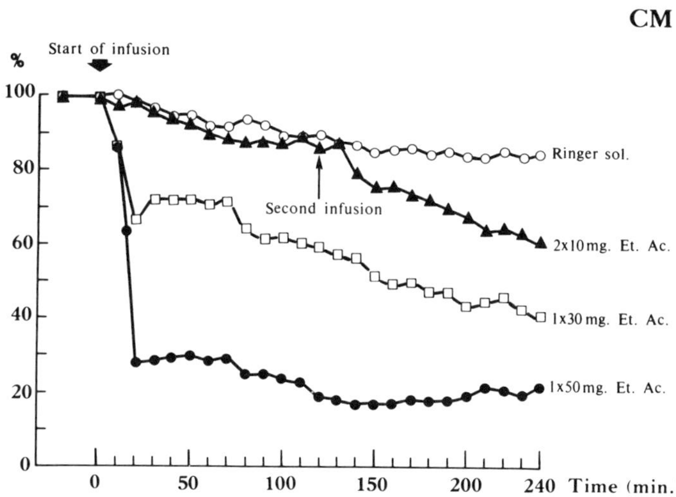

Figure 8.5 Influence of Ringer's solution and ethacrynic acid in concentrations of 2 × 10, 30, and 50 mg/kg on cochlear microphonics in the guinea pig. Ethacrynic acid and Ringer's solution were administered by i.v. infusion over a 5-min period. The 10 mg/kg infusion of EA was repeated, as indicated by the arrow and the 2 × 10 mg note on the figure. From Prazma et al.[41] Reprinted by permission of the American Medical Association.

dependent on the pO_2 of the blood. Prazma and Pecorak[119] reported that an increase in arterial pO_2 to 179 mm Hg causes a smaller decline in EP, CM, and CAP than in a control group with pO_2 of 90 mm Hg. The mechanism of this important observation is currently unknown. A high pO_2 may cause cochlear vasoconstriction, oppose EA-induced vasodilation, and therefore decrease the transport of EA into the inner ear.

Because EA is a diuretic, several authors have investigated its effect on the cochlear electrolytes. A large decrease in K^+ (from 145 to 21 meq/liter) and a large rise in Na^+ (from 5.9 to 146 meq/liter) was observed in dogs after exposure to EA.[46] Similar, but smaller, changes were observed in cats by Silverstein and Yules[114] and in rats by Bosher et al.[44] They reported that these changes reached a peak at 60 min post drug administration and returned to normal levels within 3 hr. Brusilow and Gordes[45] and Cohn et al.[46] observed large changes of electrolyte concentration in dog endolymph without a change in EP. In guinea pigs treated with EA, however, the EP declined substantially, but endolymph K^+ decreased very little.[45,48–49] To eliminate the systemic effects, I perfused EA (in a concentration of $10^{-3}M$ in Ringer's solution) through the perilymphatic space of the scala tympani of the guinea pig for 10 min; control Ringer's solution was then perfused for the next 5 min. K^+, EP, and CM were continuously recorded. After a short latency EP began to decline gradually; however, K^+, as recorded by ion-sensitive electrodes, declined only slightly (Figure 8.3).

The effect of EA on enzyme activity in the cochlea was investigated by Kaku et al.[120] By histochemical means they demonstrated a decrease in the activity of respiratory enzymes (succinic dehydrogenase and diphosphopyridine nucleotide diaphorase) in the OHC and the stria vascularis. However, during the same experiments ATPase activity did not change. This and more recent evidence indicates that Na/K ATPase activity and P-creatine levels are not substantially affected by EA.[43,82]

The ototoxic action of EA may be mediated by adenylate cyclase inhibition. Thalmann et al.[82] saw that the inhibition curve in the EP after EA administration *in vivo* overlapped with the *in vitro* inhibition curve of strial adenylate cyclase by EA. Cyclic AMP enhances electrolyte and water transport in the toad bladder, rabbit ileum, and kidney. Therefore the adenylate cyclase of the stria vascularis that produces cAMP may be responsible for the action of EA on strial function in the inner ear. The exact mechanism of ototoxic action of EA is presently unresolved, however.

Because a large portion of EA is metabolized to cysteine EA, the toxicity of this component has also been investigated. It has been suggested that the cysteine adduct of EA may actually be the ototoxic component of EA metabolism.[101] Its effect on the generation of cochlear potentials has been investigated in cats by Brown and McElwee,[121] who report that the onset of the decline in cochlear potentials after a single intravenous or intra-arterial bolus injection of EA was delayed by 10 to 15 min. This delay was thought to be caused by the conversion of EA to its cysteine adduct. In subsequent experiments, Brown[122a,122b] found that cysteine EA caused an immediate depression of CAP and that it was more potent than EA in its effect on CAP. The higher toxicity of cysteine EA than EA has also been reported in guinea pigs by Fox and Brummett.[123] Earlier, the direct effect of EA on cochlear potentials was investigated by direct perfusion through the cochlea[48] of the guinea pig (Figure 8.3). In this experiment $10^{-3}M$ EA was infused into the perilymphatic space of the scala tympani for 10 min and was subsequently removed by washing for 5 min with Ringer's solution. After a short latency period the EP began to decline gradually to negative EP values. This process continued even after NaEA had been washed away with Ringer's solution. Thus the toxic effect does not have to be only the result of action of the cysteine adduct if this conversion does not occur directly in the cochlea. The rapid depression of the vestibular responses without a latent period was documented in the cat by Mathog.[124] The depression of vestibular responses he observed were more rapid than that reported ealier for the auditory system in cats. In his study, however, EA was administered intravenously over a 1-min period, whereas in the Prazma study[41] it was injected over 5 min.

In my opinion, and in my experience with EA in the guinea pig, the onset and slope of cochlear potential depression depends on the rate of drug administration. In the past I have done experiments in which one group received 30 mg/kg of EA in a 5-min i.v. infusion and another group received the same dose by slow i.v. infusion over a 60-min period. After 30 mg/kg of EA received in 5 min EP declined from +70 to +19.3 mV at the twentieth minute (Figure 8.4). When the same dose was slowly infused during 60 min EP gradually declined from +78.5 to +69 mV at the 180th minute (Figure 8.6). Thus after 30 mg/kg of EA EP declined for 50.7 mV after a 5-min infusion and only about 9.5 mV after a 60 min infusion. In a comparison of these experiments it is seen that a slower infusion over 60 min causes a significantly smaller decline of EP than when the same dose is administered

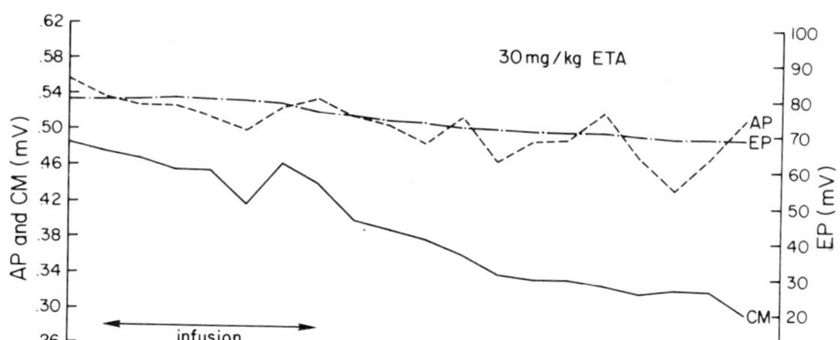

Figure 8.6 The effect of ethacrynic acid administration over 60 min by i.v. infusion on the endocochlear potential (EP), cochlear microphonics (CM), and the nerve action potential [CAP (AP)] in guinea pigs.

over a 5-min period. The smaller depression of EP, however, is probably also affected by a lower level of EA in blood and tissue because the *T* 1/2 of EA is less than 60 min. Therefore, before completing the 60-min infusion some of the drug will have been excreted. Nevertheless, these experiments document that the onset and magnitude of EA action is also dependent on the rate of its administration.*

The effect of EA on the auditory threshold was also investigated by a conditioning technique[125,126] and by recording auditory-evoked potentials.[127–128] Ernstson[126] showed transient elevation of the auditory threshold immediately after i.p. drug administration in guinea pigs. Walloch et al.[128] reported depression of potentials in guinea pigs at all recorded frequencies after i.v. administration (over a 10-min period) of 45 mg/kg EA. This depression occurred between 30 min and 2 hr after injection and was greater in the higher frequencies. Similarly, a dose-related elevation of the auditory threshold in conditioned cats was observed by Youngblood et al.[125]

The morphological changes after EA administration were located primarily in the stria vascularis. An increase in thickness of the stria vascularis caused by vacuolization, edema, and intracellular accumulation of fluid was seen 10 min to 6 hr after drug administration.[44,112,128–130] Certain differences in the description of ultrastructural changes in the stria vascularis exist. Quick and Duvall[129] described destruction of intermediate cells in the guinea pig that were found intact in the rat[44] and mouse.[130] Nakai[130] observed vacuolization of the marginal cells in the mouse; 2 to 4 hr after drug injection cytoplasmic changes in the marginal cells developed which later evolved into multivesicular bodies and large membrane-bound bodies that contained osmiophilic material. Reduced numbers of basal processes of marginal cells have also been reported in the guinea pig.[132] Dilatation of intracellular spaces in the stria vascularis was reported in the rat, cat, and guinea pig by Bosher et al.,[44] Silverstein and Yules,[114] Quick and Duvall,[129] and Matz and Hinojosa.[133] Dilatation of capillaries in the stria vascularis and prominentia spiralis in guinea pigs was noted by Dilling et al.[117] and Brummett et al.[132]

In contrast to the excessive changes observed in the stria vascularis, minimal alterations usually occur in the organ of Corti. Swelling and clumping of the mitochondria in the hair cells was described by Silverstein and Yules[114] and Quick and Duvall.[129] However, destruction of OHC in the cat and

*Editor's Note. The question of the latent period before cochlear potential depression after i.v. EA in the cat is not answered by this discussion because Brown and McElwee[121] and Brown[122a,122b] made their intravenous and intra-arterial drug injections over a 5 to 10 sec period, followed by a 5 sec wash period. This time period is much shorter than even the 1 min time period that Mathog[124] used in his vestibular study. We suspect that a species difference in the effect of EA on the auditory system of the cat and guinea pig is responsible for this apparent discrepancy. Indeed, Brown (unpublished observations) has also found that little if any latent period after i.v. EA occurs in the guinea pig. The discrepancy between no latent period occurring in the vestibular system of the cat after i.v. EA and one occurring in the auditory system of the same species cannot presently be explained.

mouse, particularly in the basal turn and the first part of the second turn, was described by Mathog et al.[112] and Nakai.[130]

Silverstein and Begin[131] and Brummett et al.[132] reported that after a single 30 mg/kg dose of i.v. EA in cats and 40 mg/kg in guinea pigs full recovery of CM and CAP occurred within 48 hr, even when mild edema and cystic changes were present in the stria vascularis for 24 to 48 hr and up to 2 1/2 months, respectively.

The ototoxicity of EA was also investigated in chronic experiments in guinea pigs by Crifo[134] with shiver audiometry. He observed that repeated i.p. administration of EA (1 mg/kg/day) caused hearing loss after 5 to 10 days and that this increase in threshold persisted for 30 days after treatment. Morphological changes were seen as vacuolization in the apical portion of the marginal cells. Conversely, Mathog and Matz,[127] who recorded evoked responses (AER) from cats, observed that the onset, duration, and magnitude of the depression of AER were dose-dependent and that all depressions were reversible even in cats treated chronically for two months. The effect of chronic treatment is therefore still unresolved and will require more attention in the future.

Reports of vestibular dysfunction after EA administration are much less frequent than those of hearing impairment. Matz et al.[104] reported bilateral hearing loss in patients who received 50 mg EA (i.v.) but vestibular caloric testing revealed bilaterally normal responses. On the other hand, dizziness and vertigo were reported after EA administration by Maher and Schreiner,[40] Pillay et al.,[107] and Matz.[135] Ataxia and destructive changes in the vestibular end organ of mice were reported after administration of 25 mg/kg of EA.[130] Reduction of vestibular nystagmus to caloric stimulation after i.v. administration of EA (20 mg/kg) to experimental animals was also observed 30 sec to 20 min postinjection.[136] Morphological changes, such as vacuolization and protrusion of cytoplasm in Type I and Type II hair cells in the vestibular end organ, were observed by Matz.[135] Mathog[124] reported that EA produced rapid depression of vestibulo-occular reflexes when given i.v. to cats in doses greater than 20 mg/kg. This depression usually returned to normal within 30 min. The optokinetic-induced eye displacements were stable and habituation from repetitive caloric stimulation was not affected by the drug. Ampullar endolymphatic potential, however, was reduced only if the dose of EA was increased to 70 mg/kg and a maximum depression (−30 mV) was reached after a 100 mg/kg dose. This low vestibular sensitivity to EA may be caused by the lower degree of vascularization in the ampullae than in the stria vascularis.[137]

In conclusion, the effect of EA on the vestibular system has been documented in animals and humans. The apparent lower incidence of vestibular dysfunction after treatment with EA and other LD may be related to the fact that those patients who require acute treatment with LD are usually bedridden; therefore vestibular dysfunction may go undetected. They may also be related to the fact that the vestibular system has no compartmentalized vascular structure such as the stria vascularis. EA does not attain high vestibular concentrations so long as the drug is not administered in a high dose and at a high rate of infusion.

8.3.2 Furosemide

Chemical Properties

Furosemide (FUR) is distributed under the trade name Lasix®. Its chemical name is 4-chloro-*N*-(2-furylmethyl)-5-sulfamoyl-O-anthranilic acid. The pure drug has a low solubility in water, approximately 2.5% in solutions of pH 7.0, but is more soluble in alkaline solutions. In the body about 80% of the drug is bound to plasma protein.

Absorption, Distribution, and Excretion

Furosemide is well absorbed from the gastrointestinal tract and after i.m. administration. Maximum human serum concentrations are reached at 30 min after i.m. administration and about 60 to 90 min after oral administration.[138] The serum *T* 1/2 in the dog is 4 hr after oral administration. In man the serum *T* 1/2 is 90 min after receiving the drug by mouth and only 30 min after i.v. injection. Peters et al.[138] reported that FUR does not concentrate in the kidney but it was later found that the kidneys actively accumulate FUR in concentrations much higher than in serum.[139] The kinetics of FUR in serum, CSF, cochlear fluids, and the aqueous humor were investigated in chinchillas that received a single i.v. injection of 100 mg/kg FUR.[140] Elimination of the drug from these fluids paralleled that in the serum, except in the perilymph in which the *T* 1/2 was approximately four times longer. When the chinchillas received 25 mg/kg i.v. twice a day for five days and 100 mg/kg on the last day no significant accumulation of FUR in the cochlear fluids was detected.

Renal excretion is the main route of FUR elimination. About 90% of an administered dose is eliminated by glomerular filtration and by active tubular secretion. A small fraction is excreted in the feces. The usual oral dose for adults is 20 to 80 mg given as a single dose with a subsequent dose 6 to 8 hr later. The parenteral dose for adults is usually 20 to 40 mg in a single injection (i.m. or i.v.). A marked diuresis usually appears within 20 to 60 min after the injection. The oral dose for children is calculated on the basis of body weight (2 mg/kg).

Mechanism and Site of Action

It has been demonstrated repeatedly that the principal place of FUR action is in the ascending limb of the loop of Henle.[2,89,141] Furosemide administered into the lumen of the renal tubule in concentrations of 10^{-5} to $10^{-6}M$ inhibits active Cl^- transport in the thick limb of Henle's loop.[2] Additional effects have been demonstrated on ion transport in the proximal tubule.[85,141–144] Because the major site of Na^+ and Cl^- reabsorption is in the thick ascending limb, its inhibition leads to large diuresis.

The molecular mechanism of FUR diuretic action has not been resolved. Originally it was reported that FUR and EA inhibit Na/K ATPase.[11,145] This mechanism, however, has been questioned by Williamson,[13] Martinez-Maldonado et al.,[14] and others. The main objection is that Na/K ATPase is blocked only by high concentrations of FUR or EA which do not correspond to the usual serum levels. It has also been observed that FUR inhibits glycolysis[15,16,97,146] and the activity of carbonic anhydrase.[85,147] Lactate accumulation and oxygen consumption was inhibited by FUR only in the presence of Na^+.[148] It appears that inhibition of glycolysis itself has no direct effect on ion transport and diuresis. When glycolysis was inhibited by iodoacetate there was no impairment of Na^+ reabsorption.[96] Furthermore, Ferguson[149] observed that FUR antagonizes adenylate cyclase. Thus it is obvious that the main site of FUR action is in the ascending loop of Henle, where transport of Na^+ and Cl^- is inhibited. Although we recognize FUR's site of action, we do not know its actual molecular mechanism. Several modes have been suggested but there is still a lot of disagreement regarding them.

Adverse Reactions

In addition to the diuretic and adverse effects on hearing, the most frequent side effects of FUR are electrolyte disturbances, volume depletion, hyperuricemia, hyperglycemia, skin rash, nephrotoxicity, and hepatotoxicity. It appears that FUR is less diabetogenic than the thiazide diuretics. Glucose tolerance tests are not usually influenced in normal patients. In rats, however, a single dose of FUR causes a decrease in glucose tolerance after loading with glucose and depresses the hypoglycemic effect of insulin.[150] Also, large doses of FUR, particularly those administered i.v., cause decreased blood pressure in rabbits and cats. As in thiazides, FUR enhances the hypotensive effect of vasodilator drugs. In addition, FUR potentiates the effects of succinylcholine in animals.[151,152] Furthermore, FUR penetrates the placenta, and because of its teratogenic potential it is contraindicated during pregnancy.

Permanent damage to the kidney by FUR has been postulated as a result of hypovolemia and renal anoxia. On the other hand, McMurty and Mitchell[153] saw renal lesions similar to FUR damage produced by the nondiuretic furan analog of FUR. Earlier, Mitchell et al.[154] observed that furosemide-induced hepatic necrosis was the result of a hepatotoxic metabolite of FUR. They also reported that the furan ring of FUR is metabolically activated to an arylated intermediate by cytochrome P-450 in hepatic microsomes. These metabolites, similar to those toxic to the kidney, may cause permanent damage to the inner ear, but they may not be responsible for the acute immediate decline of cochlear potentials.

OTOTOXICITY

Hearing loss after i.v. administration of FUR has in most instances been only temporary and is usually associated with renal failure.[59,155–160] Permanent hearing loss as a result of treatment with FUR was observed in anoxic patients who developed postoperative respiratory obstruction and oliguria secondary to hypotension.[161–162] In most patients the authors described high-frequency hearing loss. Ototoxic reactions were found more frequently when diuresis did not occur after the initial dose; FUR was subsequently administered repeatedly in rapid succession.[162] Thus most of these ototoxic conditions were the result of decreased renal function. More than 80% of all LD, including FUR, are excreted by the kidney. Therefore in patients with lowered renal function the serum level of FUR rises and may cause damage to the inner ear.

The mechanism of FUR action in the inner ear was investigated by Thalmann and coworkers[163] and Brusilow,[164] who observed a large decline in the EP after administration of FUR into the perilymphatic space. At the same time Na/K ATPase and P-creatine remained at normal levels.[163] When FUR-intoxicated ears were subjected to ischemia, however, the ischemic decline of ATPase and P-creatine was markedly reduced. The authors[163] suggested that FUR interferes with energy utilization.

A temporary decline in CM in cats was demonstrated after they had received 10 and 30 mg/kg of FUR i.v.[112,122b] These animals usually recovered within 30 minutes. In addition, loss of tuning sharpness of fibers with characteristic frequencies in the range of 7 to 30 kHz was caused by 20 mg/kg i.v. FUR.[165]

Federspil and Mausen[166] investigated morphological changes in the cochlea after a single i.v. administration of FUR (200 mg/kg) and after treatment with low doses (15, 30, and 60 mg/kg) for 30 to 40 days and after a single dose of 50 mg/kg in nephrectomized guinea pigs. None of the above procedures caused any morphological changes in the inner ear. Ultrastructural changes in the guinea pig stria vascularis after high doses (200 mg/kg) of i.v. FUR are similar to those encountered after EA with dilatation of intercellular spaces and degeneration of intermediate cells.[167a]

In conclusion, temporary hearing loss in man after treatment with FUR has been reported many times. This functional change has been reproduced in animal experiments and is demonstrated as a decline in CM, CAP, EP, and/or evoked potentials.[67b] The morphological changes induced by FUR are similar to those induced by EA and indicate that these two drugs may share a common site and mechanism of ototoxic action.

8.3.3 Bumetanide (BUM)

Chemical Properties

Bumetanide is a derivative of benzoic acid, 3-butylamino-4-phenoxy-5-sulfamoylbenzoic acid. Among numerous synthesized diuretics by Feit[168] and his group, bumetanide was chosen for its high activity and low toxicity.

Absorption, Distribution, and Excretion

Bumetanide is rapidly and almost completely absorbed from the gastrointestinal tract after oral administration. The diuresis it produces lasts 3 to 4 hr; the peak is reached in the first hour. It is quickly eliminated from the body. Its *T* 1/2 in serum after oral administration is 1.5 hr. More than 83% of BUM is excreted by the urine; the remainder, in the feces. The majority is excreted unchanged, but some metabolites of the butyl side chain were identified by Halladay et al.[169] Greater metabolization of BUM was described in rats.[170] Bumetanide is usually 30 to 60 times more potent a diuretic than FUR when given i.v. and has been reported to be 100 times more active when given orally.[170,171] Comparative studies in edematous patients have shown that 1 mg of BUM is as active as 60 mg of FUR. A ratio of effectiveness of 1/40 or more has been documented many times; however, in one instance it was reported that 8 mg of BUM was less effective than 250 mg of FUR.[172a] This apparent discrepancy is due to the fact that the higher the dose of BUM that is necessary to produce diuresis in patients, the lower the BUM/FUR dose ratio.[172b]

The diuretic activity of BUM varies with the species. The lowest oral diuretic dose of BUM was found in dogs and was 0.005 mg/kg; in rabbits it was 0.1 mg/kg, 0.5 mg/kg in mice, and 30 mg/kg in rats.[173]

Mechanism and Site of Action

Bumetanide causes a large diuresis with loss of Na^+, Cl^-, and water. Similarly, as in other loop diuretics, it primarily affects the Na^+ and Cl^- transport in the ascending limb of Henle's loop. When applied to the tubular lumen, it suppresses the positive lumen potential even in the absence of Na^+ (NaCl replaced by choline chloride).[174] Similarly, BUM inhibits active ion transport in isolated frog skin[175] and in red blood cells.[176] It is 60 to 200 times stronger than FUR as an inhibitor of Cl^- transport in amphibian cornea.[177]

In humans[178] probenecid blocks a major part of the diuresis evoked by 0.5 mg BUM i.v., but does not affect a dose of 3.0 mg i.v. This suggests that although the major action of BUM is in the loop of Henle, it also causes a significant alteration of ion reabsorption in the proximal tubule. It has been repeatedly reported that BUM, like FUR, does not inhibit ATPase[175,179] but inhibits the cyclic AMP system[180] and glycolysis.[176] Bumetanide is also a significant inhibitor of ouabain-insensitive transport of Na^+. This ouabain-insensitive transport is considered by some as an exchange diffusion, rather than a second active pump.[56,57] However, the possibility of a second active pump has been suggested in the kidney[54] and in the salivary gland.[181] External Na^+ was found to be unnecessary for the inhibitory effect of BUM and FUR in red cells[182] and in the kidney,[174] with evidence being presented of ouabain-insensitive Na^+ movements that can be blocked by FUR.

The effect of BUM on synthesis of prostaglandins has also been investigated.[9,183] Bumetanide (0.24 mg/kg i.v.) increases kidney volume by 20% and thus increases subcapsular hydrostatic pressure. It also increases renal blood flow, as well as excretion of Na^+ and Cl^-; this effect can be suppressed by pretreatment with indomethacin. These experiments support the hypothesis that prostaglandins also play a role in the diuretic action of BUM.

Adverse Reactions

Acute toxicity in mice was characterized by tremor and jumping convulsions. Intravenous LD_{50} in mice was determined as 330 mg/kg.[170] In patients prolonged therapy over 7 to 14 weeks with daily oral doses of 0.25 to 4.0 mg BUM, plus potassium supplement, caused asymptomatic hyperuricemia and, in one patient, decreased carbohydrate tolerance.[184] Another side effect described was mild to moderate muscle pain and stiffness, especially localized in the neck and particularly apparent in oliguric patients receiving high doses.[172,185]

OTOTOXICITY

The ototoxic effects of BUM were extensively studied by Brown and his coworkers,[186–188a,189–190] who compared the adverse effect of BUM with EA, the cysteine adduct of EA, and FUR. The i.v. dose-response curves of these drugs in cats were parallel in doses of 1 to 50 mg/kg, but the absolute ototoxic potency of BUM was approximately 6.5 times that of FUR. However, because the diuretic activity of BUM is 40 to 60 times higher than FUR, its ototoxic potency is only 0.11 to 0.16 that of FUR. After i.v. administration of BUM (1 to 30 mg/kg) the EP and CAP rapidly declined.[188a,188b] In cats and guinea pigs the effect was similar and about 6.5 times higher than FUR.[189] In dogs the absolute toxicity was considered to be approximately five times that of FUR.[190]

Morphological changes after BUM administration were investigated by Santi et al.[191] In their experiments on chinchillas a single i.v. injection of BUM (18 mg/kg) caused an increase in the thickness of the stria vascularis of 20 to 28 μm. The strial edema extended from the hook to the apex. In transmission electron microscopy the stria vascularis showed changes similar to those described after EA and FUR administration. They also found that the marginal cells were swollen and bulged into the endolymphatic space.

There is little data about the effect on hearing in man. Bourke,[192a] however, reported that BUM was well tolerated in three patients in which FUR caused ototoxic reactions (FUR 160 to 500 mg/day; BUM 4 to 12 mg/day). Furthermore, in a recent symposium only a few instances of ototoxicity that appeared to be causally related to BUM among the several hundred patients given the drug,[192b] were reported.

8.4 MERCURIAL DIURETICS

8.4.1 Mechanism of Action

Calomel (Hg_2Cl_2) was first used as a diuretic in the sixteenth century. Because of its cathartic effects and the uncertainty of its resorption from the intestine, it was subsequently replaced by organomercurials. When organomercurials are administered parenterally they are rapidly absorbed and quickly excreted. They react with thiol groups in the body and are excreted as the cysteine complex. Approximately 50% of the injected mercury is recovered in the urine within 3 hr and almost all, within 24 hr. The diuresis generated by mercurial diuretics can be prevented or terminated by dimercaprol (BAL), a detoxicant for heavy metal poisoning. The mechanism of mercurial action is, in part, similar to that of loop diuretics. In micropuncture studies it has been seen that mersalyl inhibits active Cl^- transport in the ascending limb of Henle's loop,[88] probably by interfering with adenylate cyclase[20] and Na/K ATPase.[193] Mercurials inhibit reabsorption of Na^+ and Cl^-, depress secretion of K^+, spare HCO_3^-, and therefore have a tendency to produce metabolic alkalosis. Other findings of their action are inconsistent (see review by Suki et al.[194]). The usual dosage of a commonly used mercurial, mercaptomerin sodium, is 1 ml (40 mg of Hg^{2+}) given i.m. or s.c., but may vary from 0.2 to 2.0 ml/day.

8.4.2 Adverse Reactions

Mercurial diuretics may cause hypersensitivity reactions (flushing, dermatitis, pruritis), gastrointestinal reactions (nausea, vomiting, diarrhea), bone marrow depression (neutropenia, agranulocytosis), and transient azotemia. They may also provoke cardiac arrhythmias if administered too rapidly.

Direct ototoxicity by the organomercurial diuretics has not been reported, but neurotoxicity of mercury compounds has been known since the middle ages. Hearing impairment and vertigo were found in 80% of the patients with Minamata disease (chronic poisoning with methylmercury).[195] Hearing loss was observed mainly at the later stage, probably as a result of retrocochlear lesions.[196] Cochlear morphological changes have also been investigated after mersalyl, methylmercury hydroxide, and mercury chloride ($HgCl_2$) administration by Thalmann et al.,[82] Falk et al.,[197] and Anniko and Sarkady,[198] respectively. Acute intoxication with mercurials affects both afferent and efferent nerve endings and the OHC.[198] Direct perfusion of the cochlea with $5 \times 10^{-4}M$ mersalyl caused swelling of the OHC, vacuolization of the cytoplasm, and clumping of chromatin along the nuclear membrane, but the junctions between the cells were still normal when observed 30 min after perfusion. When the dose of mersalyl was increased to $1 \times 10^{-3}M$, the OHC were in the process of destruction and the intercellular spaces in the stria vascularis were widened. This was apparent specifically between the marginal and intermediate cells, with shrinking of the cytoplasm of intermediate cells.[82] The chronic effect of mercurial poisoning was investigated by Falk et al.,[197] Anniko and Sarkady,[198] and von Westernhagen.[199] Falk et al.,[197] and Anniko and Sarkady[198] discovered damage to the OHC in the apical part of the cochlea; the greatest damage was in the third row. Metabolic disturbances in the hair cells and stria vascularis were reported by von Westernhagen.[199]

The acute effect of mercurials on ion transport was investigated by Stupp and Rauch,[200] who observed a marked reduction in $^{42}K^+$ transport from the scala vestibuli to the scala media when mersalyl was perfused through the scala vestibuli for 5 to 10 min at concentrations of 10^{-4} to $10^{-1}M$. Enzymes such as Na/K ATPase and adenylate cyclase are also significantly inhibited. The I_{50} of stria vascularis Na/K ATPase was about $8 \times 10^{-6}M$ for mersalyl, several times lower than the I_{50} for the EP ($5 \times 10^{-5}M$). The adenylate cyclase of the stria vascularis and the organ of Corti was inhibited by mersalyl at concentrations even lower ($I_{50} = 5 \times 10^{-6}M$ and $9 \times 10^{-7}M$), respectively (see the review by Thalmann et al.[201]).

The effect of mercurials on the generation of cochlear potentials was examined by Thalmann et al.[82] Perfusion of perilymphatic space with $HgCl_2$ and mersalyl caused a dose-dependent decrease in EP and CM. A faster reduction of cochlear potentials was observed after administration of $HgCl_2$ than after mersalyl.

In conclusion, direct ototoxicity by mercurial diuretics has not been reported. Hearing loss, however, is common among people chronically intoxicated with methylmercury. The destruction of OHC and decline of cochlear potentials after perfusion of the perilymphatic space with mercurials in animals has also been reported on numerous occasions.

8.5 INHIBITORS OF CARBONIC ANHYDRASE

A large number of sulfonamides capable of suppressing carbonic anhydrase have been tested. Most effective are acetazolamide, methazolamide, and ethoxzolamide. These agents have played an important role in the study of the fundamental physiology of fluid formation. Acetazolamide is the most commonly used of these drugs; it is readily absorbed from the gastrointestinal tract and peak serum concentration appears within 2 hr. It does not undergo metabolic alteration and is completely excreted by the kidney within 24 hr.

8.5.1 Mechanism of Action

Carbonic anhydrase catalyzes the hydration of carbon dioxide to carbonic acid. When carbonic acid dissociates to form H^+ and HCO_3^- these ions become available to the transporting systems. Acetazolamide produces inhibition of H^+ secretion in the proximal tubule and increases delivery of nonreabsorbable sodium bicarbonate to the thick ascending limb of Henle's loop. This results in a limited increase in the excretion of water and electrolytes.

Carbonic anhydrase has been found in many different tissues, including the renal cortex, gastric mucosa, eye, pancreas, CNS, and the inner ear. Formation of aqueous humor and spinal fluid is decreased after carbonic anhydrase inhibition.[202] Although there is a large amount of carbonic anhydrase in renal tissue, more than 99% of the enzyme must be inhibited before an effect becomes apparent in renal function.

The participation of carbonic anhydrase in cochlear fluid generation was described by Erulkar and Maren,[203] Maren et al.,[204] and Maren.[205] This has been confirmed by purification of carbonic anhydrase from the membranous lateral wall of the cochlea (stria vascularis, spiral ligament, and spiral prominance) by Drescher.[206]

Prazma[207] was able to demonstrate for the first time that carbonic anhydrase inhibition affected generation of the EP. During hypercapnia EP increased by about +6 mV. This elevation was inhibited by pretreatment with methazolamide or acetazolamide (Figure 8.7).

8.5.2 Adverse Reactions

After large doses patients exhibit drowsiness, paresthesias, flushing, thirst, headache, dizziness, anorexia, and vomiting. Hearing loss in man after treatment with these drugs has not been reported. However, administration of acetazolamide has been demonstrated to decrease the number of vacuoles in the stria vascularis in experimental animals.[208] In addition, a decline in CAP after high doses of acetazolamide has been described by Silverstein and Yules in experimental animals.[114]

8.6 OTOTOXIC INTERACTION OF LOOP DIURETICS AND AMINOGLYCOSIDES

Toxic interaction of loop diuretics and aminoglycoside antibiotics (AmAn) has been suggested by several authors.[58,104,105,108] They have observed that

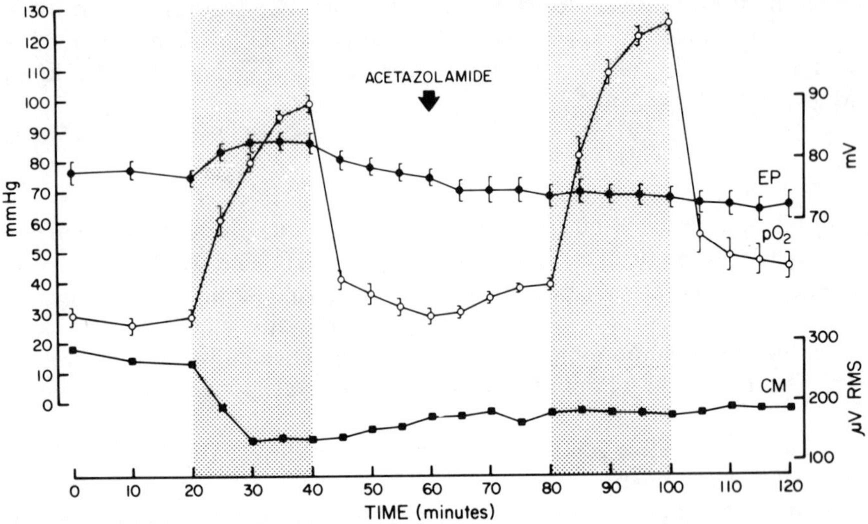

Figure 8.7 The effect of acetazolamide on hypercapnia-induced changes in EP and CM. Hypercapnia was generated by animals breathing 10% CO_2–90% O_2 in intervals (20–40 and 80–100 min) marked by the shaded area. The endocochlear potential (EP) in mV, endocochlear PO_2 (PO_2) in mm Hg, and cochlear microphonics (CM) in μV rms were recorded before and after acetazolamide administration (heavy arrow). Vertical bars represent the standard error of mean. From Prazma.[206] Reprinted by permission of the American Physiological Society.

some of their patients developed hearing losses after treatment with recommended doses of EA. These patients had also, in the past or at the same time, received AmAn treatment. This interaction has been confirmed in experiments by several authors.[113,209–213] The interaction of AmAn and LD has been tested in several different experiments: acute experiments after low- and/or high-dose combinations and in chronic experiments in which guinea pigs were treated for two weeks with AmAn and, on the last day, received 1 dose of LD.

In guinea pigs, we[209] combined low doses of i.v. kanamycin (KA) (50 mg/kg) with 10 mg/kg of i.v. EA. In the first group 50 mg/kg of KA was injected alternately with 10 mg/kg of EA, twice, at 1-hr intervals. During the 240 min of the experiment EP and CAP did not significantly change but the CM gradually declined to about 40% of the original value by the end of the 4-hr experiment. When the dose of KA was increased to 100 mg/kg and twice alternated with 10 mg/kg of EA at 1-hr intervals CM gradually declined during the entire experiment; in addition, a steep decrease in EP and CAP followed the second injection of EA at 180 minutes. In another series of acute experiments in guinea pigs, doses of the drugs were increased. Kanamycin was given s.c. at 400 mg/kg, which was followed in 2 hr by a single i.v. injection of EA at 40 mg/kg or FUR at 50 to 100 mg/kg.[113,210] Single doses of KA did not produce a decline in the CM and the CM decrease after EA or FUR was reversible. When drugs from both groups were administered several hours apart the CM declined to zero.[113,210,214a] In chronic experiments two groups of guinea pigs were treated for 14 days with KA (50 or 100 mg/kg/day i.m.), and, on the last day, the animals received 1 dose of EA (10 mg/kg i.v.). The decline in CM and EP did not occur in the group that received a low dose of KA but only in the group that received the higher dose of KA (100 mg/kg/day) and the dose of EA (10 mg/kg) on the last day of treatment. Therefore toxic interaction has been demonstrated by administering low and high doses of the two classes of drug in acute and chronic experiments. Kinetic studies of interaction between EA and GE have shown that EA facilitates gentamicin penetration into the scala media, whereas it does not affect the perilymphatic concentration of GE.[214b] This facilitation, however, could be due to nothing more than a permeability breakdown as the ototoxicity progresses; it requires further investigation.

Fox et al.[215] also documented the interaction of AmAn and LD by transmission electron microscopy. Damage to the guinea pig organ of Corti after combination treatment with KA (400 mg/kg s.c.) and EA (40 mg/kg i.v.) exceeded the effects of the individual drugs. As early as 2.5 hr after receiving the second drug the OHC exhibited a change in shape, clumping of nuclear chromatin, and alteration of membranes along their apical surfaces. After 6 hr the OHC were rounded and the endoplasmatic reticulum was missing in several places. By 24 hr many OHC were completely destroyed. Makai[213] found that the harmful effect of combining EA and 3,4-dideoxykanamycin B was greater than expected from the simple addition of the effects of the two drugs; that is, a synergistic interaction occurred. Severe disintegration and loss of OHC, IHC, and nerve fibers were observed in all turns.

Not only the auditory system but also the vestibular system is affected by the combination of AmAn and LD as reported by Mathog and Capps.[212] Their experiments, however, indicated that a combination of streptomycin and EA appears to be additive rather than synergistic.

In conclusion, it has been demonstrated repeatedly that the ototoxic effects of both drugs are cummulative in animals and man. Hawkins et al.[211] has shown that ototoxic interaction occurs if the AmAn (KA) precedes the LD (EA). Furthermore, Brummett et al.[216] demonstrated that cochlear damage results if EA is administered during a time range of 2 hr before and up to 8 hr after a dose of KA. From other experiments we know that both drugs affect the organ of Corti *and* the stria vascularis; however, the major actions of the AmAn are in the hair cells and the major actions of the LD are in the stria vascularis. It seems that each group, when acting alone, affects not only a different area of the cochlea but probably different enzymatic systems. The overlap in their cochlear sites of action could be important in the potentiating effect observed when these two groups of drugs are combined and should be more thoroughly investigated in the future.

REFERENCES

1. J. B. Hook and H. E. Williamson, *J. Pharmacol. Exp. Ther.*, **148,** 88 (1965).
2. M. Burg, L. Stoner, J. Cardinal, and N. Green, *Am. J. Physiol.*, **225,** 119 (1973).
3. J. R. Clapp, G. A. Nottebohm, and R. R. Robinson, *Am. J. Physiol.*, **220,** 1355 (1971).
4. B. R. Edwards, P. G. Baer, R. A. L. Sutton, and J. H. Dirks, *J. Clin. Invest.*, **52,** 2418 (1973).
5. M. Goldberg, in *Handbook of Physiology*, American Physiological Society, Bethesda, Md., Section 8, 1973, pp. 1003–1031.
6. R. W. Berliner, J. H. Dirks, and W. J. Cirksena, *Ann. N.Y. Acad. Sci.*, **139,** 424 (1966).
7. H. E. Williamson, W. H. Bourland, and G. R. Marchland, Prostlandins, **8,** 297 (1974).
8. M. D. Bailie, J. A. Barbour, and J. B. Hook, *Proc. Soc. Exp. Biol. Med.*, **148,** 1173 (1975).
9. U. B. Olsen, *Acta Pharmacol. Toxicol.*, **37,** 65 (1975).
10. K. Abe, N. Irokawa, M. Yasujima, M. Seino, S. Chiba, Y. Sakurai, K. Yoshinaga, and T. Saito, *Circ. Res.*, **43,** 254 (1978).
11. D. E. Duggan and R. M. Noll, *Arch. Biochem. Biophys.*, **109,** 388 (1965).
12. J. F. Hoffman and F. M. Kregenow, *Ann. NY Acad. Sci.*, **137,** 566 (1966).
13. H. E. Williamson, *Proc. 4th Int. Cong. Nephrol.*, **2,** 144 (1969).
14. M. Martinez-Maldonado, N. T. Tsaparas, C. Inagaki, and A. Schwartz, *Pharmacol. Exp. Ther.*, **188,** 605 (1974).
15. E. E. Gordon and M. DeHartog, *J. Gen. Physiol.*, **54,** 650 (1969).
16. S. Klahr, J. Yates, and J. Bourgoignie, *Am. J. Physiol.*, **221,** 1038 (1971).
17. R. H. Bowman, J. Dolgin, and R. Coulson, *Am. J. Physiol.*, **224,** 1200 (1973).
18. D. R. Ferguson and B. R. Twite, *Naunyn Schmiedeberg's Arch. Pharmacol.*, **281,** 295 (1974).
19. D. R. Ferguson and B. R. Twite, *Naunyn Schmiedeberg's Arch. Pharmacol.*, **287,** 111 (1975).
20. H. Ebel, *Naunyn Schmiedeberg's Arch. Pharmacol.*, **281,** 301 (1974).
21. G. von Bekesy, *J. Acoust. Soc. Am.*, **24,** 72 (1952).
22. C. A. Smith, O. Lowry, and M. L. Wu, *Laryngoscope*, **64,** 141 (1954).
23. I. Tasaki and C. S. Spyropoulos, *J. Neuro. Physiol.*, **22,** 149 (1959).
24. W. Kuijpers, A. C. van derVleuten, and S. L. Bonting, *Science,* **157,** 949 (1967).
25. F. M. Matschinsky and R. Thalmann, *Laryngoscope*, **77,** 292 (1967).
26. T. Konishi, R. A. Butler, and C. Fernandez, *J. Acoust. Soc. Am.*, **33,** 349 (1961).
27. T. Konishi and E. Kelsey, *Acta Otolaryngol.*, **65,** 381 (1968).
28. J. Prazma, *Acta Otolaryngol.*, **67,** 631 (1969).
29. T. Konishi and M. Mendelsohn, *Acta Otolaryngol.*, **69,** 192 (1970).
30. W. Kuijpers and S. L. Bonting, *Pfluegers Arch.*, **320,** 348 (1970).
31. B. M. Johnstone, *Acta Otolaryngol.*, **60,** 113 (1965).
32. S. K. Bosher and R. L. Warren, *Proc. R. Soc. London*, **171,** 227 (1968).
33. J. Prazma, *Acta Otolaryngol.,* **68,** 53 (1969).

34a. P. M. Sellick and B. M. Johnstone, *Prog. Neurobiol.*, **5,** 337 (1975).

34b. S. K. Bosher, *J. Physiol.*, **293,** 329 (1979).

35. T. Konishi and P. E. Hamrick, *Acta Otolaryngol.*, **86,** 176 (1978).
36. C. V. Ilberg, *Arch. Klin. Exp. Ohren Nasen Kelhkopfheilkd.*, **190,** 426 (1968).

37. R. Hinojosa, *Acta Otolaryngol. Suppl.*, **292,** 1 (1971).
38. S. T. Sitko, D. Strelioff, and V. Honrubia, *Trans. Am. Acad. Ophthalmol. Otolaryngol.*, **82,** 328 (1976).
39. V. Honrubia, D. Strelioff, and S. T. Sitko, *Ann. Otol. Rhinol. Laryngol.*, **85,** 697 (1976).
40. J. F. Maher and G. E. Schreiner, *Ann. Intern. Med.*, **62,** 15 (1965).
41. J. Prazma, W. G. Thomas, N. D. Fischer, and M. J. Preslar, *Arch. Otolaryngol.*, **95,** 448 (1972).
42. S. Paloheimo and R. Thalmann, *Arch. Otorhinolaryngol.*, **217,** 347 (1977).
43. W. Kuijpers and D. P. C. Wilberts, *J. Otolaryngol.*, **38,** 321 (1976).
44. S. K. Bosher, C. Smith, and R. L. Warren, *Acta Otolaryngol.*, **75,** 184 (1973).
45. S. W. Brusilow and E. Gordes, *J. Clin. Invest.*, **52,** 2517 (1973).
46. E. S. Cohn, E. H. Gordes, and S. W. Brusilow, *Science*, **171,** 910 (1971).
47. P. M. Sellick and B. M. Johnstone, *Pfluegers Arch.*, **352,** 339 (1974).
48. J. Prazma, Presented at 83rd meeting of Acoustical Society of America, Buffalo, NY, April 18–21, 1972, p. 23.
49. I. Melichar and J. Syka, *Hear. Res.*, **1,** 35 (1978).
50. R. Thalmann, J. Kusakari, and T. Miyoshi, *Laryngoscope*, **83,** 1690 (1973).
51. G. Whittembury, *J. Gen. Physiol.*, **51,** 303 (1968).
52. G. Whittembury and J. Fishman, *Pfluegers Arch.*, **307,** 138 (1969).
53. O. H. Petersen, *J. Physiol. London*, **208,** 431 (1970).
54. G. Whittembury and F. Proverbio, *Pfluegers Arch.*, **316,** 1 (1970).
55. G. Giebisch, L. P. Sullivan, and G. Whittembury, *J. Physiol.*, **230,** 51 (1973).
56. H. Lubowitz and R. Whittam, *J. Physiol.*, **202,** 111 (1969).
57a. M. J. Dunn, *J. Clin. Invest.*, **49,** 1804 (1970).
57b. R. D. Brown, "Comparative Acute Cochlear Toxicity of Intravenous Bumetanide and Furosemide in the Pure-Bred Beagle," Perspectives on Bumetanide: A Symposium, in Press. *J. Clin. Pharmacol.*
58. W. D. Meriwether, R. J. Mangi, and A. A. Serpick, *J. Am. Med. Assoc.*, **216,** 795 (1971).
59. A. Heidland and M. E. Wigand, *Ann. Intern. Med.*, **73,** 858 (1970).
60. K. E. Kim, G. Onesti, J. H. Moyer, and C. Swartz, *Am. J. Cardiol.*, **27,** 407 (1971).
61. A. N. Brest, G. Onesti, R. Seller, O. Ramirez, C. Heider, and J. Moyer, *Am. J. Cardiol.*, **16,** 99 (1965).
62. B. A. Carter, *Lancet II*, 1127 (1965).
63. Y. Conway and G. Leonetti, *Circulation*, **31,** 66 (1965).
64. H. Lyons, V. W. Pinn, S. Cartell, J. J. Cohen, and J. T. Harrington, *N. Engl. J. Med.*, **288,** 124 (1973).
65. J. G. G. Ledingham and R. I. S. Bayliss, *Clin. Pharmacol. Ther.*, **6,** 474 (1965).
66. F. L. Lieberman and T. B. Reynolds, *Gastroenterology*, **49,** 531 (1965).
67. J. Bergstrom and E. Hultman, *Acta Med. Scand.*, **180,** 363 (1966).
68. A. W. Jorgensen and O. H. Sorensen, *Acta Med. Scand.*, **188,** 179 (1970).
69. M. Goldberg, *Ann. N.Y. Acad. Sci.*, **139,** 443 (1966).
70. J. H. Laragh, P. J. Cannon, W. B. Stason, and H. O. Heinemann, *Ann. N.Y. Acad. Sci.*, **139,** 453 (1966).
71. M. G. Goldner, H. Zarowitz, and S. Akgun, *N. Engl. J. Med.*, **262,** 403 (1969).
72. O. Mustala and S. Toivonen, *Ann. Med. Exp. Biol. Fenn.*, **54,** 75 (1965).
73. W. P. V. Jackson and M. Nellen, *Br. Med. J.*, **2,** 333 (1966).

74. S. Toivonen and O. Mustala, *Br. Med. J.*, **1,** 920 (1966).
75. E. Lebacq and M. Marco, *Rev. Fr. Etud. Clin. Biol.*, **12,** 160 (1967).
76. O. O. Anderson and I. Persson, *Br. Med. J.*, **11,** 798 (1968).
77. N. Samaan, C. T. Dollery, and R. Fraser, *Lancett II*, 1244 (1963).
78. J. S. Charnock and A. F. Almeida, *Biochem. Pharmacol.*, **21,** 647 (1972).
79. R. W. Epstein, *Biochem. Biophys. Acta*, **274,** 119 (1972).
80. E. E. Daniel, A. M. Kidwai, K. Robinson, D. Freeman, and S. Fair, *J. Pharmacol. Exp. Ther.*, **176,** 563 (1971).
81. K. H. Beyer, J. E. Baer, J. K. Michaelson, and H. F. Russo, *J. Pharmacol. Exp. Ther.*, **147,** 1 (1965).
82. R. Thalmann, I. Thalmann, I. Ise, and S. Paloheimo, *Laryngoscope*, **87,** 699 (1977).
83. M. Goldberg, D. K. McCurdy, E. L. Foltz, and L. W. Bluemle, Jr., *J. Clin. Invest.*, **43,** 201 (1964).
84. R. Gussin and E. J. Cafruny, *J. Pharmacol. Exp. Ther.*, **153,** 148 (1966).
85. J. B. Puschett and M. Goldberg, *J. Lab. Clin. Med.*, **71,** 666 (1968).
86. J. H. Stein, C. B. Wilson, and W. M. Kirkendall, *J. Lab. Clin. Med.*, **71,** 654 (1968).
87. J. P. Rado, L. Szende, J. Tako, and L. Borcely, *J. Clin. Pharmacol.*, **10,** 375 (1970).
88. M. Burg and N. Green, *Kidney Int.*, **4,** 245 (1973).
89. J. H. Dirks and J. F. Seely, *Am. J. Physiol.*, **219,** 114 (1970).
90. R. M. Komorn and E. J. Cafruny, *Science*, **143,** 133 (1964).
91. R. M. Komorn and E. J. Cafruny, *J. Pharmacol. Exp. Ther.*, **148,** 367 (1965).
92. J. R. Sachs and L. G. Welt, *J. Clin. Invest.*, **47,** 949 (1968).
93. P. J. Bentley, *J. Physiol. London*, **195,** 317 (1969).
94. J. Bourgoignie, S. Klahr, J. Yates, L. Guerra, and N. S. Bricker, *Am. J. Physiol.*, **218,** 314 (1970).
95. C. I. Inagaki, M. Martinez-Maldonado, and A. Schwartz, *Arch. Biochem. Biophys.*, **158,** 421 (1973).
96. R. H. Bowman, J. Dolgin, and R. Coulson, *Am. J. Physiol.*, **224,** 416 (1973).
97. V. D. Jones and E. J. Landon, *Biochem. Pharmacol.*, **16,** 2163 (1967).
98. E. E. Gordon, *Biochem. Pharmacol.*, **17,** 1237 (1968).
99. S. P. Banerjee, V. K. Khanna, and A. K. Sen, *Mol. Pharmacol.*, **6,** 680 (1970).
100. G. V. Irons, Y. H. Kong, Jr., W. M. Ginn, Jr., and E. S. Orgain, *J. Am. Med. Assoc.*, **194,** 1348 (1965).
101. W. J. Schneider and L. Becker, *Arch. Intern. Med.*, **117,** 715 (1966).
102. G. J. Matz and R. F. Naunton, *J. Am. Med. Assoc.*, **206,** 2119 (1968).
103. E. Hanzelik and M. Peppercorn, *Lancet*, **1,** 416 (1969).
104. G. J. Matz, D. D. Beal and L. Krames, *Arch. Otolaryngol.*, **90,** 152 (1969).
105. R. H. Mathog and W. J. Klein, *J. Engl. J. Med.*, **280,** 1223 (1969).
106. P. S. Ng, C. E. Conley, and T. S. Ing, *Lancet*, **1,** 673 (1969).
107. V. K. G. Pillay, F. D. Schwartz, K. Aimi, and R. M. Kark, *Lancet*, **1,** 77 (1969).
108. A. H. Johnson and C. H. Hamilton, *South. Med. J.*, **63,** 511 (1970).
109. F. D. Schwartz, V. K. Pillay, and R. M. Kark, *Am. Heart J.*, **79,** 427 (1970).
110. T. Yipintsoi and V. Thongmitr, *J. Med. Assoc. Thai.*, **49,** 615 (1966).
111. A. Barrillon and J. Felix, *Presse Med.*, **78,** 2283 (1970).
112. R. H. Mathog, W. G. Thomas, and W. R. Hudson, *Arch. Otolaryngol.*, **92,** 7 (1970).
113. B. A. West, R. E. Brummett, and D. L. Himes, *Arch. Otolaryngol.*, **98,** 32 (1973).

114. H. Silverstein and R. B. Yules, *Laryngoscope*, **81,** 873 (1971).
115. A. Kohonen, T. Jauhiainen, and J. Tarkkanen, *Acta Otolaryngol.*, **70,** 187 (1970).
116. J. A. McCurdy, J. G. McCormick, and J. A. Harrill, *Arch. Otolaryngol.*, **100,** 143 (1974).
117. J. M. Dilling, T. Nakashima, and J. B. Snow, *Arch. Otolaryngol.*, **98,** 183 (1973).
118. R. Thalmann, T. Miyoshi, J. Kusakari, and I. Thalmann, *Audiology*, **12,** 364 (1973).
119. J. Prazma and J. Pecorak, *J. Clin. Invest.*, **55,** 840 (1975).
120. Y. Kaku, J. C. Farmer, and W. R. Hudson, *Arch. Otolaryngol.*, **98,** 282 (1973).
121. R. D. Brown and T. W. McElwee, Jr., *Toxicol. Appl. Pharmacol.*, **22,** 589 (1972).
122a. R. D. Brown, *Neuropharmacology*, **12,** 967 (1973).
122b. R. D. Brown, *Toxicol. Appl. Pharmacol.*, **31,** 270 (1974).
123. K. E. Fox and R. E. Brummett, *Fed. Proc.*, **33,** 271 (1974).
124. R. H. Mathog, *Laryngoscope*, **87,** 1791 (1977).
125. J. W. Youngblood, E. S. Cohn, and D. W. Warfield, *Surg. Forum*, **20,** 476 (1969).
126. S. Ernstson, *Acta Otolaryngol.*, **73,** 476 (1972).
127. R. H. Mathog and G. J. Matz, *Laryngoscope,* **83,** 977 (1973).
128. R. A. Walloch, J. Anthony, and N. Gibbons, *Laryngoscope*, **84,** 256 (1974).
129. C. A. Quick and A. J. Duvall, *Laryngoscope*, **80,** 954 (1970).
130. Y. Nakai, *ORL.*, **33,** 366 (1971).
131. H. Silverstein and R. Begin, *Laryngoscope*, **84,** 976 (1974).
132. R. Brummett, C. A. Smith, Y. Ueno, S. Cameron, and R. Richter, *Acta Otolaryngol.*, **83,** 98 (1977).
133. G. J. Matz and R. Hinojosa, *Surg. Forum.*, **24,** 488 (1973).
134. S. Crifo, *Arch. Otolaryngol.,* **206,** 27 (1973).
135. G. J. Matz, *Laryngoscope*, **86,** 1065 (1976).
136. R. M. Levinson, M. J. Capps, and R. H. Mathog, *Ann. Otol. Rhinol. Laryngol.*, **83,** 223 (1974).
137. J. Kusakari and R. Thalmann, *Laryngoscope*, **86,** 132 (1976).
138. G. Peters and F. Roch-Ramel, in *Handbook of Experimental Pharmacology*, Springer, Berlin, 1969, pp. 386–405.
139. G. H. Hirsch, A. P. Pakuts, and A. J. Bayne, *Biochem. Pharmacol.*, **24,** 1941 (1971).
140. L. Rybak, T. Green, S. K. Juhn, T. Morizono, and B. L. Mirkin, *Abstr. Res. For. Am. Acad. Otol.*, Las Vegas, September 9, 1978.
141. T. M. Morgan, M. Tadokoro, D. Martin, and R. W. Berliner, *Am. J. Physiol.*, **218,** 292 (1970).
142. T. J. Burke, R. R. Robinson, and J. R. Clapp, *Kidney Int.*, **1,** 12 (1972).
143. P. Deetjen, *Arch. Ges. Physiol.*, **284,** 184 (1965).
144. F. G. Knox, F. S. Wright, S. S. Howards, and R. W. Berliner, *Am. J. Physiol.*, **217,** 192 (1969).
145. U. Schmidt and U. C. Dubach, *Nephron*, **7,** 447 (1970).
146. T. Yoshida and J. Metcoff, *Proc. Ann. Meeting, Am. Soc. Nephrol. 4th*, Washington, D.C., 88 (1970).
147. H. W. Radke, G. Rumrich, E. Kinne-Saffran, and K. Ullrich, *Kidney Int.*, **1,** 100 (1972).
148. L. P. Sullivan, J. M. Tucker, and M. J. Scherbenske, *Am. J. Physiol.*, **220,** 1316 (1971).
149. D. R. Ferguson, *Br. J. Pharmacol.*, **27,** 528 (1966).
150. K. Formanek and T. Kenner, *Br. J. Pharmacol.*, **26,** 27 (1966).
151. E. Reyes and G. D. Appelt, *J. Pharm. Sci.*, **61,** 562 (1972).

152. T. O. Morgan, *Drugs*, **15,** 151 (1978).

153. R. T. McMurty and J. R. Mitchell, *Tox. Appl. Pharmacol.*, **42,** 285 (1977).

154. J. R. Mitchell, S. D. Nelson, W. Z. Potter, H. A. Sasame, and D. J. Iollow, *J. Pharmacol. Exp. Ther.*, **199,** 41 (1976).

155. G. H. Schwartz, D. S. David, R. R. Riggio, K. H. Stenzel, and A. L. Rubin, *N. Engl. J. Med.*, **282,** 1413 (1970).

156. D. S. David and P. Hitzig, *N. Engl. J. Med.*, **284,** 1328 (1971).

157. T. Vargish, R. Benjamin, and L. Shenkman, *Ann. Intern. Med.*, **72,** 761 (1970).

158. P. S. Venkateswaran, *Br. Med. J.*, **4,** 113 (1971).

159. L. Bergstrom, P. Jenkins, and I. Sando, *Ann. Otol. Rhinol. Laryngol.*, **82,** 555 (1973).

160. S. I. Rifkin, A. M. D. Quesada, M. J. Pickering, and D. L. Shires, *South. Med. J.*, **71,** 86 (1978).

161. R. H. Lloyd-Mostyn and I. J. Lord, *Lancet*, **2,** 1156 (1971).

162. C. A. Quick and W. Hoppe, *Ann. Otol. Rhinol. Laryngol.* **84,** 94 (1975).

163. J. Kusakari, I. Ise, T. H. Comegys, I. Thalmann, and R. Thalmann, *Laryngoscope*, **88,** 12 (1978).

164. S. Brusilow, *Can. J. Physiol. Pharmacol.*, **1,** 42 (1976).

165. R. Klinke and E. F. Evans, *Pfluegers Arch.*, **347,** Suppl. R53 Abstr. (1974).

166. P. Federspil and H. Mausen, *Monatsschr Ohrenheilkd Laryngorhinol.*, **107,** 256 (1973).

167a. C. A. Quick and W. Hoppe, *Ann. Otolaryngol.,* **84,** 94 (1975).

167b. R. D. Brown and A. M. Feldman, *Ann. Rev. Pharmacol. Toxicol.*, **18,** 233 (1978).

168. P. W. Feit, *J. Med. Chem.*, **14,** 432 (1971).

169. S. C. Halladay, I. G. Sipes, and D. E. Carter, *Clin. Pharmacol. Ther.*, **22,** 179 (1977).

170. E. H. Ostergaard, M. P. Magnussen, C. K. Nielsen, E. Eilertsen, and H. H. Frey, *Arzneim. Forsch.*, **22,** 66 (1972).

171. M. R. Cohen, E. Hinsch, R. Vergona, J. Ryan, S. J. Kolis, and M. A. Schwartz, *J. Pharmacol. Exp. Ther.*, **197,** 697 (1976).

172a. K. J. Berg, A. Tromsdal, and T. E. Wideroe, *Eur. J. Clin. Pharmacol.*, **9,** 265 (1976).

172b. P. W. Feit, panel discussion, Perspectives on Bumetanide: A Symposium, *Clin. Pharmacol. Therap.*, in Press.

173. M. P. Magnussen and E. Eilertsen, *Nauyn Schmiedeberg's Arch. Pharmacol.*, **282,** Suppl. R61 (1974).

174. M. Imai, *Eur. J. Pharmacol.*, **41,** 409 (1977).

175. H. J. Kramer, *Pharmacology*, **14,** 481 (1976).

176. H. Lubowitz, *J. Pharmacol. Exp. Ther.*, **203,** 92 (1977).

177. M. C. McGahan, T. Yorio, and P. J. Bentley, *J. Pharmacol. Exp. Ther.*, **203,** 97 (1977).

178. A. F. Lant, Postgrad. Med. J., **51,** Suppl. 6, 35 (1975).

179. M. Gemba and K. Nishimura, *Jpn. J. Pharmacol.*, **27,** 205 (1977).

180. D. R. Ferguson and B. R. Twite, *Br. J. Pharmacol.*, **49,** 288 (1973).

181. F. Proverbio, J. W. L. Robinson, and G. Whittembury, *Biochem. Biophys. Acta*, **211,** 327 (1970).

182. J. S. Wiley and R. A. Cooper, *J. Clin. Invest.*, **53,** 745 (1974).

183. U. B. Olsen, *Acta Pharmacol. Toxicol.*, **40,** 430 (1977).

184. D. L. Davies, A. F. Lant, N. R. Millard, A. J. Smith, J. W. Ward, and G. M. Wilson, *Clin. Pharmacol. Ther.*, **15,** 141 (1974).

185. M. F. Cuthbert, *Postgrad. Med. J.*, **51,** Suppl. 6, 51 (1975).

186. R. D. Brown, *Fed. Proc.*, **34,** 722 (1975).

187. R. D. Brown, *Neuropharmacology*, **14,** 547 (1975).

188a. R. D. Brown, *Toxicol. Appl. Pharmacol.*, **38,** 137 (1976).

188b. J. Kusakari, J. Kambayashi, I. Ise, and K. Kawamoto, *Acta Otolaryngol.*, **86,** 336 (1978).

189. R. D. Brown, *Pharmacologist*, **18,** 183 (1976).

190. R. D. Brown, J. E. Manno, E. A. Daigneault, and B. R. Manno, *Toxicol. Appl. Pharmacol.*, **48,** 157 (1979).

191. P. A. Santi and A. J. Duvall, *Abstr. Midwinter Res. Meeting Assoc. Res. Otolaryngol.*, February 1, 1978, p. 14.

192a. E. Bourke, *Lancet*, **1,** 917 (1976).

192b. I. H. Tuzel, Adverse Experiences; Perspectives on Bumetanide: A Symposium, *J. Clin. Pharmacol.*, in Press.

193. B. R. Nechay, *Ann. N.Y. Acad. Sci.*, **242,** 501 (1974).

194. W. N. Suki, G. Eknoyan and M. Martinez-Maldonado, A. *Rev. Pharmacol.*, **13,** 91 (1973).

195. L. T. Kurland, S. N. Faro, and H. Siedler, *World Neurol.*, **1,** 370 (1960).

196. K. Mizukoski, M. Nagaba, Y. Ohno, K. Ishikava, M. Aoyagi, Y. Watanane, I. Kato, and H. Ino, *Ann. Otol. Rhinol. Laryngol.*, **37,** 74 (1975).

197. S. A. Falk, J. K. Haseman, R. Klein, and M. K. Falk, *Laryngoscope*, **83,** 1769 (1973).

198. M. Anniko and L. Sarkady, *Acta Otolaryngol.*, **85,** 213 (1978).

199. B. von Westernhagen, *Arch. Klin. Exp. Ohren Nasen Kehlkopfheilkd*, **193,** 70 (1969).

200. H. Stupp and S. Rauch, *Arch. Klin. Exp. Ohren Nasen Kehlkopfheilkd*, **186,** 106 (1966).

201. R. Thalmann, I. Ise, B. A. Bohne, and I. Thalmann, *Acta Otolaryngol.*, **83,** 221 (1977).

202. T. H. Maren, *Physiol. Rev.*, **47,** 595 (1967).

203. S. D. Erulkar and T. H. Maren, *Nature*, **189,** 459 (1961).

204. T. H. Maren, E. R. Swenson, and A. D. F. Addink, *Ann. Otolaryngol.*, **84,** 847 (1975).

205. T. H. Maren, *J. Exp. Zool.*, **199,** 317 (1977).

206. D. Drescher, *Proc. Nat. Acad. Sci. USA*, **74,** 892 (1977).

207. J. Prazma, *Am. J. Physiol.*, **235,** 317 (1978).

208. R. L. Johnson and H. H. Spoendlin, *Ann. Otol. Rhinol. Laryngol.*, **75,** 127 (1966).

209. J. Prazma, J. P. Browder, and N. D. Fischer, *Ann. Otol. Rhinol. Laryngol.*, **83,** 111 (1974).

210. R. E. Brummett, J. Traynor, R. Brown, and D. Himes, *Acta Otolaryngol.*, **80,** 86 (1975).

211. J. E. Hawkins, D. M. Marques, C. S. Clark, and R. E. Preston, *J. Acoust. Soc. Am.*, **57** (S1), 560 (1975).

212. R. H. Mathog and M. J. Capps, *Ann. Otol. Rhinol. Laryngol.*, **86,** 158 (1977).

213. Y. Nakai, *Laryngoscope*, **87,** 1548 (1977).

214a. R. E. Brummett, R. T. Brown, and D. L. Himes, *Arch. Otolaryngol.*, **105,** 240 (1979).

214b. P. Tran-Ba-Huy, C. H. Manuel, and O. Sterkers, *Abstr. 3rd* Midwinter Res. meeting Assoc. Res. Otolaryngol., Florida, 1980, p. 61.

215. K. E. Fox, N. J. Russell, and R. E. Brummett, *Fed. Proc.*, **37,** 502 (1978).

216. R. E. Brummett, R. T. Brown, and D. L. Himes, *Arch. Otolaryngol.*, **105,** 240 (1979).

CHAPTER 9

Miscellaneous Ototoxic Agents

DENNIS L. KISIEL, Ph.D.

Director
Cleveland Hearing and Speech Center
Cleveland, Ohio

RICHARD P. BOBBIN, Ph.D.

Associate Professor of Otorhinolaryngology and Pharmacology
Department of Otorhinolaryngology
Kresge Hearing Research Laboratory of the South
Louisiana State University Medical Center
New Orleans, Louisiana

CONTENTS

9.1 INTRODUCTION

This chapter is divided into agents that exert an ototoxic effect because of their physical properties (physical agents) and those that are ototoxic because of their chemical nature (chemical agents). Varying amounts of data which range from almost none to entire books devoted to the subject have been obtained for these agents. Discussion of each agent, when possible, includes (1) its cochlear site-of-action, (2) the morphological, physiological, and biochemical changes it produces, and (3) its postulated mechanism-of-action. No attempt is made to discuss the methodologies involved in the research articles cited or the physiology of the auditory system. The reader is referred to Chapter 2 for a succinct review of auditory physiology. Auditory research methods are discussed in a number of excellent, readily available texts.[1,2]

9.2 PHYSICAL AGENTS

9.2.1 Temperature

A review of the literature generally reveals an absence of changes in the cochlear microphonic (CM) with localized reductions in cochlear temperature as large as 50°C.[3-7] Butler et al.,[8] however, found CM change to be linearly related to the log of temperature. These authors showed that CM decreased by about 6 dB over a 10° range of 35.8 to 25.8°C. Dallos[1] related the differences in the Butler[8] and Coats[4] studies to the method of reducing temperatures in the two investigations. Butler et al.[8] reduced body temperature with an ice pack, whereas Coats[4] manipulated cochlear temperature only. Dallos' explanation may not be accurate because Drescher[6,7] demonstrated no change in CM amplitude with reductions in body temperature from 39 to 29°C.

Coats[4] examined the effect of temperature on the compound VIII nerve action potential (CAP) amplitude and latency. Results of his investigation revealed a linear relationship between them. Butler et al.[8] demonstrated the elimination of the low intensity segment of the CAP amplitude input/output function with a reduction in body temperature from 35.8 to 25.8°C. This phenomenon supports the two-population theory of CAP generation. (See the discussion of the sharpening filter in the coverage of CAP in Chapter 2.) Stockard et al.[9] observed increased I-III, III-IV/V, and I-IV/V interwave latencies in the auditory-evoked responses of patients with impaired thermoregulation mechanisms.

An investigation by Drescher[6,7] demonstrated the effect of temperature on reduction of CM during and after intense-sound exposure. Apparently the rate of intense-sound-induced reduction of CM is decreased at lower temperatures, increased at higher. CM recovery is inhibited at lower temperatures, enhanced at higher. Drescher related the temperature-dependent changes in CM amplitude during and after intense-sound exposure to processes of energy metabolism and/or structural changes that do not affect normal physiological function.

9.2.2 Noise

Continuous Noise

In an attempt to explicate the effects of intense sound on the cochlea, investigators have generally subscribed to three theories: mechanical, vascular, and metabolic. The first of these, the mechanical theory, attributes pathological changes in the cochlea to mechanical stress developed within or on the organ of Corti structures.

Lim and Melnick[10] discussed four possible mechanisms for sensory-cell damage caused by mechanical forces. The first of these mechanisms suggests that the force of intense fluid eddies on the cochlear partition can potentially rupture Reissner's membrane and cause endolymph and perilymph to mix. This may result in damage to the sensory cells or secondary atrophy of the stria vascularis.[11-13] Lawrence and Yantis[11] and Eldredge et al.[13] have confirmed the possibility of rupture of Reissner's membrane by intense acoustic stimulation in the guinea pig, whereas Ward and Duvall[12] failed to observe ruptures in this cochlear structure. It is speculated that the differences noted in Reissner's membrane are due to the exposure stimulus of 123 dB SPL used by Ward and Duvall,[12] as opposed to an exposure level of 130 to 150 dB SPL in the former studies. Spoendlin[14] maintains that mechanical damage to the cochlea is not caused until intensities of 130 dB SPL are reached; this suggests that the ruptures of Reissner's membrane are not merely dissection artifacts.[11,13]

Second, Lim and Melnick[10] suggest that intense basilar-membrane motion can also result in rupture of the reticular lamina.[15-18] Bohne[16] originally described three different graduations of injury. In all three types of injury endolymph diffuses into the organ of Corti from the scala media and leads to the degeneration of the sensory cells via the toxic effect of K^+ ions on cell membranes normally exposed to a low-potassium environment.

Other investigators have presented evidence contrary to the second theory: that ionic changes in the cochlear duct result from exposure to intense sound. Lim and Melnick[18] and Spoendlin[19] have presented light and electron microscopic data that suggest that supporting cell processes close off holes made in the reticular lamina by intense sound and prevent the mixture of endolymph and perilymph. In addition, Davis and associates[20] found that the reticular lamina maintained its integrity even when compromised by the collapse of the rods of Corti and supporting cells.

The third mode of action of damaging mechanical force on the cochlear duct involves the detachment of the rest of the organ of Corti from the basilar membrane. Lurie[21] found that brief exposures to pure tones at intensities of approximately 148 dB SPL resulted in detachment of hair cells from the basilar membrane. Davis and associates[20] noted the separation of fibers of the cells of Deiter from the basilar membrane as a consequence of exposure to pure tones ranging from 138 to 147 dB SPL. Fissures appearing along the junction of the cells of Hensen and Claudius were prominent in the second and third turns when maximal damage was reported in these locations. Beagley[15] described detachment of the reticular lamina at the Hensen-Deiter cell junction in his post-mortem observations of the state of a guinea pig cochlea exposed to a 500-Hz, 120-dB SPL tone for 20 min. Rupturing of the heads of the pillar cells bordering the tunnel of Corti have been reported by a number of investigators.[14,20] The tympanic lamina (the epithelial cells on the scala tympani side of the basilar membrane) has been observed in huge cell clusters after it has been detached from the basilar membrane,[19] as has herniation of the basilar membrane.[22]

Lim and Melnick's[10] fourth hypothesis of the effect of mechanical force on the cochlea states that the tectorial membrane may be separated from the hair cells, again as the result of intense fluid motion. Assuming that the effective or physiological stimulus of the sensory receptor cells is a shearing displacement of the stereocilia, detachment of the tectorial membrane from the hair cells would therefore result in an increase in threshold. The reported "cracking," buckling, and confluence of the sensory hairs with frequent detachment of the plasma membrane may be taken as evidence of a forcible detachment of the tectorial membrane from the hairs.[19]

According to the vascular theory of the effect of intense sound on the end organ, impaired microcirculation in the ear results in a lack of oxygen that causes a reduction in the number of key enzymes and/or metabolites of the sensory cells in the cochlea.[23-26] Lawrence et al.[23] observed constriction of the vessels in the vas spirale of guinea pigs due to intense-sound exposure (sufficient to depress CM from 10 to 30 dB). Hawkins[24] and Lipscomb and Roettger[26] observed similar changes in vestibular and cochlear tissues of rats. Large gaps between endothelial cells of blood vessels and an appreciable thickening of capillary walls were frequently noted. Hawkins[24,25] observed capillary vasoconstriction and loss of cells in the suprastrial portion of the spiral ligament in guinea pigs and chinchillas.

Hawkins[24,27] suggested two possible mechanisms for the observed vasoconstriction in the cochlea exposed to intense sound. The first mechanism implicates the reduced endolymphatic oxygen tension which is observed subsequent to intense-sound exposure as the mediator of the local vasoconstriction. The second proposed mechanism suggests that adrenergic innervation of the cochlea plays a role in the vasoconstriction observed on intense-sound exposure.

This alternative was investigated by Bobbin and Gondra[28] in their study of the effect of reserpine on hair-cell scarring caused by intense-sound exposure. Among the many properties of reserpine is its ability to deplete norepinephrine from tissue receiving sympathetic autonomic innervation. Because the drug was found to have no effect on hair-cell scarring induced by a 4-kHz, 126-dB SPL, 30-min tone exposure, these authors concluded that changes in the caliber of cochlear blood vessels were not mediated by the sympathetic nervous system.

Kellerhals[29] observed the capillaries of the stria vascularis of guinea pigs exposed to gunshots to be densely packed with a nearly homogeneous, highly viscous mass. Animals pretreated with low-molecular-weight dextran to diminish blood viscosity suffered fewer hair-cell losses than those exposed only to intense sound. Kellerhals concluded that the protective effect of low-molecular-weight dextran provided indirect evidence of the existence of pathogenic microcirculation in the cochlea following acute acoustic trauma.

Universal agreement does not exist for the role of vascular disturbances in the degeneration of the cochlear duct due to intense-sound exposure.[30] Duvall et al.[31] examined the stria vascularis of chinchillas exposed to a 700-Hz to 2.8-kHz band of noise at 123 dB SPL for 15 min, commencing as early as 5 min after cessation of the exposure stimulus. Although these authors noted extensive hair-cell damage at this time, vessel collapse was not apparent. The conclusion was that the effect of intense sound is primarily on the hair cells and only secondarily on the strial blood vessels. Perlman and Kimura[32] failed to observe constriction or rupture of blood vessels in the stria or spiral ligament, despite use of exposure intensities as high as 153 dB SPL.

The metabolic theory of the effect of intense sound on the cochlea proposes that sensory-cell damage is due to alterations on enzyme systems and energy-reserve stores and the reduction of metabolites.[10,17,18,33] The vesiculation and eventual vacuolization of the endoplasmic reticulum and the swelling of associated mitochondria of the hair cell observed as a response to intense acoustic stimulation are indirect evidence of interference with enzyme systems responsible for the production of lipids, proteins, glucose, glycogen, nucleic acids, and other metabolites.[34–36] A number of theories account for the modus operandi of intense sound on enzyme systems in the cochlea; for example, Kraus and his coworkers[37] observed a stimulation of RNA synthesis in the hair cells of the basal turns of guinea pigs exposed to white noise at 85 dB SPL. These authors speculated that the use of sound greater than 85 dB SPL could cause a depletion of this key molecule and result in inhibition of transmitter formation.

Another more widely accepted view of how intense sound disrupts the normal metabolic state of the cochlea suggests that an anoxic state is induced by acoustic hyperstimulation. Spoendlin[19] compared the swelling of the afferent dendrites to the inner hair cells of guinea pigs exposed to high levels of intense sound with the same type of alteration encountered in cases of severe ischemia. Depletion of glycogen and succinic dehydrogenase stores in the hair cells has been made apparent after intense acoustic stimulation.[38,39] Because it is now known that the hair cells rely on anaerobic and aerobic processes for their energy, a depletion of succinic dehydrogenase and glycogen would presumably greatly alter hair-cell function.[40]

A disarrangement, or confluence, of stereocilia and deformities of the cuticular plate have been reported by a number of investigators.[12,18,19] Spoendlin[19] suggests that these alterations of the stereocilia could be a result of metabolic as well as mechanical effects of intense-sound exposure in that they are similar to analogous effects found in cochleas damaged by toxic substances.

Some investigators have proposed that the mechanism of action of intense sound on the cochlea depends on the type of sound to which the ear is exposed. Thus Spoendlin and Brun[33] suggest that acoustic trauma is due to metabolic loss up to 130 dB; above 130 dB damage is induced mechanically. Stockwell et al.[41] suggest that mechanical stress produces damage at high-frequency sound exposures, whereas metabolic deficiencies account for damage observed in response to those of low-frequency sound. Other investigators have suggested that a combination of these theories could adequately explain histological and biochemical variations in the cochlea after intense-sound exposure (e.g., see Spoendlin[14]).

Studies of the effect of intense sound on the cochlea have contained examinations of anatomical, behavioral, and electrophysiological variations due to intense acoustic stimulation. Evidence accrued in recent years has suggested that hair-cell counts from surface preparations are at best only a first-order approximation of the functional status of the cochlea. Bohne et al.[42] observed that a few intense-sound-exposed chinchillas had fewer missing hair cells than nonintense-sound-exposed controls, yet they had lower cochlear potentials. It was only on an electron microscopic evaluation of the cochlear tissue of the intense-sound-exposed chinchillas that various types of ultrastructural damage were observed that could have accounted for the reduced cochlear potentials. Eldredge and Miller[43] reported that a chinchilla with only a slight deviation from normal sensitivity had profound losses of outer hair cells. Eldredge et al.[44] observed decreases in the CM and CAP in chinchillas with small cochlear lesions and normal behavioral thresholds.

Ward and Duvall,[12] in a discussion of histological correlates of permanent threshold shift (PTS) and temporary threshold shift (TTS), observed that chinchillas with PTS had concurrent total loss of inner hair cells in the first and second turns, whereas chinchillas with TTS had only outer hair-cell losses. Alexander and Githler[45] noted a poor correlation between impaired cochlear structures and CM sensitivity when CM losses were reduced less than 30%, when compared to preexposure norms. Their histological preparations were largely within normal limits, whereas CM losses were significantly poorer than those seen in the normal ear. The authors concluded: "When little anatomical change is evident and the electrical audiogram is significantly depressed, it is our belief that the electrical audiogram is a more reliable indicator of the true condition of the peripheral auditory apparatus."

Henderson et al.[46] exposed chinchillas to high levels of impulse noise that produced large, behaviorally measured TTSs that recovered within 30 days. These animals had nearly complete degeneration of outer hair cells in the region of 8 to 12 mm from the base of the cochlea. On the basis of their results Henderson questioned the practice of evaluating the effects of intense sound on the function of the cochlea by the use of behaviorally determined threshold procedures. Eldredge[47] found poor matches between behavioral audiograms and narrow wedges of hair-cell loss in the chinchilla.

Pinheiro et al.[48] also discussed the problems in detecting small hair-cell losses with behavioral-conditioning techniques. In the monkey they found a poor correlation between hair-cell losses as large as 50% and behaviorally determined threshold shifts. Pinheiro et al.[48] attributed the inability of the behavioral audiogram to detect small cochlear lesions to a redundancy of nerve innervation in the cochlea,[49] spread of fields of excitation as a function of stimulus intensity,[50] and the possible existence of regions of hypersensitivity bordering areas of depressed hearing sensitivity.[51]

Electrophysiological potentials have been widely used to study the effect of intense sound on the cochlea. The CM and CAP have been most extensively investigated with comparatively little attention addressed to the cochlear endolymphatic potential (EP). Although it is well known that EP affects the magnitude of CM, few studies have addressed themselves to the changes in EP after intense-sound exposure.[52–57] The Benitez et al.[56] study revealed no change in EP, but simultaneous losses of sensitivity for CAP and CM in chinchillas exposed for seven days to an octave band of noise centered at 500 Hz with an intensity of 95 dB SPL. Johnstone and Sellick's[57] study revealed an increase in EP following high levels of intense-sound exposure similar to the increase seen after perfusion of the scala tympani with 0.1% procaine solution or K^+.[58,59]

Changes in CM as a result of intense-sound exposure have been of interest to investigators for at least four reasons:

1 The need to understand the physiological processes underlying behavioral changes due to intense-sound exposure before their effects on threshold can be interpreted is apparent.[60]

2 Because the hair cells, peripheral auditory nerve fibers, and central-auditory structures may be viewed as elements in a series circuit, changes in CM caused by intense-sound exposure are reflected in the magnitudes and latency of the CAP and brainstem potentials.[56]

3 Because CM is not normally considered a fatiguable response, losses as a consequence of intense-sound exposure can be studied independently of decrements of response due to adaptation.[61]

4 The CM loss and recovery curves share many similarities to the corresponding behavioral TTS curves and reasonably good correlations with behavioral thresholds have been observed.[62]

Tonndorf and Brogan[63] demonstrated three different types of change in CM after intense-sound exposure: (1) shift of CM responses to a lower pseudothreshold level (sensitivity), (2) change in maximum output with no change in sensitivity, and (3) a combination of these changes. Davis and associates[20] showed a shift in sensitivity and a decrease in the maximum output due to intense-sound exposure; the relative loss of voltage is the same at all SPLs. A parallel shift in sensitivity, combined with a reduction in maximum voltage, is illustrated in Figure 9.1. Other nonmonotonic, input/output functions have also been observed in response to high-intensity-sound exposures.[64]

Change in the maximum output of CM after intense-sound exposure has generally been shown to be less than the corresponding shift in sensitivity of the same measure.[20,56,64–66] Shifts in sensitivity for various intense-sound exposure paradigms are illustrated in Figure 9.2. The significance of changes in CM sensitivity and maximum output of CM was summarized by Benitez et al.[56] These authors suggested that changes in the conductive mechanism of

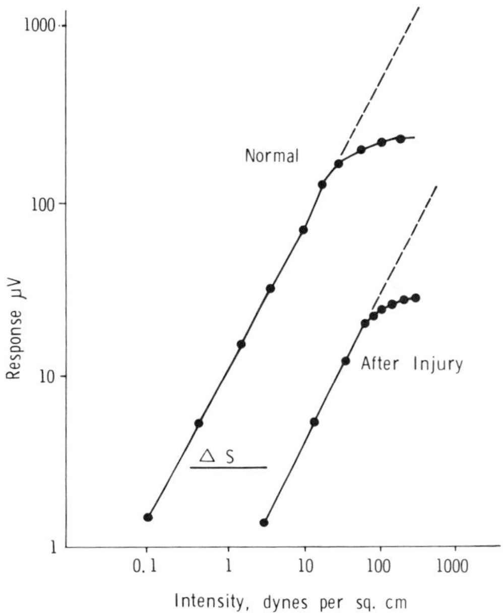

Figure 9.1 Amplitude of 5-kHz CM before and after overstimulation with a 7-kHz tone. Note that 1 dyne/cm² = 86 dB SPL (see Chapter 2 for more discussion). (This figure is a modification of an original illustration by Wever and Lawrence.[65])

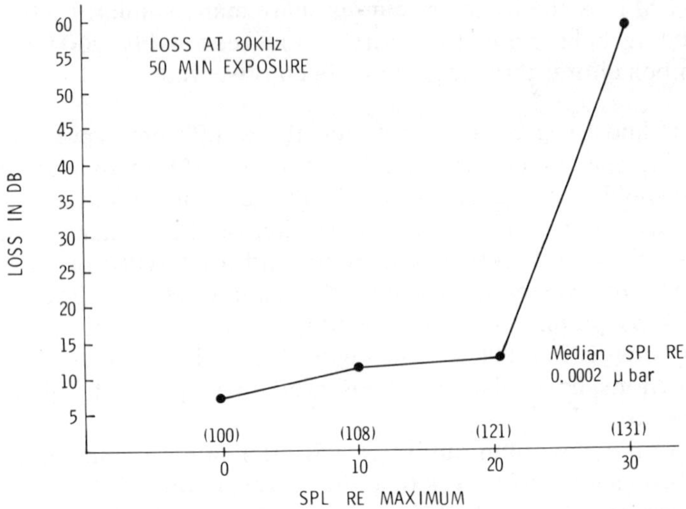

Figure 9.2 Mean shift of sensitivity (loss in dB) following 50 min of exposure to a 5-kHz tone at four exposure intensities. The numbers in parentheses represent median exposure intensities in dB SPL (reference pressure equal to 0.0002 μbar or 0.0002 dynes/cm^2; that is, SPL RE: 0.0002 μbar). Beneath these numbers the exposure intensities are expressed in terms of the additional dB SPL above those necessary to evoke a maximum CM magnitude (i.e., SPL RE: MAXIMUM). See Chapter 2 for more discussion. (From Price.[60])

the middle and inner ears are responsible for changes in CM sensitivity. With increased impedance in the middle or inner ears energy transfer would presumably be reduced, thus causing a shift to the right of the CM input/output curve (shift in CM sensitivity toward higher intensities). Changes in maximum output of CM were considered due to a decrease in the EP or any mechanism that would cause a decrease in the range of resistance of modulation of the current at the hair-bearing surface of the hair cells. Changes in the maximum output of CM are presumably easier to interpret, because reversible fatiguability (overloading) and irreversible losses are the sole mechanisms by which this measure may change. Interpretation of irreversible changes in CM, however, is complicated by the possibility of a primary EP reduction and a secondary CM reduction as opposed to a primary CM reduction. In light of these difficulties in interpretation of the maximum output and sensitivity of CM these measures may be considered as no more than ". . . limited indicators of the detailed mechanisms involved with acoustic trauma. . . ."[62]

Similarities noted between the loss and recovery curves of CM and TTS would seem to warrant increased investigation of CM in studies of the effect of intense sound on the cochlea. The growth of TTS and the loss of CM sensitivity appear to depend on the duration and intensity of exposure in a similar manner. The linear functions that relate the recovery of CM sensitivity and TTS with duration also appear to be similar. Space considerations preclude a detailed discussion of the relation of CM and CAP to TTS or PTS. Durrant[62] reviews this area quite cogently in a recent publication.

Few investigators have examined the long-term recovery of CM in cases of severe acoustic trauma.[11,15,67] In the Lawrence and Yantis[11] study 32 guinea pigs were exposed to two different levels of intense sound (135 and 150 dB SPL) for equivalent durations. The CMs were recorded from the round window immediately before and after intense-sound exposure and at 56 days postexposure. As in TTS studies and studies of transient changes in CM sensitivity, the amount of recovery was independent of initial sensitivity shift. In addition, the degree of initial loss did not predict whether an ear would recover or continue to lose its function.

Alexander and Githler[68] investigated the recovery of CM in the guinea pig from exposure of jet engine noise. Results indicated that the recovery of CM was a complicated process dependent on healing of cells, the return of minimally damaged cells to normal functioning, and a delayed degeneration of sensory epithelia that occurred as late as six weeks postexposure. Beagley[15] observed appreciable recovery of CM over a 14-day period in guinea pigs exposed to 500-Hz tones for 20 min. Recovery was related to the percentage of the transient CM depression caused by a "split" between the cells of Deiter and Hensen.

The CAP has not received so much attention from investigators as CM in attempts to elucidate the effects of intense-sound exposure on the cochlea. Early studies regarding the merits of the CAP were rather pessimistic. Davis and associates[20] criticized CAP as being too "labile" for monitoring the effects of acoustic trauma, both during exposure and in the recovery period. Eldredge et al.[44] argued that the inordinately reduced voltages are reflective of a loss of synchrony of neural firing and of neural units. With this interpretation CAP may be viewed as the most sensitive index of cochlear functioning. Davis and associates[20] and Eldredge et al.[44] emphasized that CAP was a weighted response reflective of neural activity from the basal turn of the cochlea and as such was not sensitive to local activity. This viewpoint is no longer tenable because the use of narrow-band masking, filtered clicks, and tone bursts in clinical electrocochleography has demonstrated that nerve fibers originating from the first and second cochlear turns may contribute to CAP.[44,69,70]

With a judicious choice of stimuli and control of stimulus parameters CAP can be useful in monitoring the effect of intense sound on the cochlea. As shown with CM, various similarities between recovery of CAP from intense-sound exposure and TTS have been demonstrated.[71,72] Eldredge et al.[44] noted a closer rank-order correlation between loss of the component of the CAP masked by a 6-to-8-kHz noise band and hair-cell loss than the corresponding relation between CM depression and anatomical injury. These authors concluded that N_1 peak voltages as a function of SPL may be the most sensitive index of hair-cell loss, as responses can be obtained over a wider range than with CM.

Mitchell et al.[73] investigated the effect of acoustic overload that causes TTS in guinea pigs. They concluded that the anatomical site of these transient behavioral threshold shifts was at the level of the VIII nerve. The basis for this conclusion was that N_1 was depressed and no change was noted in the CM. An example of changes in the input/output amplitude function of the N_1 component of the CAP after intense-sound exposure is illustrated in Figure 9.3. On the other hand, Benitez et al.[56] noted a closer numerical correspondence between asymptotic TTSs and the CM loss in the second and third turns than between the CAP depression and TTSs, which suggests that behavioral transient hearing loss has an underlying peripheral cochlear substrate.

Impulse Noise

The magnitude and location of cochlear lesions caused by exposure to impulse noise appear to be governed by complex interactions of amplitude, duration, critical level, number of impulses, temporal pattern of impulse, and microstructure.[74] Nevertheless, certain features are shared with trauma caused by continuous noise; for example, damage to the outer hair cells of the "hook" region of the cochlea (the extreme basal portion) has been reported for both impulse and continuous noise exposure.[75,76] A second "notch" of outer hair-cell damage 8 to 10 mm from the base of the cochlea was reported in rhesus monkeys after exposure to impulse noise.[75] Relatively normal segments of hair cells were present basalward and

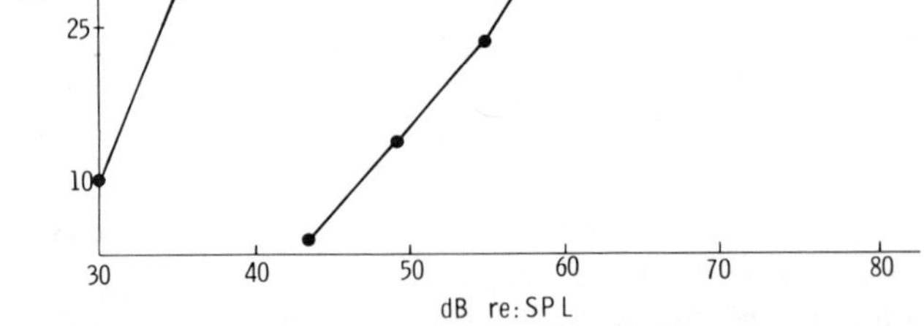

Figure 9.3 N_1 amplitude evoked with a 6-kHz tone before and after a 15-min exposure to a 6-kHz tone at 105 dB SPL (dB reference pressure equal to 0.0002 dyne/cm^2; that is, dB RE: SPL. See Chapter 2 for more discussion). Left arrow points to baseline function (before exposure); right arrow points to postexposure function. (Adapted from an original illustration by Mitchell et al.[73])

apically from the 8-to-10-mm locus. Similar sharply delineated loci of hair-cell destruction have been observed after continuous noise exposure. The locus of damage in the chinchilla cochlea reported by Henderson et al.[46] as a consequence of impulse-noise exposure was shifted apically in relation to the 8-to-10-mm lesion site reported by Jordan et al.[75] The difference in the two studies is related to the duration of stimulus used in the two investigations. Shorter duration impulses are generally reported to cause greater damage to the cochlear base than the longer.[74,77] Inner hair cells are generally intact after either type of intense-sound exposure.[46,75] Impulse noise apparently causes a greater loss of myelinated nerve fibers than continuous noise.[75,77] A study by Kellerhals et al.[78] revealed that impulse noise caused heavy damage to the organ of Corti which resulted in subsequent retrograde degeneration of peripheral neurons, spiral ganglion cells, and finally the fibers of the acoustic nerve.

Neither impulse nor continuous noise exposures seem to obey the dictum of the equal-energy hypothesis uniformly. Eldredge and Covell[79] compared the effect of a pure tone and narrow band noise of equal overall sound pressure on cochlear potentials. Contrary to expectation, the narrow band with a lower dB-spectrum level caused greater change than the pure tone. The authors hypothesized that peak energy of the signal was a more relevant parameter than "equal energy" in determining losses of cochlear potentials. Henderson and Hamernik[74] reviewed a variety of violations of the equal-energy hypothesis for impulse noise.

A comprehensive review of the psychoacoustic and physiological effects of impulse noise on man are beyond the scope of this review. Excellent current reviews are available.[74,80,81] Among the more important differences noted between impulse and continuous noise exposures were the loss and recovery patterns that developed after each type of acoustic insult. Ward[82] and Ward et al.[83] postulated that the TTS grows linearly with exposure time following impulse noise exposure. Recovery functions have been reported to be linear in time and triphasic in shape.[82]

It has been observed with continuous noise that little relation exists between experimentally produced TTS and PTS.[75,84] The large magnitude of TTS produced by small numbers of impulses has been suggestive of the mechanical factors that underlie their effect on the cochlea.[74,83]

9.2.3 Interaction of Different Types of Intense Sound

Dichotomous results have been reported in the literature with respect to combinations of intense sound. Low levels of impulse and steady-state noise in combination have resulted in lower magnitudes of TTS than that produced by intense-sound exposure alone. The protective effect was assumed to be mediated by the acoustic reflex.[85,86] This scientific evidence presumably lends credence to the often-mentioned fallacy that continued intense-sound exposure "toughens" ears and makes them more resistant to intense sound. Henderson and Hamernik[74] indicated that high-intensity-level combinations of impulse and steady-state noise could result in a large PTS and concommitant reduction of hair cells. Each noise exposure alone resulted in negligible effects on cochlear potentials and behavioral measures.

9.2.4 Vibration

Low-frequency vibration of the body or head has reportedly been shown to affect the auditory and vestibular systems. Guignard and Coles (cited in reference 87) studied the effect of whole-body vibration and intense sound on the hearing of human subjects. Vibration alone caused few changes in threshold acuity. A facilitatory effect (improved acuity) was even noted at one frequency (2 kHz). In addition, vibration prevented the TTS caused by injurious intense-sound levels. Jauhiainen et al.[87] conducted a similar investigation with guinea pigs as subjects. In their paradigm these authors subjected 10 guinea pigs to whole-body vibration (10 cps, 6-mm amplitude) for 48 hr. Monitoring of CM after the control period revealed the physiological correlate of increased sensitivity reported in Guignard and Coles' investigation. Jauhiainen et al.[87] speculated that the enhancing effect may have been due to the protective influence of the acoustic reflex threshold at 2000 and 4000 Hz and/or a sensitization of the cochlea somehow related to hyperventilation and increased O_2 consumption during vibration exposure. Results from an investigation by Yokoyama et al.[88] were at variance with the data from the Guignard and Coles study. Their study revealed greater threshold shifts and delayed recovery time from a combined vibration and intense-sound exposure than from intense sound alone. Yokoyama et al.[88] speculated that an interaction of intense sound and vibration could result in physical displacement of auditory, thoracic, and abdominal organs, thus causing a disturbance in homeostasis for autonomic function, or their interaction could mechanically interfere with the cochlear vasculature.

At least two investigations in the literature have indicated the effect of low-frequency vibration on the vestibular system.[89,90] Aantaa et al.[89] investigated the integrity of the vestibular system of 49 workers in a room in which diesel engines were being tested. Forty-five (45) percent of the workers exhibited vestibular dysfunctions in the form of spontaneous nystagmus, lowered caloric excitability, or pathology in rotary tests. The authors speculated that lesions were apparent in the peripheral vestibular system as a result of low-frequency (10 Hz) vibration of the air which set up resonance vibrations in the skull. Lackner and Graybiel[90] induced vertical and horizontal nystagmus experimentally by applying a hand-held physiotherapy vibrator to various positions on the skull. These authors deduced that both horizontal and vertical semicircular canals were stimulated by vibration of this type.

9.3 CHEMICAL AGENTS

9.3.1 Metabolic Poisons

Anoxia

Reduction of the oxygen supply to the cochlea has shown marked effects on the cochlear potentials. Historically, the effect of oxygen on hearing has been known as early as 1904 when Aggazzotti (as reported in Wever et al.[91]) found a dulling of threshold activity as a result of atmospheric changes. Anoxic conditions have been experimentally induced by methods such as clamping the trachea, respiration of expired air, and inspiring air with reduced O_2 concentration.[91–95] None of the above studies, however, maintained the general physiological state of the test animal.[1]

Local (cochlear) anoxic effects were first produced by Perlman et al.[96] by occluding the anterior inferior cerebellar artery and interrupting cochlear blood flow. Konishi et al.[97] also used this technique in their investigations of the effect of anoxia on cochlear potentials. Misrahy et al.[98] introduced a method of inducing localized hypoxia in the cochlea. In this method a mixture of glucose and glucose oxidase was injected into the scala media of the cochlear turns. The resulting enzymatic oxidation of glucose consumed local supplies of O_2 and reduced CM amplitude.

A review of the literature reveals that reductions in CM, CAP, summating potential (SP), and EP all occur after a period of prolonged anoxia. Only a single report by Bornschein and Gernandt[92] claimed that a differential reduction of the N_1 and N_2 neural components of CAP, without permanent diminution of CM, would occur as a result of reduction of O_2 levels of the cochlea. These authors demonstrated complete recovery of CM with continued reduction of the CAP and anoxic guinea pigs, provided that the initial diminution of CM did not exceed 10 dB.

Using the condition of anemic anoxia in cats, Sugar and Gerard[99] reported the O_2 requirements of various central nervous system generators in terms of three parameters: survival time, recovery time, and revival time. Survival time was defined as the interval between the initiation of O_2 deprivation and the elimination of potentials. Conversely, recovery time was defined as the period between the return of normal inspiratory function and the reemergence of potentials. Revival time represented the longest period of O_2 deprivation after which a return toward baseline levels could be detected.

Survival time, recovery time, and revival time depend on complex interrelationships of variables such as the length of O_2 deprivation, percentage of O_2 in inspired air, method of inducing anoxic states, initial depression of cochlear potentials, general physiological state of the preparation, circulatory adjustments, and changes in arterial O_2. With respect to survival time, the consensus in the literature is that CM and SP are most resistant to conditions of hypoxia in the cochlea.[92,95,97] Wever et al.[91] reported a reduction in the amplitude of CM after inspiration of air containing 4% O_2. Under conditions of extreme deprivation reductions in CM amplitude have varied from 49 to 80% of preexposure values.[91] Survival times reported in the literature are in the order of 40 to 50 sec.[96-97] Most investigators have described a biphasic reduction in CM. The initial precipitous decline in CM is generally attributed to that portion of the potential dependent on normal metabolic functioning of the cochlea.[100]

A rapid decrease in SP amplitude has been reported during anoxia followed by a polarity reversal. During recovery polarity has been observed to return to normal but amplitude often remained reduced.[97,101] A correlation between EP recovery and SP-polarity reversal has been noted.[97] An overshooting period of the neural potentials, the N_1 and N_2 components of CAP, has been observed coincidentally with an increase in SP magnitude.[95] Konishi et al.[97] argued that the dual polarity changes in SP that occur rapidly after interruption of O_2 supply are evidence of interference with metabolic processes in the cochlea.

Investigations have shown that N_1 and N_2 reduce earlier and recover later than SP, EP, or CM.[95,97] N_1 is reportedly more resistant than N_2 to O_2 deprivation.[95] Bornschein and Gernandt[92] removed N_1 and N_2 selectively from the composite CM-neural recording by repeated anoxic exposures. Fernandez and Alzate[95] were unable to replicate these findings. In regard to the rapid diminution of the neural potentials by anoxia Konishi et al.[97] argued that the stimulating event for the cochlear nerve fibers, and not their capacity to fire, was the critical factor in N_1 reduction. These authors cited the ability of peripheral nerve fibers to fire when electrically stimulated, even after long periods of anoxia had been in effect.

Dichotomous results are present in the literature with regard to anatomical lesions caused by prolonged O_2 reduction. Falbe-Hansen et al.[102] found no evidence of lesions in guinea pigs and cats deprived of O_2. Lawrence et al.[93] reported on the sites of lesion in the organ of Corti of guinea pigs with inspired low-concentration O_2 (0.5%) at repeated intervals. Although the basal turn usually sustained the greatest amount of damage, there were otherwise no fixed patterns of change. Lesions of the supporting cells preceded hair-cell damage. The greatest amount of degeneration occurred in an animal that had experienced respiratory difficulties as a consequence of respirator dysfunction. Histological preparation of the organ of Corti revealed a collapsed structure with Reissner's membrane covering a misshapen mass of epithelial cells over the entire length of the basilar membrane. Bohne[16] varied periods of anoxia to investigate the effect of ischemia. After the longest anoxic period (2 hr) degeneration was observed in myelinated nerve fibers in the osseous spiral lamina, radial tunnel fibers, and nerve fibers in the inner spiral bundle. Inner hair cell degeneration was more advanced than outer hair cell damage, the opposite of the conditions observed in noise damage. Thalmann and his colleagues have reviewed the effects of biochemically or mechanically produced ischemia in a number of publications.[103-105] A summary of their work indicates that the stria vascularis is more susceptible than the organ of Corti to O_2 deprivation. Strial P-creatine and ATP levels decline even faster than CM or EP during O_2 reduction. ATP levels in the organ of Corti, on the other hand, are hardly affected by O_2-deprivation periods as long as 3 min. Thalmann and his colleagues related this phenomenon to the high glucose and glycogen stores in the organ of Corti, which especially in the apical turns, relies heavily on anaerobic processes. The greater accumulation of succinic dehydrogenase in the basal turn suggests that oxidative processes are more important here.[106]

Cyanide

Cyanide acts effectively as a metabolic inhibitor of oxidative processes in the cochlea.[107-109] After perfusion of the perilymphatic spaces with 50 m*M* cyanide (dissolved in Ringer's solution) an apparent reversible reduction of EP and CM and CAP, with partial recovery, occurs. In Konishi and Kelsey's[108] investigation the organ of Corti potential was reduced from its preperfusion levels of −80 to −100 mV to −25 to −70 mV following cyanide perfusion. Subsequent anodal polarization enhanced CM amplitude. Konishi and Kelsey interpreted their experimental results as evidence that the negative potential of the anoxic scala media was a depolarization potential of the hair cells. Perfusion of the scala tympani with cyanide was more effective in depressing the cochlear potentials than perfusion of scala vestibuli. On this basis the authors reasoned that the stria vascularis was probably not the site of action, because the stria is equally accessible from either scala. The data also suggested that the basilar membrane may be more permeable to cyanide than Reissner's membrane. It should also be noted, however, that Prazma has placed a different interpretation on the data of Konishi and Kelsey (see Chapter 8). This suggests that the stria is *not* equally accessible from either scala.

Thalmann et al.[105] commented that Konishi and Kelsey's[108] experimental techniques resulted in marked charge gradients in perilymph and stria vascularis. Using lower concentrations of cyanide and higher flow rates than Konishi and Kelsey, Thalmann et al.[105] established a high correlation between EP reduction and ATP and P-creatine levels in the stria vascularis, which confirmed the action of cyanide on the strial respiratory process.

Iodoacetate

Iodoacetate, a powerful inhibitor of glycolysis, decreases CM when perfused through the perilymphatic space.[105,110] In addition to reducing the CM to 10% of its original amplitude, iodoacetate application (1 m*M*) resulted in reduced ATP levels, especially in the apical turns. Thalmann et al.[105] suggested that the dependence of ATP reduction on the cochlear turn supports the theory that oxidative processes are more prominent in the basal turn, whereas the apical turns depend on glycolytic processes. Further evidence that confirmed the sites of glycolytic and oxidative processes was Thalmann's observation[105] that the negative organ of Corti potential of the basal turn declined only slightly at a time when large reductions of EP and CM were present after perilymphatic perfusion with iodoacetate.

Heavy Metals

Heavy metals are listed routinely in the literature as ototoxic agents, generally without research support. Among the metals considered as ototoxic are arsenic, cadmium, lead, mercury, zinc, gold, and manganese.

Deafness, tinnitus, and vertigo are infrequent symptoms of arsenical poisoning in man and animals. Rosenwasser[111] discussed a case that involved a man who had been given intravenous injections of arsenic for treatment of depression, following which he developed a unilateral hearing loss of sudden onset. Gradual recovery came after termination of therapy. Arsphenamine (salvarsan) has been used historically in the treatment of lues and trypanosomiasis.[112] Kobrak,[113] among others, described the paradox of assessing the ototoxicity of a drug used to treat a disease known to cause a sensorineural hearing loss. Taylor[114] cited a few cases in which hearing loss resulted from treatment of nonsyphilitic diseases with arsenicals.

Arsenicals have caused injury to the vestibular system of man and animals. Ross and Lederer[115] observed both salvarsan and neosalvarsan to be toxic for the vestibular system when injected into the middle ear. Ehrlich[116] discovered a vestibular disturbance in waltzing mice after arsacetin administration. Johansen[117] reported vestibular disturbances in guinea pigs, but other investigators failed to detect vestibular disturbances or pathology in arsenical poisoning. Tschirren[118] and Miyamoto[119] failed to detect any morphological or physiological abnormalities in atoxyl and/or arsacetin poisoning.

In addition to vestibular disturbances, arsenical intoxication has caused abnormalities of the auditory system. Miyamoto[119] and Werner,[120] in a discussion of the effect of atoxyl on the guinea pig ear, found marked degeneration of the epithelial layer of the stria vascularis and a collapsing of the organ of Corti caused by a depression of Reissner's membrane which, in the late stages, appeared collapsed on the remnants of the cochlea. Degenerative changes of the spiral ganglion and modiolar nerve fibers were also reported. Similar effects of atoxyl were reported by Nakaruma,[121] Ozeni,[122] and Ruedi.[123] Anniko and Wersall[124] showed by electron microscopy that the intermediate and marginal cells of the stria vascularis become swollen and vacuolated within 12 hr of atoxyl administration. These cells were eventually extruded into the endolymphatic space which left wide pericapillary spaces around the strial vasculature. These authors stressed the need for further investigation to determine whether hair-cell and/or neural degeneration was correlated with strial pathology.

Causse et al.[125] studied the effect of arsacetin on the cochlea. Among their findings were loss of Preyer's reflex, reduction of CM, and delayed vestibular disturbances. Osler[126] and Leonard et al.[127] reported marked histopathological changes in the organ of Corti and stria vascularis after arsacetin administration which included collapse of Reissner's membrane, disruption of supporting cells, evidence of pyknotic nuclei in the external outer hair cells, and vacuolization of the cells of Hensen. Injury to the hair cells did not occur without accompanying stria vascularis pathology.

Vertigo and ataxia are frequently cited as symptoms of lead encephalopathy, a central nervous system syndrome that results from ingestion of lead.[128,129] Taylor[114] stated, without further documentation, that deafness resulting from lead poisoning could be of central origin due to vascular deficiencies or the result of an ototoxic effect on the spiral ganglion at the peripheral level.

Ototoxicity resulting from mercury intoxication, which included the triad of vertigo, deafness, and tinnitus, was reported as early as the sixteenth century by Serapius (cited by Westernhagen[130]). Wyss (cited in reference 114) reported the case of two chemists who were deaf and blind at death as a result of mercurial poisoning. As in arsenical intoxication, deafness attributed to mercury, when used in treatment of lues, may have been a symptom of the disease process. In 1953 an outbreak of a neurological disorder was reported in the Minamata Bay area of Japan as a result of the ingestion of methyl mercury from contaminated fish. The clinical features of 121 documented cases of mercurial poisoning were parasthesias of the extremities, ataxia, dysarthria, aphasia, deafness, and blurring of vision from visual-field constriction.[131,132] In a supporting animal study of the effect of acute methyl mercury intoxication on the guinea pig cochlea pathological features noted included degeneration of outer hair cells in the organ of Corti 2½ turns from the base of the cochlea.[133]

Dinitrophenol

Dinitrophenol (DNP), a specific inhibitor of oxidative phosphorylation, has reduced the EP and the ATP and P-creatine levels of the stria vascularis, whether the drug was applied by perilymphatic perfusion or by the vascular route. Reductions in EP occurred only for high concentrations of DNP (1 mM) when the agent was applied by perfusion through the perilymph.[104] A concentration as low as $10^{-6}M$ was sufficient to cause a depression of EP when DNP was injected into the cochlear vasculature. Thalmann et al.[105] speculated that the discrepancy between the concentrations of DNP necessary to decrease the EP and the high strial phosphate levels support the stria vascularis as the locus for action of salicylates, another potent inhibitor of oxidative phosphorylation. Subsequent electrophysiological and biochemical investigations of the action of salicylates have not confirmed this supposition, however. Panayiotopoulos and Stopp[134] demonstrated reduction of CAP, CM, SP, and the cochlear after potential, following perilymphatic perfusion with DNP.

Carbon-Based Compounds

A review of the literature revealed inconclusive evidence of the ototoxic properties of carbon-based compounds such as the solvent carbon tetrachloride and gases, carbon monoxide and carbon disulfide. Histological lesions, as well as perceptive deafness, have been reported in people exposed to carbon tetrachloride.[135] Vertigo, tinnitus, and deafness have been cited as symptoms of carbon monoxide (CO) poisoning; the hearing loss, however, has usually been transitory in nature.[114] Rutenberg (cited in reference 114) reported hemorrhages in the cochlear vasculature as a result of CO intoxication in mice, guinea pigs, and cats. Ruttin (cited in reference 114) reported on three clinical cases of CO poisoning which resulted in vestibular disorders and hearing loss ranging from a slight sensorineural loss to a profound hearing loss. Taylor[114] mentioned temporary deafness, vertigo, and tinnitus as sequelae of carbon disulfide poisoning. Deafness was reportedly the most persistent of the triad of symptoms. Evidence given in a study by Girardi et al.[136] refuted data from previously cited studies. Evaluating the results of their research, these authors concluded that CO, carbon disulfide, and carbon tetrachloride have differential effects on the vestibular and auditory symptoms. These agents never impaired the social hearing level of patients while affecting the vestibular system, presumably through their affinity for the nucleoreticular substance of the brainstem.

Cancer Treatment Drugs

Nitrogen mustard is an alkylating agent used as a cancer chemotherapeutic drug. When administered by the technique of whole-body perfusion it has ototoxic properties.[137–141] Conflicting reports are present in the literature concerning ototoxic effects on the cochlea.[140,141] Schuknecht,[140] in his histological examination of the cochlea of a patient with a bilateral sensorineural hearing loss as a sequela of nitrogen mustard therapy, discovered organ of Corti shrinkage with no hair-cell damage. In a behavioral experiment with cats Cummings[141] produced severe hearing losses by carotid perfusion with nitrogen mustard. Histological studies revealed severe losses of basal and middle-turn inner and outer hair cells.

A number of reports of hearing loss in patients treated with 6-aminonicotinamide (6A-N) for malignant neoplasms[142–144] have been published. As with nitrogen mustard and *cis*-diammine dichloroplatinum (II) intoxication, the resulting high-frequency loss is reversible after the termination of drug therapy.

A study by Kornfield et al.[145] on mice identified lesions of the sprial ligament, epithelium of the external spiral sulcus, and hair cells of the lower basal and upper second turns following 6A-N administration. Bobbin[146] was unable to demonstrate any evidence of cochlear pathology in guinea pigs after 10-mg/kg intraperitoneal injections of 6A-N.

Ototoxicity of *cis*-diammine dichloroplatinum (II) has been evaluated clinically and in experimental animal models.[147,148] The latter investigation revealed loss of the Preyer reflex and destruction of basal-turn outer hair cells with limited destruction of inner hair cells and inner and outer pillar cells following single dosages of 6, 9, 12, or 18 mg/kg of *cis*-diammine dichloroplatinum (II) in the guinea pig.

Because *cis*-diammine dichloroplatinum (II) and 6A-N do not share the same anticancer mechanism and lesions caused by the latter drug appear to be more extensive than those caused by the platinum derivative, it would be premature to speculate on a possible cochlear mechanism for either agent.[145–147]

Tetrodotoxin

One of the model substances used by membrane physiologists is tetrodotoxin, an agent that blocks passive movement of Na^+ across cell membranes.[149] Konishi and Kelsey[108] and Katsuki et al.[150] demonstrated an irreversible decline of CAP after perilymphatic perfusion with tetrodotoxin. The EP and CM were not affected if low concentrations were used. The investigations cited above confirm the supposition that CM generation depends on a different ionic mechanism than that required for the CAP. They also confirmed findings from other sense organs in which the receptor potential was not affected by tetrodotoxin.[151]

Konishi and Kelsey's[108] investigation showed a differential reduction of the low-intensity segment of the CAP function after tetrodotoxin administration, an effect similar to that seen after intense sound exposure, cooling of the cochlea, and intoxication with agents such as procaine. The differential reduction of the low-level segment of the CAP curve presumably reflects the destruction of outer hair cells.

9.3.2 Miscellaneous Chemical Agents

Dimethylsulfoxide

Two reports on the ototoxicity of dimethylsulfoxide appeared in the mid-1960s.[152,153] Lebo et al.[152] examined the effect of chronic application of topical dimethylsulfoxide to the external auditory meati of 10 volunteer convicts. Subjects were evaluated at intervals ranging from 2 to 74 days; they failed to report lethargy, tinnitus, vertigo, changes in auditory acuity, nausea, or gustatory disturbances. Serial audiometric examinations revealed no significant changes in pure-tone thresholds. There was also an absence of any characteristic variation of the normal bacterial flora of the external auditory meatus. Herd et al.[153] reported on a six-year-old girl with dermatomyositis whose skin wounds were treated with an ointment consisting of 1% neomycin and 11% dimethylsulfoxide. One and a half months after treatment the child suffered complete loss of VIII cranial nerve function, vertigo, and nystagmus. Herd et al. concluded that the VIII nerve dysfunction was caused by neomycin ototoxicity exacerbated by increased cutaneous absorption brought about by dimethylsulfoxide.

Nicotine and Tobacco

The paucity of literature on the effect of nicotine and tobacco on the cochlea is highlighted by Larson et al.[154] and Larson and Silvette.[155,156] Despite the lack of research support for the deleterious effect of nicotine and/or tobacco on hearing, physicians have recommended that patients with hearing problems stop smoking[157,158] and nicotine is listed as an ototoxic drug by reviews of cochlear literature.[159,160]

In a review of the late nineteenth and early twentieth century literature Maffei and Miani[161] enumerated numerous audiovestibular deficits purportedly the result of chronic tobacco "intoxication." The list included "general hearing disturbances," tinnitus, vertigo, and vestibular disturbances with accompanying spontaneous nystagmus. Maffei and Miani[161] investigated the effect of tobacco smoke on guinea pigs treated acutely, subacutely, and chronically. Although levels of tobacco smoke inhaled and pathologies present varied considerably by group, the marked alterations included vascular thrombosis, hemorrhages, and edema, mild rarefaction and intercellular edema in the spiral ganglion, vacuolization and cytoplasmic swelling in the organ of Corti, and mucosal atrophy of the Eustachian tube.

Two studies found cochlear pathology in animals treated chronically with nicotine, as cited by Larson et al.[154] Kostencki (cited in reference 162) was unable to find any effect of acute or chronic nicotine treatment on the hearing organ of rabbits. Bobbin and Gondra's[162] paradigm used both chronic and acute nicotine exposures. Acute nicotine exposures, at a dosage of 1 mg/kg, i.v., produced a rise in blood pressure and changes in heart rate but no decrease in cochlear potentials. Reductions in EP, CM, and CAP occurred only in cardiovascular collapse. Intracochlear perfusion with a 10-m*M* nicotine solution (pH 7.2) resulted in a slight reduction of the magnitude of the upper segment of the CAP input/output functions and a 10-dB shift in sensitivity. No changes were seen in EP or CM.

Treatment of guinea pigs with nicotine for 20 days at daily dosages of 1, 5, 10, and 20 mg/kg i.p. produced no change in the amplitude input/output functions of CM or CAP recorded 21 days after the last dosage. An examination of hair-cell scarring, as seen in the surface preparations of Engstrom et al.,[163] revealed no significant differences between the degree of hair-cell damage from saline and from the various dosages of nicitone. Treatment of guinea pigs with nicotine plus exposure to intense sound also demonstrated a lack of effect of nicotine on hair-cell scarring in the cochlea. Because various drugs have exacerbated the effect of intense sound on the cochlea, the failure to show an interaction of nicotine and intense sound emphasizes the absence of toxicity of chronic nicotine exposure on the auditory end organ.

9.3.3 Miscellaneous Therapeutic Agents

Anesthetic Agents, Sedatives, and Tranquilizers

Few reports of the effects of anesthetics on cochlear potentials have appeared in the literature. Henricksen and Merlis[164] reported an elevation in the auditory threshold of cats for high- and low-frequency tones following Nembutal® anesthesia. These authors related these changes to a depression of the respiratory rate and not to temperature decreases or the level of anesthetic per se. Wilpizeski et al.[165] reported that the ototoxicity of ethacrynic acid was enhanced by barbiturate anesthesia as observed in the elevation of the visual-detection level for CM.

Numerous investigators have failed to observe changes in the late auditory-evoked potentials after sedative or anesthetic administration.[166–170] On the other hand, Rapin and Graziani[171] found that the administration of 5 mg of pentobarbital per kilogram of body weight to infants produced fast activity in the ongoing EEG record and obscured the late auditory potentials. Price and Goldstein[167] noted high-voltage background activity and increased background noise activity following Sodium Pentothal® administration. Burian et al.[172] reported changes in response latency and amplitude without threshold elevation after the administration of halothane, meprobamate, chlorprothixene, chlorpromazine, and pentobarbital. Strange[173] evaluated the effects of Atosil®, Nembutal®, Mandrax®, and Valium® on the late auditory-evoked response. Atosil® affected responses the least because it appeared to reduce their amplitude by only 20 to 30% up to 1½ hr after administration. Karnahl and Benning[174] found that Mandrax® and Valium® produced more marked changes in the cortical auditory responses than Atosil®.

It is a clinical axiom that sedatives and/or anesthetics have little or no effect on the early auditory responses.[175] Bobbin et al.[176] found no latency changes in the brainstem-evoked response of guinea pigs following ketamine or Nembutal® administration. Stockard et al.,[177] however, reported temperature-independent changes in wave I-V interwave latencies following enflurane anesthesia.

Overdosages of sedatives, especially barbiturates, are known to cause vestibular symptoms that mimic central pathology of electronystagmography (ENG) tests. Eviatar and Goodhill[178] reviewed the effects of Nembutal® on the vestibular system in detail.

A number of investigations have evaluated the effect of central depressants on the acoustic middle-ear reflex in rabbits. Borg and Moller[179] found that alcohol and pentobarbital have a depressive effect on the middle-ear reflexes of man. Threshold elevation and a decrease in reflex magnitude were much greater for the crossed than for the ipsilateral reflexes. These authors concluded that this differential effect was mediated by nonauditory input into the middle-ear muscles from the reticular formation.

In a clinical investigation Richards et al.[180] demonstrated that pentobarbital had no effect on the intra-aural muscle reflexes at dosages used for the management of convulsive and behavioral disorders. Borg and Moller[181] evaluated the effect of pentobarbital-sodium (Nembutal®, Abbott), enibomal-sodium (Narcotal®, Astra), urethane, urethane-chloralose, and lidocaine (Xylocaine®, Astra) on the middle-ear muscle reflex in animals. All anesthetics, except for the topical anesthetic lidocaine, elevated the contralateral reflex by a greater amount than the ipsilateral reflex. The magnitude of the threshold shift was related to the effect of the anesthetic on the central nervous system. Robinette et al.[182] were unable to demonstrate any effect of secobarbital on static or relative compliance measures, reflex thresholds, or gradient measures in a clinical population.

Alcohol

There is anatomical evidence of central pathology as a sequela of chronic alcoholic intoxication. Pathological foci have been found in the hypothalamus, third ventricle, and periaqueductal gray of chronic alcoholics.[183] Victor et al.[184] described various gross central nervous system changes in the brains of alcoholics with Wernicke-Korsakoff syndrome; degenerative changes included convolutional atrophy, enlargement of third and lateral ventricles, and the inferior colliculus. Small, circumscribed lesions were also reported in the medial geniculate body.

Basili and Tobin[185] examined the performance of non-Korsakoff alcoholics on a battery of central auditory tasks which included the Token Test of DeRenzi and Vignolo, Pitch Pattern Recognition by Pinheiro, Interaural Intensity Difference for Sound Lateralization by Pinheiro and Tobin, and Low Pass Filtered Speech from Willeford's battery. These tasks assess the integrity of the auditory central nervous system from the brainstem to the auditory cortex. Statistically significant differences were seen from control scores for alcoholics on the Low Pass Filtered Speech and Pinheiro's Pitch Pattern Test. These results are symptomatic of brainstem and/or auditory-cortex pathology. Spitzer[186] examined the central auditory function of 15 non-Korsakoff alcoholics on a variety of tasks, which included the Performance Intensity for Phonetically Balanced Words (PIPB) function, Staggered Spondaic Words (SSW), and Synthetic Sentence Index (SSI) with ipsilateral and contralateral competing messages. Although variability was high on nearly all measures, only one alcoholic performed within normal limits on all tasks.

Investigations of the effect of alcohol on the Acoustic Reflex Threshold (ART) have been conducted by Spitzer,[186] Borg and Moller,[187] Cohill and Greenberg,[188] and Robinette and Brey.[189] Borg and Moller[187] examined changes in acoustic impedance before and after oral administration of ethyl alcohol which raised blood level concentrations from 0.02 to 0.15%. Among the authors' major findings were the following:

1 There were no frequency-dependent effects in elevations of the acoustic reflex.

2 The contralateral and ipsilateral reflexes appeared to be equally susceptible to the influence of ethyl alcohol.

3 A blood concentration of 0.13% was necessary to raise the acoustic reflex threshold by 10 dB. A similar elevation (11 dB) was seen by Cohill and Greenberg[188] in patients who had consumed 30 ml of alcohol. Robinette and Brey[189] reported blood levels of 0.15% to raise the reflex threshold at 500 Hz by about 4 to 5 dB.

4 Ethanol did not change the slope of the crossed and uncrossed reflexes. This indicates that there was no greater reduction of the amplitude of the acoustic reflex at suprathreshold as opposed to threshold levels. Robinette and Brey[189] found ARTs to be elevated at 500 Hz after ingestion of enough alcohol to raise blood levels from 0.09 to 0.15%. In addition to elevation of threshold, reflex magnitudes decreased and TTS caused by concomitantly applied noise increased. Spitzer[186] found 27 absent reflexes among her chronic alcoholic population compared with seven in her normal population.

Reports of sensorineural hearing loss (peripheral hearing loss), tinnitus, and auditory hallucinations have been largely anecdotal in nature.[190–192] A histopathological examination of the temporal bones of 16 alcoholics failed to confirm a peripheral site of lesion.[193] Studies on pure-tone sensitivity of alcoholics were equally as inconclusive; for example, Nordahl[194] found that in a population of 83 institutionalized alcoholics only 17% had a sensorineural hearing loss. The author speculated that age, occupational hearing loss, and/or socioacousis could be factors in the segment of the population with pure-tone losses. On the other hand, Montanti and Paterni[195] discovered sensorineural hearing loss in 15 of 16 alcoholics.

There have been only a few investigations of the effect of alcohol ingestion on the late components of the auditory-evoked response reported in the literature.[196] These investigations reported central nervous system dysfunction at the cortical level. Stockard et al.[197] reported on the brainstem-evoked response of two chronic alcoholics with diagnosed cases of central pontine myelinolysis. Reductions in wave V amplitude and longer conduction times were correlated with severity of the clinical manifestations of the central nervous system disorder. Prolongation of wave I–V interwave latency has been reported in chronic alcoholic intoxication and a decrease in this latency period during withdrawal.[198]

Vertigo is commonly reported as a presenting symptom by acute and chronic alcoholics. As discussed by Aschan et al.,[199] the effects of alcohol intoxication probably originate at the vestibular periphery and cause a positional alcohol nystagmus I or II, depending on head position.

Anti-Inflammatory Agents and Analgesics

Although there is considerable documentation of the ototoxicity of salicylates, there is a great deal of confusion in the literature with regard to site of action, reversibility of effect(s), and modus operandi. In high therapeutic dosages salicylates, particularly in the form of aspirin, have been known to cause hearing loss, tinnitus, and vertigo, usually of a transient nature.[200–204] Reports of hearing loss of a permanent nature have also been reported.[205–209] Although a permanent hearing loss cannot be discounted as a şequela of salicylate ototoxicity, many of these reports must be suspected because of simultaneous treatment with another ototoxic agent, inadequate means of assessing hearing loss, and hearing loss resulting from a coexisting disease entity.

Waltner[207] reported a bilaterally symmetrical 50-to-60 dB sensorineural hearing loss and recruitment in a patient who had ingested 200 aspirins to alleviate rheumatitis pain. There was a nearly equal threshold elevation at all frequencies, a finding replicated by Myers et al.[210] Two days after the termination of aspirin treatment the patient reported a recovery of hearing and alleviation of tinnitus. Vestibular tests were also normal at this time. At seven days posttreatment auditory thresholds had returned to normal. McCabe and Dey[202] found that hearing loss after salicylate intoxication was as much as 20 dB greater for the high tones (6 kHz), compared with low-frequency tones (250 Hz). Falbe-Hansen[200] reported both conductive and high-frequency perceptive loss as symptoms of salicylate toxicity. He drew an analogy to Meniere's syndrome and suggested that salicylates caused an increased secretion of perilymph which resulted in elevated labyrinthine pressure that impeded normal movement of the round and oval windows. Falbe-Hansen's conclusions are not supported by the high-frequency losses reported because of the characteristic low-frequency tilt to the audiogram of patients with Meniere's.

Bernstein and Weiss[204] administered a battery of peripheral and central auditory and vestibular tests to patients with rheumatoid arthritis who were administered acetylsalicylic acid as part of a therapeutic regimen. Tests administered included sweep frequency Bekesy audiometry, tests of phonetic-balance word discrimination, filtered speech, and caloric testing. Results of the test battery supported a peripheral (cochlear) site of action of the toxic agent.

Silverstein et al.[211] evaluated the effect of a single intraperitoneal infusion of salicylate (350 mg/kg) on CM and CAP of the cochlea of the cat. Two to three hours after salicylate infusion the sensitivity of CM increased by as much as 25 dB, in addition to a 40% reduction of CM amplitude and a 70% reduction of CAP voltage. Mitchell et al.[212] were unable to replicate the finding of Silverstein et al.[211] They did, however, find a transient reduction in CAP sensitivity (threshold). These authors concluded that salicylate's site of action may be presynaptic at the synapse or postsynaptic. Gold and Wilpizeski[213] found a 10-to-13-dB increase in sensitivity of response recorded from the cochlear nucleus after salicylate intoxication. These authors suggested inappropriately that this evidence confirmed a cochlear site of action of salicylate. Thalmann[104] reported an absence of effect of dosages up to 500 mg/kg of sodium salicylate on EP and only a slight effect on CM. The low-intensity segment of the CAP input/output curve, however, was eliminated with only slight reductions in the magnitude of the high-level response.[214]

A great deal of controversy in the literature surrounds the effect of salicylate on cochlear structures. A number of investigations have reported that salicylates cause degenerative changes in the spiral ganglion.[215–217] Covell's[218] experimental studies on salicylate intoxication revealed damage to the mitochondria of the outer hair cells and scala vestibuli. He did not observe ischemic changes in the caliber of the stria vascularis blood vessels. Vascular hemorrhages and constriction have been observed on post-mortem fixation in a variety of intralabyrinthine locations, which include capillaries of the suprastrial spiral ligament, stria vascularis, and basilar membrane.[217] Other investigators have shown no evidence of pathology of the auditory or vestibular structures following salicylate poisoning.[203] A recent report by Aly et al.[219] revealed a loss of Reissner's membrane and flattening of the epithelial elements of the organ of Corti of the guinea pig after daily oral ingestion of 0.13 gm/kg dosages of salicylates for two months.

There is evidence that salicylate affects at least three groups of cellular enzymes[220]; for example, it is now known that salicylates uncouple oxidative phosphorylation, although there is still conjecture regarding their site of action. Lutwak-Mann[221] identified salicylate-induced inhibition of succinic dehydrogenase, cytochrome oxidase, and other enzymes in liver slices. Salicylates are known to affect transamination and dehydrogenation, but whether the levels attained in the cochlear tissues are sufficient to inhibit the respective enzyme systems is a matter of conjecture.[111] Silverstein et al.[211] reported that an elevation of glucose and a decrease in malic dehydrogenase correlated with elevations of serum levels of sodium salicylate and decreased CM and CAP output from the cochlea.

Because of the well-documented high metabolic rate of activity of the stria vascularis and the marked effect of 2,4-dinitrophenol, another inhibitor of oxidative phosphorylation on the EP,[223] it was once believed that the stria vascularis was the locus of action of salicylates. Thalmann,[104] however, was unable to find evidence of reduced ATP and P-creatine levels or EP losses following salicylate administration. Other investigators were unable to find alterations in the organ of Corti, auditory nerve, or spiral ganglion at dosages up to 400 mg/kg. Thalmann[104] suggested that the site of salicylate action was at the infranuclear region of the hair cells and/or the postsynaptic nerve endings, both rich in mitochondria but not accessible to standard biochemical analyses with existing techniques.

Among the side effects of indomethacin, a nonsteroidal inflammatory agent used in the treatment of rheumatoid arthritis and related disorders, are dizziness, vertigo, and temporary hearing loss.[224,225] Hawkins[112] suggested that the mode of action of the salicylates was to inhibit prostaglandin synthetase, thus effecting prostaglandin synthesis and the caliber of the cochlear vasculature. Brune et al.[222] demonstrated a similar action of indomethacin on prostaglandin synthetase. Brown and Feldman[226] suggested that indomethacin application may upset the homeostasis of the cochlear fluids in a similar manner to its known action on cerebrospinal fluid.

Antihistamines

Wood et al.[227] reviewed the side effects of a variety of antihistamines used as antimotion sickness drugs. Both diphenhydramine (Benadryl®) and dimenhydrinate (Dramamine®) reportedly cause dizziness and vertigo. Other antihistamines, such as meclizine and cyclizine, were considered superior because of their milder side effects. Douglas[228] enumerated a number of undesirable central nervous system side effects of antihistamines, including tinnitus.

Diuretics Other than Loop Diuretics

Mercurial diuretics have several features in common with "loop diuretics"; for example, the susceptibility of renal adenylate cyclase and Na/K ATPase to both groups of drugs, a renal site of action, and an effect on the EP and CM of the cochlea.[229]

A number of marked differences in the action of mercurial and loop diuretics on the cochlea, however, include the following anatomical, electrophysiological, and biochemical variations:

1 Marked reduction of the negative organ of Corti potential by mercurial diuretics.
2 Degeneration of membranes of outer hair cells and obliteration of fluid spaces in the organ of Corti by mercurial diuretics.
3 Interference with strial Na/K ATPase by mercurials. Thalmann et al.[229] concluded that the action of the mercurial diuretics on the cochlea

results from complex mechanisms such as interference with enzyme generation and use at the strial level and gross morphological alterations at the hair-cell level.

Local Anesthetics and Topically Applied Agents

Clinical reports of hearing loss following nonaural, topical application of the aminoglycosides have reemphasized their ototoxicity. Neomycin induces ototoxicity following topical administration to the skin of burn patients[230] and following rectal or colonic irrigation.[231] Aminoglycosides are particularly well absorbed from bronchial,[232] intrapleural,[233] and intraperitoneal sites.[234] The use of local anesthetics for middle-ear surgery has been well documented.[235,236] Numerous studies have cautioned against their use because of the nonreversible alterations of auditory function. Athough most investigations use the method of topical administration to the external auditory meatus or middle ear (usually round window), other studies have been performed with parentally administered drugs; for example, whereas intramuscular lidocaine or mepivacaine produced no change in cochlear electrical activity,[237] intravenously administered procaine was reported to cause considerable increases in auditory thresholds.[238] Increased intralabyrinthine pressure was implicated as the probable cause of the change in auditory sensitivity.

Reversible and nonreversible changes in CM and CAP input-output curves were indicated after the application of local anesthetics to the round window. These changes included shifts in sensitivity and reduction in maximum output of both classes of potential. Recovery of function and magnitude of loss appeared to be related to concentration and number of applications; for example, Rahm et al.[235,236] demonstrated reversible changes in cochlear response with procaine hydrochloride (2%) and hexylcaine hydrochloride (1%) and permanent losses with hexylcaine hydrochloride (5%) and cocaine (10%). Strother et al.[239] demonstrated a 6-dB decrease in CM amplitude after a single cocaine application (10%) and a 10-dB reduction after lidocaine (0.5%). Following a second application of cocaine (10%), CM output was reduced 38 dB.

Epinephrine has been applied separately[240,241] and with local anesthetics.[237,242] No deleterious effects have been reported on the organ of Corti that appear to be due to epinephrine, regardless of the method of application of epinephrine.

Perfusion of the perilymph with lidocaine decreases CM and CAP; the effect on CAP is approximately four times greater than the effect on CM.[243] The low-intensity segment of the CAP input/output curve was eliminated after lidocaine perfusion without affecting the high intensity portion of the curve, a phenomenon analogous to recruitment. CAP was rapidly depressed when 0.05 to 0.1% procaine was introduced into the scala tympani[59]; CM was depressed when procaine was applied to scala media or scala tympani.

The EP was reportedly increased after procaine perfusion into either labyrinthine chamber. From these results the authors concluded that procaine interfered with K^+ permeability. Reduction of endolymph K^+ has been shown to eliminate the ionic asymmetry of endolymph and perilymph necessary for CM production. Potassium-rich endolymph is important to the sensitivity of the hair cells to sound stimulation, production of CM, and the inhibitory effect of procaine.[59]

Intratympanic Ototoxicity of Antibiotics and Miscellaneous Drugs

The effects of systemic administration of aminoglycosides on the ear are well documented. Fewer accounts of ototopical applications are available.[244]

Schuknecht[245] studied the effect of streptomycin injected into the auditory bullae of cats. As would be expected, auditory and vestibular symptoms produced were dose-dependent. Cats given an injection of 0.50 g in a 1 cm^3 of water experienced a severe disequilibrium reaction that consisted of nystagmus, falling, nausea, vomiting, and ataxia. Animals given a 0.25-g injection of streptomycin in saline experienced a less severe equilibrium problem. Histological examination of the auditory and vestibular systems demonstrated a severe hair-cell loss in the cristae and maculae of the vestibule and degeneration of hair cells in the basilar turn of the organ of Corti. Davis and associates[20] confirmed Schuknecht's observation of outer hair-cell reduction with streptomycin application. Schuknecht[245] also demonstrated ablation of vestibular and auditory function in humans treated with streptomycin injections (intratympanic, 0.125 g/cm^3) for amelioration of symptoms of Meniere's disease.

Many authors have voiced concern over the possibility of otic trauma induced by intratympanic therapy with commercially available drugs that contain neomycin.[246] Results of experimental studies do not uniformly confirm this supposition. Mittelman[244] was unable to discover any histological evidence of cochlear damage following round-window application of neomycin in guinea pigs. Riskaer et al.[247] corroborated Mittelman's finding in a behavioral study of the ototoxic effects of neomycin applied to the external and middle ear of guinea pigs. On the other hand, Kohonen and Tarkkanen[248] found that application of relatively low, multiple concentrations of neomycin caused varying hair-cell degeneration patterns. Brummett et al.[146] demonstrated hair-cell loss and reduced CM following multiple neomycin and polymyxin-B application.

Mittelman[244] reviewed the effects of topical application of gentamicin on the cochlea. Two experimental investigations with animals revealed dose-related changes in the vestibular sensory epithelia and cochlear hair cells.[249,250] Federspil[251] was unable to obtain evidence of ototoxicity of gentamicin in a clinical group of 19 patients treated for radical cavity infections and otitis externa.

Unlike aminoglycosides, neurotoxic polymyxins and tetracyclines are not ototoxic when given systemically.[252] Polymyxin-B, choramphenicol, and erythromycin, however, have all been shown to have ototoxic properties when applied topically.[246,248,252–254]

Interaction of Intense Sound with Drugs

Experimental paradigms that involve the administration of drugs before or following intense-sound exposure have produced varying results. Drugs have been shown to potentiate the effect of intense sound, to protect the ear from injurious levels of sound, and to have no interaction with intense sound.[255] Exposure to high levels of industrial and recreational intense sound in modern society has promulgated interest in the interaction of antibiotics and intense sound.[256,257]

Dayal et al.[256] investigated the effect of incubator noise (68 to 72 dB) on kanamycin-treated guinea pigs. Using the surface-preparation technique to evaluate the status of hair cells, they showed an interaction of drug dosage and intense sound. These authors suggested that nontoxic dosages of kanamycin ''sensitized'' the hair cells to damage from subsequent intense-sound exposure. Darrouzet and Sabrenho[258] showed an order effect in their study of the reaction of the cochlea to intense sound and kanamycin. These authors demonstrated that intense sound followed by kanamycin treatment were more injurious to the cochlea than the reverse order of ototraumatic agents. Vernon et al.[259] found no interaction between kanamycin and acoustic overloads.

Jauhiainen et al.[260] studied the effect of intense sound and neomycin on guinea-pig cochlear anatomy and electrophysiological potentials. Greater losses of cochlear potentials and hair cells were evident in the drug-plus-intense-sound group at all frequency (250 Hz to 4 kHz)–intensity (60 to 100 dB SPL) combinations. On the other hand, Hawkins et al.[261] found a slight interaction between neomycin and acoustic overloads only when excessively intense sound levels were used.

Woodford et al.[257] were unable to demonstrate an interaction between sodium salicylate and various TTS-producing intense-sound paradigms. Vernon et al.[259] failed to expose interaction between intense-sound exposure and ethacrynic acid. Vernon's investigation was designed to maximize any possible potentiation effect of the combination of drug and intense sound rather than to examine a possible protective effect afforded the ear by pretreatment with a diuretic.

Bobbin et al.[262] investigated the interaction of aminooxyacetic acid (AOAA) and in intense-sound exposure (127 dB SPL and 4 kHz for 30 min). Decreased permanent hair-cell damage revealed by surface preparations of the drug-plus-intense-sound group indicated that AOAA provided the cochlea with a protective effect. Bobbin explained his results within the framework of an adaptation of Davis' battery model. Davis' model was extended by suggesting that excess current flow (apparently K^+) occurs dur-

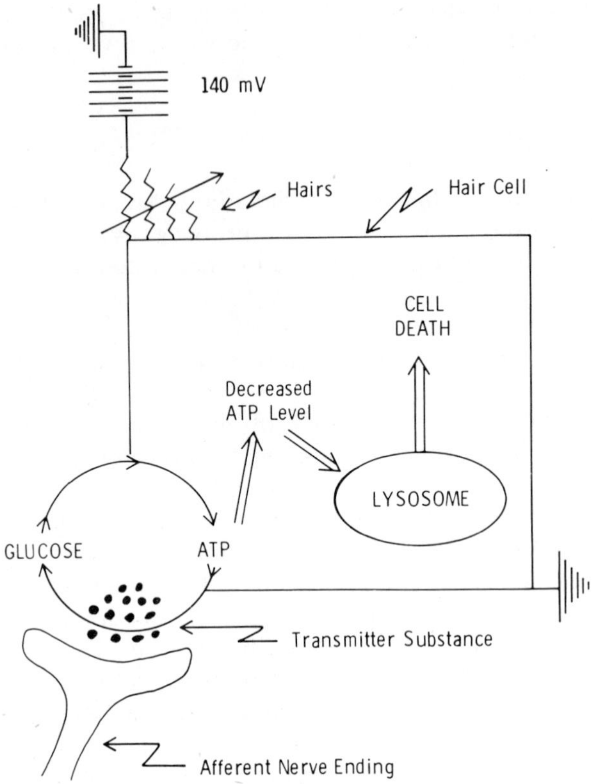

Figure 9.4 Bobbin et al.'s[262] model of the effect of intense sound on the cochlea (see text for detail).

ing hair-cell-damaging–intense-sound exposure. These abnormal current levels result in reduced ATP stores, lysosome breakdown, and eventual cell death (see Figure 9.4). Bobbin proposed that pretreatment with AOAA would result in a decreased EP, thus preventing injurious levels of current from flowing to the hair cell, therefore alleviating damage from noise. Kisiel[263] further evaluated Bobbin et al.'s[262] hypothesis of the effect of intense sound on the cochlea in his investigation of changes in round-window-recorded CM and CAP following a combined EA– or AOAA–intense sound treatment. Only differences in CM sensitivity were present when comparing the intense-sound-drug and intense-sound-alone groups. Kisiel speculated that the inability to observe other effects could be related to inadequacies of the recording technique used, the selection of the particular drugs and/or intense-sound parameters, or to the CM and CAP monitoring periods.

ACKNOWLEDGMENTS

We wish to acknowledge the assistance of Sandy Kisiel, Pam Burrell, Gae Decker, and Madeline Bobbin. Research was supported by the National Institutes of Health (Clinical Research Center Grant), USPHS NS-11647 and the Deafness Research Foundation. Laboratory facilities were provided by the Kresge Foundation.

REFERENCES

1. P. Dallos, *The Auditory Periphery: Biophysics and Physiology*, Academic, New York, 1973.
2. C. A. Smith and J. A. Vernon, *Handbook of Auditory and Vestibular Research Methods*, Thomas, Springfield, Ill., 1976.
3. C. Fernandez, H. Singh, and H. Perlman, *Acta Oto Laryngol.*, **49,** 189 (1958).
4. A. C. Coats, *Science*, **150,** 1481 (1965).
5. M. B. Meikle and J. Vernon, *J. Acoust. Soc. Am.*, **54,** 99 (1973).
6. D. G. Drescher, *Science*, **185,** 273 (1974).
7. D. G. Drescher, *J. Acoust. Soc. Am.*, **59,** 401 (1976).
8. R. A. Butler, T. Konishi, and C. Fernandez, *Am. J. Physiol.*, **199,** 688 (1960).
9. J. J. Stockard, F. W. Sharbrough, and J. A. Tinker, *Ann. Neurol.*, **3,** 368 (1978).
10. D. J. Lim and W. Melnick, *AGARD Conf. Proc.*, **171,** AGARD, Washington, D.C. (1975).
11. M. Lawrence and P. D. Yantis, *Ann. Otol. Rhinol. Laryngol.*, **66,** 595 (1957).
12. W. D. Ward and A. J. Duvall, *Ann. Otol.*, **80,** 881 (1971).
13. D. H. Eldredge, W. P. Covell, and H. Davis, *Laryngoscope*, **67,** 66 (1957).
14. H. H. Spoendlin, in *Effects of Noise on Hearing*, Raven, New York, 1976, p. 69.
15. H. A. Beagley, *Acta Oto Laryngol.*, **60,** 437 (1965).
16. B. A. Bohne, "Scar Formation in the Inner Ear Following Acoustical Injury. Sequence of Changes from Early Signs of Damage to Healed Lesion." Unpublished Doctoral Dissertation, Washington University, St. Louis, Mo., 1971.
17. B. A. Bohne, in *Effects of Noise on Hearing*, Raven, New York, 1976, p. 41.
18. D. J. Lim and W. Melnick, *Arch. Otolaryngol.*, **94,** 294 (1971).
19. H. H. Spoendlin, *Acta Oto Laryngol.*, **71,** 166 (1971).
20. H. Davis, R. W. Benson, W. P. Covell, C. Fernandez, R. Goldstein, Y. Katsuki, J.-P. Legouix, D. R. McAuliffe, and I. Tasaki, *J. Acoust. Soc. Am.*, **25,** 1180 (1953).
21. M. H. Lurie, *J. Acoust. Soc. Am.*, **11,** 420 (1940).
22. H. Voldrich, *Acta Oto Laryngol.*, **74,** 392 (1972).
23. M. Lawrence, G. Gonzalez, and J. E. Hawkins, *Am. Ind. Hyg. Assoc. J.*, **28,** 425 (1967).
24. J. E. Hawkins, *Ann. Otol. Rhinol. Laryngol.*, **80,** 903 (1971).
25. J. E. Hawkins, *Laryngoscope*, **82,** 1091 (1972).
26. D. M. Lipscomb and R. L. Roettger, *Laryngoscope*, **83,** 259 (1973).
27. J. E. Hawkins, in *Auditory System: Clinical and Special Topics, Handbook of Sensory Physiology, Vol. V/3*, Springer, Berlin, 1976, p. 707.
28. R. P. Bobbin and M. I. Gondra, *Ann. Otol. Rhinol. Laryngol.*, **85**(2), 247 (1976).

29. B. Kellerhals, *Acta Oto Laryngol.*, **73,** 249 (1972).
30. J. Durrant, in *Noise and Audiology*, University Park, Baltimore, 1978, p. 122.
31. A. J. Duvall, W. D. Ward, and K. E. Lauhala, *Ann. Otol. Rhinol. Laryngol.*, **83,** 498 (1974).
32. H. B. Perlman and R. Kimura, *Acta Oto Laryngol.*, **54,** 99 (1962).
33. H. H. Spoendlin and J. P. Brun, *Acta Oto Laryngol.*, **75,** 220 (1973).
34. H. Engstrom and H. W. Ades, *Acta Oto Laryngol. Suppl.*, **158,** 219 (1960).
35. H. H. Spoendlin, *Ann. Otol. Rhinol. Laryngol.*, **71,** 657 (1962).
36. H. A. Beagley, *Acta Oto Laryngol.*, **60,** 479 (1965).
37. H. Kraus, W. Richrath, L. Dullweber, D. Gerbig, R. Prieshof, and J. Tillman, *Acta Oto Laryngol.*, **80,** 230 (1975).
38. K. H. Vosteen, *Arch. Otorhinolaryngol.*, **172,** 489 (1958).
39. D. Ishii, T. Takahashi, and K. Balogy, *Acta Oto Laryngol.*, **67,** 573 (1969).
40. R. Thalmann, T. Miyoshi, and I. Thalmann, *Laryngoscope*, **82,** 2249 (1972).
41. C. W. Stockwell, H. W. Ades, and H. Engstrom, *Ann. Otol. Rhinol. Laryngol.*, **78,** 1144 (1969).
42. B. A. Bohne, D. H. Eldredge, and J. H. Mills, *Ann. Otol.*, **82,** 595 (1973).
43. D. H. Eldredge, J. D. Miller, *ASHA Report* **4,** 110 (1969).
44. D. H. Eldredge, J. H. Mills, and B. A. Bohne, *Adv. Otorhinolaryngol.*, **20,** 64 (1973).
45. I. E. Alexander and F. J. Githler, *J. Comp. Physiol. Psychol.*, **44,** 513 (1951).
46. D. Henderson, R. Hamernik, and R. Sitler, *Arch. Otolaryngol.*, **99,** 62 (1974).
47. D. H. Eldredge, *J. Acoust. Soc. Am.*, **510,** 84th Meeting of the Acoustical Society of America (July 1972).
48. M. Pinheiro, V. Jordan, and G. A. Luz, *Acta Oto Laryngol. Suppl.*, **312,** 31 (1973).
49. W. D. Neff, *J. Comp. Physiol. Psychol.*, **40,** 203 (1947).
50. H. F. Schuknecht, in *Neural Mechanisms of the Auditory and Vestibular Systems*, Thomas, Springfield, Ill., 1960.
51. E. C. Carterette, *J. Speech Hear. Res.*, **12,** 497 (1969).
52. G. A. Misrahy, K. M. Hildreth, E. W. Shinabarger, E. W. Clark, and E. A. Rice, *J. Acoust. Soc. Am.*, **30,** 247 (1958).
53. F. Suga, J. B. Snow, W. J. Preston, and J. L. Glomset, *Laryngoscope*, **77,** 784 (1967).
54. V. Honrubia and P. H. Ward, *J. Acoust. Soc. Am.*, **48,** 388 (1969).
55. V. Honrubia and P. H. Ward, *J. Acoust. Soc. Am.*, **47,** 498 (1970).
56. L. D. Benitez, D. H. Eldredge, and J. T. Templer, *J. Acoust. Soc. Am.*, **52,** 1115 (1972).
57. B. M. Johnstone and P. M. Sellick, *J. Oto Laryngol. Soc. Aust.*, **3,** 317 (1972).
58. T. Konishi and E. Kelsey, *J. Acoust. Soc. Am.*, **43,** 462 (1968).
59. T. Konishi and E. Kelsey, *J. Acoust. Soc. Am.*, **43,** 471 (1968).
60. G. R. Price, *J. Acoust. Soc. Am.*, **44,** 1541 (1968).
61. W. A. Rosenblith, R. Galambos, and I. J. Hirsch, *Science*, **111,** 569 (1950).
62. J. D. Durrant, in *Effects of Noise on Hearing*, Raven, New York, 1976, p. 179.
63. J. Tonndorf and F. A. Brogan, USAF Sch. Aviat. Med. Proj., #21-27-001, Rep. #6 (1952).
64. J. Tonndorf, R. W. Hyde, and F. A. Brogan, *Ann. Otol. Rhinol. Laryngol.*, **64,** 392 (1955).
65. E. G. Wever and M. Lawrence, *J. Acoust. Soc. Am.*, **27,** 853 (1955).
66. D. H. Eldredge, R. C. Bilger, H. Davis, and W. P. Covell, *J. Acoust. Soc. Am.*, **33,** 152 (1961).

67. J. E. Hawkins, L. G. Johnsson, W. C. Stebbins, D. B. Moody, and S. L. Coombs, *Acta Oto Laryngol.*, **81,** 337 (1976).

68. I. E. Alexander and F. J. Githler, *J. Comp. Physiol. Psychol.*, **45,** 381 (1952).

69. H. Davis, in *Sensory Communication*, Wiley, New York, 1961, p. 119.

70. D. C. Teas, D. H. Eldredge, and H. Davis, *J. Acoust. Soc. Am.*, **34,** 1438 (1962).

71. J. E. Pugh, M. P. Horowitz, and D. J. Anderson, *Arch. Otolaryngol.*, **100,** 36 (1974).

72. H. Sohmer and H. Pratt, *Audiology*, **14,** 130 (1975).

73. C. Mitchell, R. Brummett, and J. Vernon, *Arch. Otolaryngol.*, **103,** 117 (1977).

74. D. Henderson and R. P. Hamernik, in *Noise and Audiology*, University Park, Baltimore, 1978, p. 143.

75. V. M. Jordan, M. L. Pinheiro, K. Chiba, and A. Jimenez, *Acta Oto Laryngol. Suppl.*, **312,** 16 (1973).

76. D. B. Moody, W. C. Stebbins, J. E. Hawkins and L. Johnsson, *Arch. Otorhinolaryngol.*, **220,** 47 (1978).

77. R. P. Hamernick, D. Henderson, D. S. Dosanjh, and R. Sitler, "Impulse Noise: Some Electrophysiological and Anatomical Effects," paper read at Seventh International Congress of Acoustics, Budapest (1971).

78. B. Kellerhals, H. Engstrom, H. W. Ades, *Acta Oto Laryngol. Suppl.*, **226,** 72 (1967).

79. D. H. Eldredge and W. P. Covell, *Laryngoscope*, **68,** 465 (1958).

80. G. A. Luz, J. L. Fletcher, W. J. Travel, and J. D. Mosko, *Acta Oto Laryngol. Suppl.*, **312** (1973).

81. W. Melnick, in *Noise and Audiology*, University Park, Baltimore, p. 83, 1978.

82. W. D. Ward, *J. Acoust. Soc. Am.*, **34,** 1230 (1962).

83. W. D. Ward, W. Selters, and A. Glorig, *J. Acoust. Soc. Am.*, **33,** 781 (1961).

84. R. W. Sitler, "The Effect of Impulse Noise on the Auditory Mechanism of the Chinchilla," unpublished doctoral dissertation, Syracuse University, New York, 1972.

85. A. Cohen, G. Kylin, and P. LaBenz, *J. Acoust. Soc. Am.*, **40,** 1371 (1966).

86. J. G. Walker, *J. Sound. Vib.*, **24,** 493 (1972).

87. T. Jauhiainen, A. Kohonen, J. Tarkkanen, and M. Kaimo, *Laryngoscope*, **79,** 1950 (1969).

88. T. Yokoyama, S. Osako, and K. Yamamoto, *Acta Oto Laryngol.*, **78,** 207 (1974).

89. E. Aantaa, E. Virolainen, and V. Karskela, *Acta Oto Laryngol.*, **83,** 479 (1977).

90. J. R. Lackner and A. Graybiel, *Aerospace Med.*, **45,** 1267 (1974).

91. E. G. Wever, M. Lawrence, R. W. Hemphill, and C. B. Straut, *Am. J. Physiol.*, **159,** 199 (1949).

92. H. Bornschein and B. Gernandt, *Acta Physiol. Scand.*, **21,** 82 (1950).

93. M. Lawrence, A. Nuttall, and P. Burgio, *Ann. Otol.*, **84,** 499 (1975).

94. K. G. Wing, J. D. Harris, A. D. Stover, and J. H. Brouillette, U. S. Naval Medical Research Laboratory, Research Report 188 (1952).

95. C. Fernandez and R. Alzate, *Arch. Otolaryngol.*, **69,** 82 (1959).

96. H. B. Perlman, R. Kimura, and C. Fernandez, *Laryngoscope*, **69,** 591 (1951).

97. T. Konishi, R. A. Butler, and C. Fernandez, *J. Acoust. Soc. Am.*, **33,** 349 (1961).

98. G. A. Misrahy, E. W. Shinabarger, and J. E. Arnold, *J. Acoust. Soc. Am.*, **30,** 701 (1958).

99. O. Sugar and R. W. Gerard, *J. Neurophysiol.*, **1,** 558 (1938).

100. L. Gisselsson, *Acta Oto Laryngol.*, **2,** 106 (1954).

101. R. Goldstein, *Am. J. Physiol.*, **178,** 331 (1954).

102. J. Falbe-Hansen, E. Christensen, L. Gisselsson, H. J. Hansen, and P. M. Permm, *Arch. Otolaryngol.*, **67,** 71 (1958).

103. F. M. Matchinsky and R. Thalmann, *Laryngoscope*, **77**, 292 (1967).

104. R. Thalmann, in *The Nervous System: Human Communication and its Disorders*, Vol. 3, Raven, New York, 1975, p. 31.

105. R. Thalmann, I, Thalmann, I. Ise, and S. Paloheimo, *Laryngoscope*, **86**, 699 (1976).

106. K. L. Horn, L. R. Langley, and G. A. Gates, *Arch. Otolaryngol.*, **104**, 42 (1978).

107. H. Davis, I. Tasaki, C. A. Smith, and B. H. Deatherage, *Fed. Proc.*, **14**, 112 (1955).

108. T. Konishi and E. Kelsey, *Acta Oto Laryngol.*, **65**, 381 (1968).

109. R. Thalmann, J. Kusakari, and T. Miyoshi, *Laryngoscope*, **83**, 1690 (1973).

110. H. Bornschein and R. Thalmann, *Experientia*, **19**, 413 (1963).

111. H. Rosenwasser, *Arch. Otolaryngol.*, **15**, 284 (1932).

112. J. E. Hawkins, in *Auditory System: Clinical and Special Topics (Handbook of Sensory Physiology, Vol. V/3)*, Springer, Berlin, 1976, p. 707.

113. F. Kobrak, *Ohres. Klin. Wschr.*, **5**, 1572 (1926).

114. H. M. Taylor, *Laryngoscope*, **47**, 692 (1937).

115. E. L. Ross and L. G. Lederer, *Laryngoscope*, **47**, 555 (1937).

116. P. Ehrlich, *Berl. Klin. Wschr.*, **44**, 280 (1907).

117. H. Johansen, *Proc. Fifth Int. Congr. Otolaryngol.*, 579 (1953).

118. B. Tschirren, *Pract. Otorhinolaryngol.*, **19**, 416 (1957).

119. T. Miyamoto, *Arb. Med. Univ. Okayama*, **2**, 412 (1931).

120. C. F. Werner, in *Bau, Funktion and Krankheiten des Innenohres vom Standpunkte lines experimentellen und Vergleichenden Pathologie*, Thieme, Leipzig, 1940.

121. H. Nakaruma, *Z. Oto. Rhino. Laryngol.*, **41**, (1935).

122. J. Ozeni, *Z. Oto. Rhino. Laryngol.*, **43**, (1937).

123. L. Ruedi, *The Scientific Papers of the American Otological Society*, **88**, 993 (1951).

124. M. Anniko and J. Wersall, *Acta Oto Laryngol.*, **80**, 167 (1975).

125. R. Causse, N. Buu-Hoi, L. Goudet, and A. Hoan, *CR Soc. Biol.*, **143**, 68 (1949).

126. W. Osler, *Arsenic in Modern Medicine*, Vol. II, Lee and Leibger, Philadelphia, 1925, p. 668.

127. J. E. Leonard, T. Nakashima, and J. Snow, *Arch. Otolaryngol.*, **94**, 541 (1971).

128. N. Allen, in *The Nervous System, The Clinical Neurosciences*, Raven, New York, 1975, p. 235.

129. S. C. Harvey, in *The Pharmacological Basis of Therapeutics*, Macmillan, New York, 1975, p. 924.

130. B. Westernhagen, *Arch. Klin. Exp. Ohren Nasen Kehlkopfheilkd.*, **186**, 106 (1969).

131. O. Benesi and J. Sommer, *Handbuch der Neurolog des Ohres*, Berlin, Vol. 2, 1929, p. 787.

132. L. T. Kurland, S. H. Fargo, and H. Siedler, *World Neurol.*, **1**, 370 (1960).

133. S. A. Falk, R. Klein, J. A. Haseman, G. M. Sanders, F. A. Talleg, and D. J. Lim, *Arch. Pathol.*, **97**, 297 (1974).

134. C. P. Panayiotopoulos and P. E. Stopp, *J. Physiol.*, **210**, 495 (1970).

135. C. E. Pierangeli, *Clin. Otorinolaringoiatr.*, **11**, 1 (1959).

136. G. Girardi, C. Cis, and A. Piatti, *Arch. Ital. Otol.*, **78**, 756 (1967).

137. M. E. Conrad and W. H. Crosby, *Blood*, **16**, 1089 (1960).

138. W. Lawrence, P. Kuehn, E. T. Masle, and D. G. Miller, *J. Surg. Res.*, **1**, 142 (1961).

139. W. G. Young, A. M. Lesage, M. L. Dillon, J. M. Lee, H. A. Collaway, and J. W. Reeves, *Ann. Surg.*, **154**, 372 (1961).

140. H. Schuknecht, *Southern Med. J.*, **57,** 1161 (1964).
141. C. W. Cummings, *Laryngoscope*, **78,** 530 (1968).
142. S. G. Taylor, S. Kofman, H. H. Sky-Peck, and C. Perlia, *J. Lab. Clin. Med.*, **52,** 950 (1958).
143. F. P. Herter, S. G. Weissmann, H. G. Thompson, G. Hyman, and D. S. Martin, *Cancer Res.*, **21,** 31 (1961).
144. C. P. Perlia, S. Kofman, H. Sky-Peck, and S. G. Taylor, *Cancer*, **14,** 644 (1961).
145. M. Kornfield, L. M. Geller, D. Cowen, A. Wolf, and F. Altmann, *Exp. Neurol.*, **26,** 17 (1970).
146. R. P. Bobbin, personal communication.
147. R. W. Fleischman, S. W. Stadnicki, M. F. Ethier, and U. Schaeppi, *Toxicol. Pharmacol.*, **33,** 320 (1975).
148. M. Rozeneweig, D. D. von Hoff, M. Slavik, and F. M. Muggia, *Ann. Intern. Med.*, **86,** 803 (1977).
149. C. Y. Kao, *Pharmacol. Rev.*, **18,** 997 (1966).
150. Y. Katsuki, K. Yanagisawa, and J. Kanzaki, *Science*, **151,** 1544 (1966).
151. W. R. Loewenstein, C. A. Terzuolo, and Y. Washizu, *Science*, **142,** 1180 (1963).
152. C. P. Lebo, P. E. Poenisch, and W. S. McAfee, *Ann. Otol. Rhinol. Laryngol.*, **75,** 208 (1966).
153. J. K. Herd, A. Cramer, F. C. Hoak, and B. M. Norcross, *Pediatrics*, **40,** 905 (1967).
154. P. S. Larson, H. B. Haag, and H. Silvette, *Tobacco Experimental and Clinical Studies*, Williams and Wilkins, Baltimore, 1961.
155. P. S. Larson and H. Silvette, *Tobacco Experimental and Clinical Studies,* Suppl. I, Williams and Wilkins, Baltimore, 1971.
156. P. S. Larson and H. Silvette, *Tobacco Experimental and Clinical Studies*, Suppl. II, Williams and Wilkins, Baltimore, 1971.
157. S. L. Shapiro. *Eye Ear Nose Throat Monograph*, **43,** 96 (1964).
158. D. L. Derlacki, *The Medical Treatment of Meniere's Disease*, Saunders, Philadelphia, 1968, p. 519.
159. G. Bredberg, *Acta Oto Laryngol. Suppl.*, **236** (1968).
160. M. I. Wright, *The Pathology of Deafness*, Manchester University Press, 1971, p. 50.
161. G. Maffei and P. Miani, *Arch. Otolaryngol.*, **75,** 386 (1962).
162. R. P. Bobbin and M. I. Gondra, *Ann. Otol. Rhinol. Laryngol.*, **85,** 247 (1976).
163. H. Engstrom, H. W. Ades, and A. Andersson, *Structural Pattern of the Organ of Corti*, Almqvist and Wiksell, Stockholm, 1966.
164. G. F. Henriksen and J. K. Merlis, *Proc. Soc. Exp. Biol. Med.*, **74,** 882 (1950).
165. C. Wilpizeski, S. Isaacson, and S. Saliman, *J. Acoust. Soc. Am.*, **51,** 143 (1972).
166. M. Abe, *Tohoku J. Exp. Med.,* **60,** 47 (1954).
167. L. L. Price and R. Goldstein, *J. Speech Hear. Dis.*, **9,** 361 (1966).
168. D. T. R. Cody, D. W. Klass, and R. G. Bickford, *Trans. Am. Acad. Opthalmol. Otolaryngol.*, **19,** 81 (1967).
169. T. Suzuki and K. Taguchi, *Ann. Otol. Rhinol. Laryngol.*, **77,** 102 (1968).
170. P. Skinner and F. Antonio, *J. Speech Hear. Res.*, **12,** 394 (1969).
171. I. Rapin and L. J. Graziani, *Neurology*, **17,** 881 (1967).
172. K. Burian, G. F. Gestring, and S. Hruby, *Electroencephalogr. Clin. Neurophysiol.*, **28,** 215 (1970).
173. G. Strange, *Arch. Klin. Exp. Ohren Nasen Kehlkopfheilkd.*, **201,** 294 (1972).

174. T. Karnahl and C. D. Benning, *Arch. Klin. Exp. Ohren Nasen Kehlkophfheilkd.*, **201,** 181 (1972).

175. J. J. Stockard and F. W. Sharbrough, in *Clinical Uses of Cerebral, Brainstem and Spiral Somatosensory Evoked Potentials*, Vol. 7, Karger, Basel, 1978, p. 77.

176. R. P. Bobbin, J. May, and T. Lemoine, *Arch. Otolaryngol.*, **105,** 467 (1979).

177. J. J. Stockard, J. E. Stockard, and F. W. Sharbrough, *Am. J. EEG Technol.*, **18,** 177 (1978).

178. A. Eviatar and V. Goodhill, *Acta Oto Laryngol. Suppl.*, **237** (1968).

179. E. Borg and A. R. Moller, *Acta Oto Laryngol.*, **64,** 415 (1967).

180. G. B. Richards, O. C. Mitchell, and J. L. Speights, *Eye, Ear, Nose, and Throat Monthly*, **54,** 69 (1975).

181. E. Borg and A. R. Moller, *Acta Physiol. Scand.*, **94,** 327 (1975).

182. M. S. Robinette, D. P. Rhoads, and M. W. Marion, *Arch. Otolaryngol.*, **100,** 351 (1974).

183. J. Gilroy and J. S. Meyer, *Medical Neurology*, 2nd ed., Macmillan, New York, 1975, p. 258.

184. M. Victor, G. Collins, and R. Adams, *The Wernicke-Korsakoff Syndrome*, F. A. Davis, Philadelphia (1971).

185. A. G. Basili and H. Tobin, "Auditory Comprehension and Central Hearing Among Non-Korsakoff Alcoholics," paper delivered at the American Speech and Hearing Association Convention, San Francisco, 1978.

186. J. B. Spitzer, "Central Auditory Evaluation of Chronic Alcoholics," paper delivered at the American Speech and Hearing Association Convention, San Francisco, 1978.

187. E. Borg and A. R. Moller, *Acta Oto Laryngol.*, **64,** 415 (1967).

188. E. N. Cohill and H. J. Greenberg, *J. Am. Audiol. Soc.*, **2,** 121 (1977).

189. M. S. Robinette and R. H. Brey, *Arch. Otolaryngol.*, **104,** 31 (1978).

190. P. Courbon and J. Chapolaud, *Ann. Med-Psychol.*, **95,** 764 (1937).

191. V. J. Duchon and M. Bauer, *Prac. Otorhinolaryngol.*, **22,** 94 (1960).

192. M. M. Gross, E. Halpert, L. Sabot, and J. Polizas, *J. Nervous Ment. Dis.*, **137,** 445 (1963).

193. D. Wolff and M. Gross, *Arch. Otolaryngol.*, **87,** 350 (1960).

194. T. Nordahl, *Acta Oto Laryngol. Suppl.*, **188** (1964).

195. G. Montanti and F. Paterni, *Boll. Mal. Orecch. Gola Naso*, **83,** 500 (1965).

196. Y. Naki, *Jpn. J. Pharmacol.*, **14,** 235 (1964).

197. J. J. Stockard, V. V. Rossiter, W. L. Wiederholt, and R. M. Kobayashi, *Arch. Neurol.*, **33,** 726 (1976).

198. N. S. Chu, K. C. Squires, and A. Starr, *Arch. Neurol.*, **35,** 596 (1978).

199. G. Aschan, M. Bergstedt, and J. Stahle, *Acta Oto Laryngol Suppl.*, **129** (1956).

200. J. Falbe-Hansen, *Acta Oto Laryngol. Suppl.*, **44** (1941).

201. E. N. Meyers and J. M. Bernstein, *Arch. Otolaryngol.*, **82,** 483 (1965).

202. P. McCabe and F. Dey, *Ann. Otol. Rhinol. Laryngol.*, **74,** 312 (1965).

203. J. D. P. Grahm and W. A. Parker, *Quant. J. Med.*, **17,** 153 (1948).

204. J. M. Bernstein and A. D. Weiss, *J. Laryng. Otol.*, **81,** 915 (1967).

205. D. Schwabach, *Dtsch. Med. Wschr.*, **10,** 163 (1884).

206. W. Kirchner, *Mschr. Orenheilk.*, **17,** 85 (1883).

207. J. G. Waltner, *Ann. Otol. Rhinol. Laryngol.*, **64,** 617 (1955).

208. M. Gignoux, H. Martin, and H. Cajgfinger, *J. Fr. Oto. Rhinolaryngol.*, **15,** 631 (1966).

209. Y. P. Kapur, *Arch. Otolaryngol.*, **81,** 134 (1965).
210. E. N. Myers, J. M. Bernstein, and G. Fostiropolous, *N. Eng. J. Med.*, **273,** 587 (1965).
211. H. Silverstein, J. M. Bernstein, and D. G. Davies, *Ann. Otol.*, **76,** 118 (1967).
212. C. Mitchell, R. Brummett, D. Himes, and J. Vernon, *Arch. Otolaryngol.*, **98,** 297 (1973).
213. A. Gold and C. R. Wilpizeski, *Laryngoscope*, **76,** 674 (1966).
214. R. Thalmann, T. Miyoshi, J. Kusakari, and I. Thalmann, *Audiology*, **12,** 364 (1973).
215. H. Haike, *Arch. Ohrenh.*, **63,** 72 (1904).
216. K. Beck, *Z. F. Ohrench.*, **68,** 128 (1913).
217. M. H. Lurie, *Trans. Am. Acad. Ophthalmal. Otolaryngol.*, **40,** 375 (1935).
218. W. P. Covell, *Arch. Otolaryngol.*, **23,** 663 (1936).
219. S. Aly, S. Mousa, M. El-Kahky, A. Saleh, and A. ElMofty, *J. Egypt. Med. Assoc.*, **58,** 144 (1975).
220. J. M. Stowers, in *Salicylates, International Symposium*, Little, Brown, New York, 1963, p. 65.
221. C. Lutwak-Mann, *Biochem. J.*, **36,** 706 (1942).
222. K. Brune, M. Glatt, and P. Graf, *Gen. Pharmacol.*, **7,** 27 (1976).
223. B. M. Johnstone, in *Membranes and Transport*, Volume III, Wiley, New York, 1971, p. 167.
224. P. L. Boardman and E. D. Hart, *Ann. Rheum. Dis.*, **26,** 127 (1967).
225. H. Zeidler, J. Kalden, G. Josenhans, G. Binzus, W. Standel, S. Harting, R. Eberl, G. Tausch, H. Broll, N. Fellmann, and E. Lienhardt, *Arzneim. Forsch.*, **25,** 312 (1975).
226. R. D. Brown and A. M. Feldman, *Ann. Rev. Pharmacol. Toxicol.*, **18,** 233 (1978).
227. C. D. Wood, R. S. Kennedy, and A. Grabiel, *Aerospace Med.*, **36,** 1 (1965).
228. W. W. Douglas, in *The Pharmacological Basis of Therapeutics*, Macmillan, New York, 1975, p. 589.
229. R. Thalmann, I. Ise, and B. A. Bohne, *Acta Oto Laryngol.*, **83,** 221 (1977).
230. D. R. Kelly, E. R. Nilo, and R. B. Berggren, *New Engl. J. Med.*, **280,** 1338 (1969).
231. R. L. Fields, *Arch. Otolaryngol.*, **79,** 67 (1964).
232. V. Lorian, *Acta Tuberc. Scand.*, **42,** 149 (1962).
233. W. Leach, *J. Laryngol. Otol.*, **76,** 774 (1962).
234. P. Krahl, *Arch. Klin. Exp. Ohlen Nasen Kehlkopfheilkd.*, **182,** 591 (1963).
235. W. E. Rahm, W. F. Strother, W. L. Gulick, and J. F. Crump, *Ann. Otol. Rhinol. Laryngol.*, **68,** 1037 (1959).
236. W. E. Rahm, W. F. Strother, W. L. Gulick, and J. F. Crump, *Ann. Otol. Rhinol. Laryngol.*, **69,** 969 (1960).
237. R. Nowak and D. Dahl, *HNO (Hals-Nasen-Ohrenaerzte)*, **14,** 8 (1966).
238. F. Frutfero and A. Sarforis, *J. Fr. Oto. Rhino. Laryngol.*, **15,** 805 (1966).
239. W. F. Strother, D. E. Rahm, and J. F. Crump, *Ann. Otol. Rhinol. Laryngol.*, **73,** 141 (1964).
240. W. L. Gulick and R. A. Cutt, *Ann. Otol. Rhinol. Laryngol.*, **71,** 105 (1962).
241. W. L. Gulick, W. C. Patterson, and D. Meyers, *Ann. Otol. Rhinol. Laryngol.*, **71,** 110 (1962).
242. R. A. Cutt, *Laryngoscope*, **73,** 702 (1963).
243. V. Honrubia and P. H. Ward, *Otorhinolaryngology*, **17,** 470 (1966).
244. H. Mittelman, *Trans. Am. Acad. Ophthol. Otolaryngol.*, **76,** 1432 (1972).
245. H. F. Schuknecht, *Acta Oto Laryngol. Suppl.*, **132** (1957).

246. R. E. Brummett, R. F. Harris, and J. A. Lindgren, *Laryngoscope*, **86,** 1177 (1976).

247. N. Riskaer, E. Christensen, P. Peterson, and H. Weidman, *Acta Oto Laryngol.*, **46,** 137 (1956).

248. A. Kohonen and J. Tarkkanen, *Acta Oto Laryngol.*, **68,** 90 (1969).

249. J. Wersall, P. G. Lundquist, and B. Bjorkroth, *J. Infect. Dis.*, **119,** 410 (1969).

250. J. Webster, T. McGee, R. Carroll, and M. Williams, *Trans. Am. Acad. Ophthalmol. Otolaryngol.*, **74,** 115 (1970).

251. P. Federspil, *J. Infect. Dis.*, **119,** 465 (1969).

252. H. Stupp, K. Kupper, F. Lagler, H. Sous, and M. Quante, *Audiology*, **12,** 350 (1973).

253. E. P. D'Angelo, W. C. Patterson, and R. C. Morrow, *Arch. Otolaryngol.* **85,** 682 (1967).

254. Y. Koide, A. Hata, and R. Hando, *Acta Oto Laryngol.*, **61,** 332 (1966).

255. N. C. White and W. D. Ward, *Acta Oto Laryngol.*, **67,** 611 (1969).

256. V. S. Dayal, A. Kokshanian, and D. P. Mitchell, *Ann. Otol. Rhinol. Laryngol.*, **80,** 897 (1971).

257. C. M. Woodford, D. Henderson, and R. P. Hamernik, *Ann. Otol. Rhinol. Laryngol.*, **87,** 117 (1978).

258. J. Darrouzet and E. Sabrenho, *Rev. Bras. Cir.*, **46,** 120 (1963).

259. J. Vernon, R. Brummett, and R. Brown, *Trans. Am. Acad. Ophthalmol. Otolaryngol.*, **84,** 407 (1977).

260. T. Jauhiainen, A. Kohonen, and M. Jauhiainen, *Acta Oto Laryngol.*, **73,** 387 (1972).

261. J. E. Hawkins, D. M. Marques, and C. S. Clark, *J. Acoust. Soc. Am.*, **58** (Suppl. 1), 588 (1975).

262. R. P. Bobbin, P. S. Guth, and A. B. Mines, *Trans. Am. Acad. Ophthalmol. Otolaryngol.*, **82,** 299 (1976).

263. D. L. Kisiel, "Interaction of Intense Sound with Aminooxyacetic Acid and Ethacrynic Acid," unpublished doctoral dissertation, Memphis State University, Memphis, Tennessee, 1979.

CHAPTER 10

Pharmacology of Audiogenic Seizures

PHILLIP C. JOBE, Ph.D.

Professor of Pharmacology and Psychiatry
Veterans Administration Medical Center and
Louisiana State University
School of Medicine
Departments of Pharmacology and Therapeutics
and Psychiatry
Shreveport, Louisiana

CONTENTS

10.1 INTRODUCTION

Although one of the first references to sound-induced seizure in animals was made by Donaldson in 1924,[1] it was not until 1939 that widespread interest in this phenomenon developed.[2] At that time Maier and Glaser[3] reported that trained rats, forced by the sound of an air blast to attempt to solve an insoluble problem, experienced a tonic–clonic seizure followed by catatonia and subsequent recovery. These investigators concluded that the seizure was precipitated by conflict-induced neurosis. Later that year, however, Morgan and Morgan[4] stimulated rats with an air blast and observed that seizures were elicited in animals that were not subjected to an insoluble problem. Further investigations led Morgan[5] to conclude that the syndrome reported by Maier and Glaser[3] was induced by sound rather than neurosis. Within a short time other investigators[6–17] corroborated this observation.

Because of the apparent primacy of the auditory component in producing the convulsive reaction, Morgan and Waldman[16] suggested the phrase "audiogenic seizure" (hereafter denoted by AGS) as descriptive of the sound-induced syndrome. Other terms that have been applied to the behavior include "epileptoid seizure,"[18] "noise-fright convulsion,"[13] and "sonogenic convulsion."[19]

It is now obvious that AGS susceptibility is genetically determined.[20,21] In this regard, some strains of mice such as the DBA/2J exhibit a high incidence of AGS, whereas the C57BL/6J show a low incidence.[22] Although in Sprague Dawley rats (obtained from Sprague Dawley, Inc.) the incidence of AGS is low, strains of rats that have an extremely high incidence (> 95%) of AGS activity have been developed by the selective breeding of parents that exhibit this trait. This strain has been developed at the University of Arizona[23] and two others are currently under development at the Veterans Administration Hospital in Shreveport, Louisiana (Jobe, unpublished work) and Northeast Louisiana University in Monroe, Louisiana (Bourn and Geiger, personal communication).

10.2 AUDIOGENIC SEIZURES IN DIFFERENT ANIMAL SPECIES

Audiogenic seizures have been reported in several mammalian species, including rats,[1–5,23] mice,[24–29] rabbits,[30–33] dogs,[34] hamsters,[35] and humans.[36–39] A syndrome that appears to be an AGS has also been reported in goats[40] and a sound-induced running episode has been observed in cats[41] and chickens.[42]

As pointed out by Laird and Huxtable,[43] all species except man experience similar although not identical seizure responses when exposed to an appropriate sound stimulus. Some genetically susceptible animals will exhibit in consecutive order a startle response, quiescence, one, two, or three intense running episodes (each separated from the other by a short period of quiescence), and a clonic or tonic–clonic convulsion. After a clonic convulsion the postictal phase is often characterized by jumping, vocalizations, and finally catatonia. After a tonic-clonic convulsion the postictal phase is characterized by loss of righting reflex, respiratory depression, and muscular flaccidity.

Other susceptible animals will respond to sound stimulation only with an abbreviated form of the complete seizure described above. These animals will exhibit a startle response and one to three running episodes, but convulsions fail to occur despite prolonged stimulation. Some animals that exhibit a quiescent period after a running episode will begin to run again and will continue running throughout the period of stimulation, whereas others will remain quiescent. A few animals will experience a single running episode that lasts throughout the period of stimulation. In my laboratory I have observed that rats that continue to run become catatonic when sound stimulation is terminated.

Although the overt seizure patterns in mice and rats are quite similar, at least one difference exists: some strains of mice die in postictal respiratory depression,[29,44] whereas mortality in susceptible rats [from colonies at the University of Arizona and the Veterans Administration Hospital (in Shreveport, LA)] is negligible.[45]

Figure 10.1 describes different types of AGS observed in rats as well as an AGS response scoring system used to quantitate the intensity of seizure responses.[23] This scoring system provides a convenient way of comparing the intensity of AGS in test animals with that of corresponding control animals in experimental protocols.

In my laboratory I have observed that the typical rat will exhibit consistent responses when exposed to the seizure-provoking sound stimulus on different occasions. In most instances the range of ARS variation is not more than ± 1.0.

Other AGS scoring systems have been developed for use with mice. Included are the 5-point scale of Wilson,[46] the 4-point scales of Schreiber and Schlesinger[47] and Henry and Bowman,[48] and the 10-point scale of Alexander and Alexander.[49]

Further details regarding the seizure patterns exhibited by mice and rats have been summarized in excellent papers by Swinyard,[27] Collins,[26] and Krushninsky et al.[50]

Audiogenic seizures in rabbits[32,33] differ from those in rats[23] and mice[26] in that the tonic convulsion is characterized by dorsiflexion rather than ventriflexion of the trunk and neck. Sound-induced seizures in dogs include a tonic convulsion that is usually followed by but occasionally preceded by a running episode.[34] Death as a result of AGS is unusual in rabbits and dogs as well as rats.

In contrast to what occurs in other species, sound-induced seizures in humans have no running components. Rather they are characterized by localized neuronal discharges without motor components or by psychomotor, petit mal, or grand mal types of seizure.[51]

ARS SCORE	RESPONSE TO SOUND STIMULATION
0	No response.
1	Running only; no convulsion.
2	Two running phases separated by a refractory period; convulsive endpoint consists of clonus of forelimbs, hindlimbs, head, pinnae, vibrissae, and tail. (A)

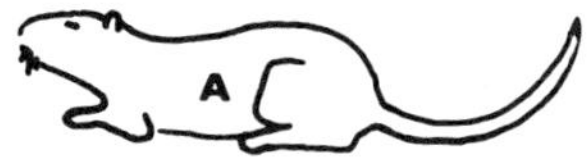

ARS SCORE	RESPONSE TO SOUND STIMULATION
3	Same as 2 except only one running phase and no refractory period.
4	Two running phases separated by a refractory period; convulsive endpoint consists of tonic flexion of neck, trunk, and forelimbs with clonus of hindlimbs. (B)

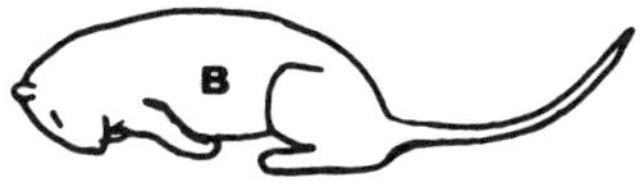

ARS SCORE	RESPONSE TO SOUND STIMULATION
5	Same as 4 except only one running phase and no refractory period.
6	Two running phases separated by a refractory period; convulsive endpoint similar to 4 except hindlimbs are in partial tonic extension (i.e., tonic extension of thighs and legs with clonus of feet). (C)

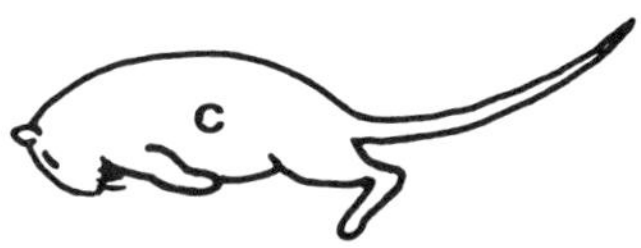

ARS SCORE	RESPONSE TO SOUND STIMULATION
7	Same as 6 except only one running phase and no refractory period.
8	Two running phases separated by a refractory period; convulsive endpoint similar to 4 except hindlimbs are in complete tonic extension (i.e., animal in maximal convulsion). (D)

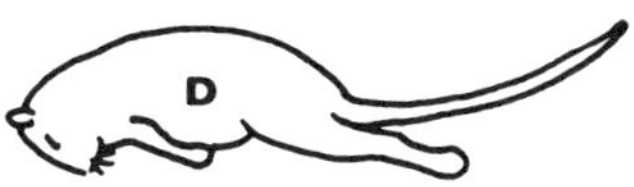

ARS SCORE	RESPONSE TO SOUND STIMULATION
9	Same as 8 except only one running phase and no refractory period.

Figure 10.1 Description of Audiogenic Response Scoring System. ARS refers to Audiogenic Response Score.

10.3 CHARACTERISTICS OF THE SEIZURE-PROVOKING ACOUSTIC STIMULUS

A review of the literature shows that among the different kinds of acoustic stimuli used to provoke seizures in animals, noise (produced by bells, jingling keys, an 8-to-16-kHz band of noise, high-frequency oscillators beating against low-frequency oscillators, and so on) is generally considered to be superior to pure tones.[52–55] At least two reports, however, indicate that AGS susceptible mice will convulse in response to pure tones[56,57] and that the incidence of seizures is as great with a pure tone of 20 kHz as with noise generated by two bells (an Edwards No. 340 6-in. bell or an Edwards No. 13-3 3-in. bell).[57] In contrast, recent observations by Duplisse[58] indicate that the AGS susceptible rat does not exhibit a seizure in response to pure tone stimulation. Some earlier reports suggest that rats will convulse during pure tone stimulation[53,59]; however, the experimental methods used make it impossible to determine the sound level or whether the animals were acoustically primed (discussed later) or genetically susceptible.

In rats and mice the commonly used acoustic stimulation modality is a bell (fire bell, doorbell, or school bell or two bells ringing simultaneously). The power spectra of these stimuli contain intensity peaks scattered from a few hundred Hz up to 50 kHz.[57,60,61] Typically, seizure provoking acoustic stimuli are delivered at intensities of 95 to 130 dB (reference; 0 dB = 0.0002 dyne/cm^2) for the duration of 30 to 120 sec; the animal is nonsusceptible (ARS = 0 in the scoring system described above) if it does not exhibit a seizure by the end of the stimulation period. When pure tones are used[56,57,62] the ranges of intensity and durations of stimuli are the same.

Observations in people who are susceptible to AGS reveal that effective acoustic stimuli include doorbells, a ringing telephone, gunshots, and voices.[39,63] Musicogenic epilepsy, a special type of human disorder in which AGS is precipitated by music, has been reported by a number of investigators.[36–39] Most individuals with musicogenic epilepsy exhibit seizures only in response to acoustic stimuli.[51]

10.4 BIOLOGICAL BASIS OF AUDIOGENIC SEIZURE SUSCEPTIBILITY

As pointed out earlier, AGS susceptibility in animals is genetically determined. Despite the plethora of studies in genetics, most of them on mice, the nature of the transmission of this trait has been the subject of considerable controversy.[21–64] Although several reports indicate a single dominant or recessive gene control, Hohenboken and Nellhaus[64] and Fuller and Collins[21] believe that the weight of the evidence suggests that AGS susceptibility is determined by a polygenic system. Regardless of the exact nature of the genetic expression, the fact that susceptibility is genetically determined implies that the etiology has biochemical, electrophysiological, and/or morphological bases.

10.4.1 Auditory Physiology, Cochlear Morphology, and Audiogenic Seizure

A large number of physiological and morphological studies have been conducted on the AGS-susceptible mouse, whereas few have been performed on the rat and almost no reports exist from studies of other species. Consequently an evaluation of the "mouse literature" is compared with findings obtained on the rat, when available.

Audiogenic Seizure Susceptibility that Exists, Because of Genetic Factors, on First Exposure to an Acoustic Stimulus

AGE OF ONSET AND DEVELOPMENT OF AUDIOGENIC SEIZURES

A prominent feature of genetically determined AGS susceptibility in mice is that these animals exhibit a seizure in response to sound only during a restricted period of the life cycle. The age of onset and development of AGS in susceptible mice appears to correlate to some extent with auditory system maturation, a process that is complete at about 15 days of age[65–68] as determined by N_1 response to a click[69] and cochlear microphonic (CM) responses.[70] In Vicari's studies[71] the incidence of AGS in mice develops from zero before 19 days of age to 60% between days 20 and 24 and finally to 88% between days 25 and 39. A marked decline in seizure incidence to 7% was observed by 59 days and followed by an abrupt fall to zero after day 79. These observations are in agreement with those reported in DBA/2J and B6D2F1 mice by Schlesinger et al.[22]

An exception to the early development of and subsequent loss of susceptibility in mice has been noted by Gates and Chen.[72] These investigators reported that BALB/C mice are nonsusceptible when young but have a high incidence of seizure at 1 to 1½ years of age. Also, once Frings and Frings mice have matured to the age at which they are susceptible to AGS they retain their susceptibility for life (E. A. Swinyard, University of Utah, personal communication).

In rats, onset of susceptibility occurs at about 16 days after birth; close to 100% of the susceptible animals respond by day 28 (P.C. Jobe, personal observations, unpublished data). AGS-susceptible rats, in contrast to most mice, retain their susceptibility and characteristic seizure intensity throughout their lives.[73]

Studies of the development of the auditory system of the normal nonsusceptible rat reveal that cochlear potentials first appear at 8 days of age,[74] whereas the first behavioral response to sound occurs between 9 and 10 days,[75] and the waves of the auditory brainstem-evoked responses assume adult shapes and latencies by 20 days of age.[76] Although amplitudes of N_1 (as observed in recordings of brainstem potentials) continue to increase for the first six months of life in the rat, no significant changes occur in latencies.[77]

RELATION TO AUDITORY PHYSIOLOGY AND MORPHOLOGY

Audiogenic-seizure-susceptible mice and rats both appear to have a cochlear abnormality. Susceptible mice of the Swiss/RB strain have a severe hearing impairment, evaluated by the Preyer reflex at all frequencies tested between 1 and 40 kHz (50-dB elevation at 15 kHz, maximal) and a severe degeneration of the outer hair cells in the base of the cochlea.[78–80] They also have reduced CM potentials. Although the N_1 response to a click stimulus appears to be normal, the dB level required to produce a 10 μV evoked response from the surface of the inferior colliculus is 20 dB greater in the susceptible Swiss/RB strain than in controls at all frequencies tested (2 to 40 kHz).[81] A probable explanation for this differential behavior of CM and N_1 is that although outer hair cells of the cochlea produce the preponderance of CM,[69] the inner hair cells receive the dominant innervation from the afferent auditory dendrites.[82] In contrast to the findings in mice, CM and N_1 are both reduced in AGS susceptible rats.[83,84]

From a developmental standpoint, evoked response thresholds of the inferior colliculus of the DBA/2J mice (to frequencies of 1 to 70 kHz) appear normal before the time of appearance of maximum susceptibility.[85] Auditory sensitivity of this genetically susceptible strain to the higher frequencies then decreases rapidly with age. Thresholds to frequencies greater than 30 kHz are not obtainable by 47 to 48 days of age and evoked response thresholds to all frequencies above 50 kHz are elevated. By 100 days of age evoked responses cannot be obtained at any frequency in the DBA/2J mice.[85] In contrast, evoked responses in 105-to-107-day-old mice from the nonsusceptible strain can still be obtained, albeit only in response to sounds of greater intensity than were used initially.

On the basis of these observations, it appears that a developmental cochlear impairment may be, at least in part, responsible for the susceptibility of certain strains of mice and rats to AGS. Furthermore, the progressive decrease in seizure intensity and susceptibility (percentage of animals exhibiting seizures) that ultimately occurs with increasing age in genetically susceptible mice may be due to advancing impairment in the auditory system of these animals; that is, auditory input into the CNS eventually becomes so drastically reduced that a convulsion cannot be initiated.

Factors other than a developmental cochlear impairment are also involved in the genetically determined expression of AGS susceptibility. Portmann et al.[79] found that two types of Swiss/RB mice can be distinguished: one group that is susceptible to AGS and another that is not. These two groups of animals have similar cochlear abnormalities but they are not completely deaf.[80] In addition, Jobe et al.[86] observed a similar grouping in his colony of AGS-susceptible rats and found that treatment of the resistant group with Ro 4-1284, a monoamine depletor, caused 60% of these animals to become susceptible, whereas controls did not become susceptible after Ro 4-1284.

Susceptibility to Audiogenic Seizure Induced by Priming

ACOUSTIC PRIMING

Acoustic priming is a process by which a nonsusceptible animal is exposed to an intense acoustic stimulus during a sensitive period of its life in order to induce susceptibility to AGS when the animal is again exposed to the stimulus days or weeks later. Acoustic priming has been observed in AGS-resistant strains of mice such as the C57BL/6J,[87] CFI,[88] and SJL,[89] as well as in the heterogenous stock maintained by the Laboratory of Behavioral Genetics in Boulder, Colorado.[90,91]

Whether a mouse will become susceptible to AGS as a result of acoustic priming appears to have, at least in part, a genetic basis. In some strains of mice 100% of the animals will exhibit AGS after priming, whereas other strains have a lower incidence and at least one strain is relatively resistant.[92] Also, mice that are resistant to priming can be selected from a priming-prone heterogenous stock.[91,93] On the basis of their studies, Deckard et al.[91] estimate that between 20 and 30% of the variability in the response of their heterogenous stock to acoustic priming can be attributed to genetic factors. These investigators also suggest that the genetic mechanisms which underlie priming-induced susceptibility to AGS are different from those that determine AGS susceptibility to the first exposure of a seizure-provoking acoustic stimulus.

Developmental studies have shown that to be effective in producing AGS susceptibility, acoustic priming must occur during a precisely defined "sensitive period" early in the life of the animal. Depending on the strain of mouse tested, acoustic priming can be performed any time between 14 and 30 days after birth, but the highest incidence of seizures occurs when the priming stimulus is administered between 16 and 25 days of age.[94] Although primed mice may retain susceptibility to AGS for three weeks (or more), various investigators have reported data indicating that two to six days between priming and reexposure to the acoustic stimulus appears to produce the highest incidence of seizures as well as the most severe.[94–97] In their investigations of heterogenous stock Deckard et al.[91] found that there was no difference between the effectiveness of priming, whether the interval to AGS test stimulus was three or seven days. According to Chen[98] and Chen et al.,[99] the minimum interval that must accrue between priming and seizure testing in BALB/C mice is about two days. Because of this time-dependent development of AGS susceptibility following the priming stimulus, Chen and

Gates[93] suggest that the priming exposure serves as a trigger for the development of the processes that underlie susceptibility.

Acoustic priming is effective, whether produced binaurally or monaurally.[89,100] When monaural priming is performed the occurrence of AGS is observed only when the primed ear is exposed to the acoustic stimulus. Thus Fuller and Collins[89] suggest that the ontological changes induced by acoustic priming are localized within the uncrossed structures of the auditory system. As an extension of this concept, Henry[100] suggests that priming could occur by a disruption of the reflexive uncoupling of the auditory ossicles or by damage to the olivocochlear bundle of Rasmussen to eliminate its centrifugal gating properties.

Although acoustic priming can be produced readily in several strains of mice, the phenomenon is not easily demonstrated in most other animals. Iturrian and Johnson[101] have successfully produced priming in the hamster. Chen and Gates,[93] however, point out that because these experiments were not systematically conducted they should not be the basis of a definitive conclusion. The possibility of priming in rats is suggested by two reports in which the investigators may have unintentionally primed a large number (40 to 60%) of the animals used for their investigations.[102a,103] Recent observations by Jobe et al.[102b] show that multiple exposures to a loud acoustic stimulus alter the onset of AGS susceptibility as well as the level of seizure severity ultimately exhibited by the developing progeny of AGS-susceptible rats. Pups exposed to an acoustic stimulus at frequent intervals become susceptible to AGS more rapidly and exhibit severer seizures than those exposed at less frequent intervals. In addition, Brown et al.[102c] reported that in very young progeny of genetically *nonsusceptible* parents multiple exposures to intense acoustic stimulation cause the appearance of susceptibility but do not independently alter seizure intensity.

A number of studies that contribute significantly to an understanding of the physiological and morphological bases of the acoustic priming phenomenon indicate that priming produces a cochlear impairment. In this regard, Henry and Saleh[104] have observed that priming causes severe degeneration of the outer hair cells in the base of the cochlea. These same investigators and Saunders et al.[61] also demonstrated that the thresholds for N_1 and CM (1 to 50 kHz) are elevated in primed mice; the greatest elevation is 25 dB at 17 kHz. Not only do most of these changes appear to be qualitatively similar to those observed in AGS-susceptible mice but N_1 can also be elicited in some of the primed mice without any indication of an accompanying CM potential. Also, the greatest impairment in CM occurs when the mice are acoustically primed during the particular day in which the strain exhibits its highest degree of susceptibility to priming.[55]

Perhaps the most significant physiological observations are that acoustic priming in mice decreases the amplitude of brainstem-evoked responses (BSER) to sounds of low intensity while increasing the amplitude of the BSER to loud sounds and producing a 15-dB decrement in the threshold of the Preyer reflex elicited by a 15 kHz acoustic stimulus (the only frequency tested).[100,104–107] On the basis of their observations Saunders et al.[61,106] proposed that priming produces cochlear hair cell damage and thereby a reduction in auditory input at a critical period after birth. According to the concept of these investigators, this ultimately results in the abnormal development of an "overrecruitment" or supersensitive state. It should be noted that this concept, known as the *auditory deprivation hypothesis,* is applied by Saunders only to acoustic priming and not to the genetically determined AGS susceptibility that occurs on first exposure to the acoustic stimulus.

OTHER TYPES OF PRIMING

The validity of the auditory deprivation hypothesis of priming has been tested in mice by several methods of producing a reduction in auditory input. The methods that do not involve the use of a loud acoustic priming stimulus include (1) unilateral and bilateral destruction of the tympanic membranes,[99,108] a technique that reduces auditory input by at least 40 dB,[109] (2) ear plugging, which produces a reduction of at least 26 dB,[110] (3) induction of otitis media,[111] and (4) chronic administration of kanamycin at doses that cause widespread outer hair cell damage while leaving the inner hair cell relatively intact.[60] As would be expected according to the auditory deprivation hypothesis, AGS susceptibility developed in response to all four of these methods.

The effectiveness of these treatments in causing AGS susceptibility appeared to be maturationally dependent, as in acoustic priming. The treatments were most effective if they were administered during an early period in the animal's life. In the kanamycin study[60] it was necessary to treat the mice with the drug between the fifth and twenty-first days of life in order to cause the appearance of AGS. When treatment was delayed and given from days 17 to 26 susceptibility did not develop and there was less outer hair cell damage than when the treatment was given to the younger animals. In addition, ear plugging at 17 days of age effectively caused priming, whereas at 28 days of age it did not.[110]

Another form of "priming," which as been reported, is due to the alcohol or barbiturate withdrawal syndrome. Prolonged treatment with either of these drugs, in doses sufficient to cause physical dependence, will cause the appearance of AGS susceptibility in mice and rats during the abstinence syndrome which develops after abrupt cessation of drug administration.[112–117]

Chen and Gates and others have stated that the basic supersensitive process in auditory deprivation may be similar to that found in withdrawal priming. The observations of Chu et al.,[116] however, show that no significant changes occur in the amplitudes of the waves of auditory BSER in rats during chronic treatment with alcohol or during the alcohol abstinence syndrome. These investigators also observed a significant increase in the latencies of the waves of BSER during chronic alcohol administration and a significant decrease in the latencies during the withdrawal period. Consequently, facilitation of conduction through the brainstem, not hyperrecruitment, would appear to be associated with withdrawal-induced AGS susceptibility.

Abnormalities in Auditory Function as a Basis for Audiogenic Seizure Susceptibility

The functional state of the auditory system is abnormal in all three types of AGS described above; that is, in seizures that occur because of (1) a genetically determined "first exposure" susceptibility, (2) acoustic deprivation, and (3) drug withdrawal. However, noteworthy functional differences exist between each of these types of AGS. Epileptiform activity has not been demonstrated in the electrocorticogram of genetically susceptible rats or mice either during an AGS episode itself or in seizure-free periods when the acoustic stimulus is not applied.* In contrast, spontaneous epileptiform EEG activity and convulsions do occur during alcohol withdrawal in rats and mice.[113,119]

In addition, the genetically susceptible mouse shows an impaired behavioral threshold to acoustic stimuli and reduced auditory input to the CNS, whereas the acoustically deprived mouse shows a hyperrecruitment phenomenon. In comparison, during the alcohol abstinence syndrome the rat exhibits facilitation of conduction through the brainstem auditory nuclei as well as hyperexcitability in cortical areas.

Because the overt motor components of seizure in the three types of AGS are not qualitatively different, it might be concluded that each of the seizures is being mediated by a common oscillator mechanism. Evidence indicates that this mechanism involves the nuclei of the primary auditory pathway, particularly the inferior colliculi and their functional connections with the reticular formation.

The importance of the inferior colliculus in the etiology of AGS is supported by reports that show that bilateral lesions of this structure completely block AGS of genetically susceptible rats and mice,[58,120] whereas bilateral lesions of the medial geniculate reduce the severity of seizure but do not block it.[121] Furthermore, in rats that exhibit an ARS = 2 when exposed to the acoustic stimulus direct electrical stimulation of the inferior colliculus produces an "audiogenic seizure," whereas stimulation of the medical geniculate does not.[58] In this regard, stimulation of the inferior colliculus

*AGS in mice and rats may be an analog of one especially important component of grand mal seizure; namely, the brain-stem component that apparently is responsible for the motor aspects of the grand mal seizure.[58,118] This concept is supported by observations that show that the electrical activity of AGS is limited to subcortical areas. Thus AGS in animals may be an appropriate model for studies designed to elucidate the inhibitory deficits that may exist in the brainstem and given rise to increased susceptibility to seizures.

produces running activity followed by convulsions, but stimulation of the medical geniculate merely causes the rat to raise its head and turn it contralaterally. As the voltage applied to the medial geniculate is increased convulsive activity on the contralateral side of the rat progresses from facial twitches to clonus of the forelimb and eventually to clonic involvement of both forelimbs. Another important observation in the animals with an ARS = 2 is that seizure thresholds to electrical stimulation of the inferior colliculus are lower than those for control rats that are not susceptible to AGS.[58]

Evidence also indicates that above a certain level of seizure severity the role of the medial geniculate becomes significant. In rats which have an ARS > 5 not only does electrical stimulation of the inferior colliculus cause an "audiogenic seizure" but stimulation of the medial geniculate produces the same result.[73] Furthermore, electroshock thresholds to focal stimulation of both nuclei are lower than corresponding thresholds in non-AGS susceptible controls.[73] Thus, it appears that the inferior colliculus is involved in the production of low-intensity AGS (ARS = 2) and that as the severity of seizure increases both the inferior colliculus and the medial geniculate are of etiological significance.

The importance of the reticular formation in the AGS process is emphasized by the observation that an abnormally low, focal electroshock seizure threshold exists in the reticular formation of rats that exhibit seizure with an ARS > 5.[73] The seizure is not typical of AGS, however, perhaps because electrical stimulation of the reticular formation with a stereotaxically placed electrode is not functionally equivalent to bombardment of selected neurons that would occur when the impulses arrive from the auditory nuclei.

In harmony with these observations and on the basis of their own findings, Kesner,[122] Maxson and Cowan,[118] and others have postulated that the necessary elements for an AGS are input from the inferior colliculi to the reticular formation, establishment of paroxysmal activity in the reticular formation, and a consequent initiation of AGS. Because it has been demonstrated that the genetically susceptible mouse has a reduced auditory input into the CNS, it is important to determine how this paroxysmal activity can be initiated despite reduced input into the auditory nuclei and finally into the reticular formation. Perhaps it may occur in a fashion somewhat analogous to suggestions made by Faingold[123] and Faingold and Caspary[124] for chemically induced convulsions in normal (non-AGS) animals. If so, the reticular formation of the immature, genetically susceptible mouse may develop abnormally (due to lack of normal auditory input) and consequently become more readily triggered into paroxysmal (oscillator) activity. Thus enhancement of auditory-evoked responses in the reticular pathways and/or reorganization of neuronal firing patterns in the reticular formation would be the developmental event(s) necessary to cause susceptibility.

This same basic hypothesis would also be applicable to the data cited above for AGS-susceptible rats. When genetically susceptible rats are grouped according to their ARS scores, those with severer seizures also have a greater number of auditory nuclei with lowered electroshock seizure thresholds. Consequently, it is apparent that the reticular formation in the rat is not the only structure that develops an abnormal responsiveness to incoming auditory impulses. Thus, in the rat it appears that some type of developmentally related compensation for reduced auditory input occurs in the auditory nuclei as well as in the reticular formation.

10.4.2 Role of Central Nervous System Neurotransmitters in Audiogenic Seizures in Genetically Susceptible Animals

Several observations link ascending and descending CNS neurotransmitter systems with AGS activity in animals. To a large extent the functional significance of the various neurotransmitters has been determined by pharmacological approaches. Pathophysiological studies that do not involve the use of drugs have also contributed to our knowledge of the area.

Investigations of the role of neurotransmitters in AGS are hampered because direct estimation in the CNS of the amount of neurotransmitters in the synaptic cleft is not possible at the present time. Even estimations of neurotransmitter turnover rates, which are often regarded as indicative of synaptic neurotransmitter content, can be misleading because an increased rate could be caused by an augmented release of transmitter into the cytoplasm of the nerve ending, where it is catabolized before it enters the cleft. As a consequence, and contrary to what is often considered to be the case, an *increased* turnover rate could coincide with a *decreased* synaptic neurotransmitter content!

Nevertheless, as pointed out by Maynert et al.,[125] appropriate use of selected pharmacological agents has provided a basis for inferring whether the amount of neurotransmitter in the synapse is increased or decreased. However, a major problem in the use of drugs in determining the role of a particular neurotransmitter in AGS is that their neurochemical effects are not restricted to one neurotransmitter. As a result of this multiplicity of drug effects, support for a hypothesis regarding the role of any one neurotransmitter system in AGS should be based on well-designed studies of drugs with diverse chemical structures. Whenever possible pharmacological studies should be coupled with physiological and pathological investigations that do not use drugs. Although none of the various studies designed to determine the role of neurotransmitters in AGS has used all of these approaches, the different studies provide a fairly broad basis for the conclusions that have emerged.

The Catecholamines, Norepinephrine (NE) and Dopamine (DA)

Numerous observations relate CNS noradrenergic neuron systems to AGS. Observations that have been made in rats and mice have some common features and consequently are at least partly compatible with the concept that NE subserves a similar inhibitory role in AGS in these two species. Although dopaminergic neurons may influence AGS in the mouse, they do not appear to do so in the rat.

RATS

Jobe[45] and Jobe et al.[23,126] have demonstrated that reduction of brain noradrenergic activity in genetically susceptible rats is associated with an increased severity of AGS. In these studies, some treatments caused simultaneous depletion of both NE and DA; thus it was not always possible to ascribe greater importance to one or the other catecholamine as an attenuator of AGS. Several observations provided evidence that NE rather than DA modulated AGS; for example, Ro 4-1284 (a benzoquinolizine that interferes with catecholamine storage and thereby reduces catecholaminergic transmission) markedly intensified AGS and depleted NE and DA 1 hr after administration; however, 4 hr later AGS enhancement was no longer apparent and the brain NE content showed definite recovery, whereas DA remained severely reduced. When repletion of these catecholamine storage sites was prevented by administration of α-methyl-p-tyrosine (a potent inhibitor of NE and DA synthesis) the pronounced effects of Ro 4-1284 on AGS and brain catecholamine content were substantially prolonged; that is, they were still present 13 hr after Ro 4-1284, the latest time interval tested in this experiment. In comparison to the combination treatment α-methyl-p-tyrosine alone caused an equally severe reduction of brain DA content at this late interval, but it produced significantly less reduction in NE and no enhancement of AGS (this lack of effect of α-methyl-p-tyrosine on AGS in rats has also been reported by Prakhe[127]).

The systemic administration of reserpine (another catecholamine storage inhibitor chemically dissimilar to Ro 4-1284) also causes a dramatic intensification of AGS intensity in rats that corresponds with maximal depletion of NE and DA content.[128] Although AGS intensity begins to return to normal before the whole-brain catecholamine content begins to increase toward pretreatment values,[128] repletion of NE storage sites in the hypothalamus correlates closely with dissipation of reserpine's effect on AGS intensity (Jobe, unpublished observations).

Observations with intracerebroventricularly (ICV; into one of the lateral ventricles) injected reserpine also contribute to an understanding of the role of NE in AGS in rats. When given by this route reserpine intensified AGS and markedly reduced brain NE content but only moderately lowered DA.[126]

On the basis of these observations Jobe et al.[23] concluded that brain noradrenergic neurons exert an inhibitory effect that tends to limit the spread of seizure discharge in the CNS. Consequently depletion of brain NE disrupts inhibitory function, allows more efficient spread of seizure activity in the brain, and thereby causes an increased severity of AGS.

Bourn et al.[129,130] have extended these observations by testing the effects of ICV administration of 6-hydroxydopamine on AGS intensity in rats. This compound was chosen for study because it exerts a relatively specific neurotoxic (degenerative) effect on catecholaminergic neurons and thereby reduces transmission at these synapses.[131] When administered alone this drug caused a significant reduction of NE content in all brain regions studied as well as a reduction in DA levels in the cortex, striatum, and hypothalamus. It also caused a significant increase in the severity of AGS. To determine whether depletion of DA or NE was most important in causing the enhancement of AGS severity, Bourn et al.[130] pretreated a group of rats with desipramine, a drug that inhibits the entry of 6-hydroxydopamine into noradrenergic but not into dopaminergic neurons (when given in this way desipramine selectively prevents the neurotoxic effects of 6-hydroxydopamine on NE containing neurons). The results of Bourn et al.[130] indicated that in desipramine pretreated rats, 6-hydroxydopamine failed to alter AGS severity or to change brain NE levels, whereas it substantially reduced dopamine stores in the cortex, striatum, hypothalamus, and the pons-medulla.

Although the mode of action of lithium carbonate on catecholamines is speculative, studies on its interaction with α-methyl-ρ-tyrosine also tend to support the concept that noradrenergic neurons influence AGS severity in rats.[132,133] A functional role of NE in AGS mechanisms is further supported by evidence obtained from investigating the interaction between Ro 4-1284 and compounds that diminish the efficiency of the NE uptake mechanism in the presynaptic neuron or that inhibit monoamine oxidase.[23,45,134] The inhibitors of NE uptake (methylphenidate, imipramine, or cocaine) produced a marked reduction in the intensity of AGS and substantially inhibited the enhancement of seizure produced by Ro 4-1284. The monoamine oxidase inhibitor, iproniazid, did not diminish seizure intensity in the dosage used; however, it markedly inhibited the capacity of Ro 4-1284 to enhance seizure. Higher doses of iproniazid alone exerted potent inhibiting effects on audiogenic and electroshock seizures.[128,135] The effects of these drugs on AGS can be explained on the basis of evidence that indicates that imipramine, methylphenidate, and cocaine produce an increase in synaptic NE by inhibiting the monoamine reuptake mechanism located in the presynaptic nerve membrane.[136-143] Furthermore, monoamine oxidase inhibitors combined with reserpine increase the rate of release and the duration of action of physiologically active catecholamines.[144,145] It has also been shown, however, that methylphenidate may produce an increase in synaptic 5-HT[146,147] and that iproniazid plus reserpine causes a large increase in the concentration of whole brain 5-HT.[128,135,148] Therefore, to determine whether the AGS-inhibiting properties of methylphenidate and iproniazid resulted, at least in part, from effects on NE metabolism, animals were pretreated with α-methyl-ρ-tyrosine.[23,45,134] After treatment with this drug the capacity of methylphenidate and iproniazid to prevent Ro 4-1284-induced enhancement of seizure intensity was substantially inhibited. Thus, it appears that an increase in synaptic NE is largely responsible for the diminished seizure activity produced by these drugs.

Intraperitoneally administered L-3,4-dihydroxyphenylalanine (L-DOPA) or NE or DA (given ICV because they do not pass the blood brain barrier when administered systemically) reduced the intensity of AGS.[45] Because L-DOPA given systemically and NE or DA given centrally increase brain NE and/or DA content,[149-153] these data indicate that increases in brain catecholamine levels are associated with a decrease in the intensity of AGS. It is possible, however, that the anticonvulsant action of DA may be related to its conversion to NE. In support of this view Jones and Roberts[154] have shown that NE given ICV completely antagonized the capacity of reserpine to enhance pentylenetetrazol-induced seizure, whereas DA given in an equimolar dose produced only a slight antagonism. As an alternative explanation for the anticonvulsant activity of DA it has been suggested that DA may interact "nonspecifically" with NE receptors.[155]

The results cited above show that there is an inverse relationship between the concentration of NE in the brain and the intensity of AGS in the rat. Furthermore, the results provide evidence for the rejection of DA as a possible mediator in AGS mechanisms and show that in the presence of low NE levels depletion of 5-HT stores is not necessary for the enhancement of seizure. Consequently it is suggested that NE, but not DA, has a central inhibitory action that serves to attenuate AGS.

In spite of the fact that these studies strongly link CNS noradrenergic neuron systems with AGS *intensity,* they do not provide the evidence required to show that the level of activity of these (or some of these) neurons also determine *susceptibility* to AGS in the rat. Recent observations of Jobe et al.,[86,156] however, do provide evidence of such a link. In these studies two types of Sprague Dawley-derived rat were used: the progeny of genetically susceptible and nonsusceptible parents. The results showed that 45 min after Ro 4-1284 (a time when monoamine depletion was maximal) the progeny of nonsusceptible parents were still nonsusceptible. In contrast, Ro 4-1284 caused a dramatic increase in susceptibility in the nonsusceptible progeny of susceptible parents (≃ 60% became susceptible). Almost 50% of these animals retained their induced susceptibility after the monoamine depleting effects of Ro 4-1284 had completely dissipated (19 days later). These observations suggest that CNS noradrenergic neurons function as determinants of AGS susceptibility in animals that also carry some other genetic factor. Nervertheless, a deficit in monoaminergic transmission is insufficient to cause susceptibility in rats not carrying this other susceptibility factor. More specific documentation is needed to substantiate this interpretation.

In summary, central noradrenergic neurons serve as attenuators of AGS *intensity* in rats and recent evidence indicates that they may also play an important role in genetically determined AGS *susceptibility.* An anatomical substrate involved in the regulation of intensity appears to be the ascending noradrenergic fibers that develop in the locus ceruleus.[157] The role of other ascending or descending noradrenergic systems in AGS intensity has not been established. No studies of the role of the individual noradrenergic neuron system as determinants of AGS *susceptibility* have been reported.

MICE

A number of excellent studies have examined the role of NE in AGS susceptibility and intensity in mice. In my view the evidence that supports a noradrenergic role in AGS in this species is more equivocal than in the rat. The following information shows the complex picture that emerges from studies in mice.

Schlesinger et al.[22,158] have shown that DBA/2J mice, which are susceptible to AGS, have significantly lower levels of NE in the brain than seizure-resistant C5JBL/6J mice, but only at 21 days of age, which corresponds to the period of maximal seizure risk in DBA/2J animals. In contrast to these selected observations several other findings of Schlesinger et al.[22,158] appear to provide no support whatever for a noradrenergic deficit as a cause of AGS susceptibility in mice; for example, at 14 days of age B6D2F1 mice are completely nonsusceptible to AGS and their brain NE levels are low. By 21 days of age these animals develop a high degree of susceptiblity and a marked increase in brain NE levels. Thus, a decrement in NE content does not appear to be responsible for the onset of susceptibility in this strain.

Another indication that brain NE levels may not be involved in regulation of AGS in mice is provided in the work of Alexander and Kopeloff.[159] These investigators determined the brain NE levels of two strains of mice: (1) 3-week-old AGS susceptible mice, derived from the Swiss strain and inbred for susceptibility for 32 to 40 generations, and (2) control non-AGS susceptible Swiss mice. Their results showed that the brain NE levels of the susceptible animals were no different than the levels of the nonsusceptible strain.

The interpretation of the pharmacologic data presented by Schlesinger et al.[158] is also equivocal. In an effort to test their hypothesis that reduced synaptic NE levels cause the appearance of AGS susceptibility these investigators studied the effect of two drugs (tetrabenazine and reserpine) that cause depletion of brain NE by inhibiting incorporation of this amine into the storage vesicles. At times when maximal depletion of NE occurred AGS susceptibility was not enhanced. Instead some degree of anticonvulsant effect was observed. These investigators suggest that some dynamic aspect of monoamine metabolism is more important in affecting seizure susceptibility than are steady-state levels of NE. In their view this concept is supported by the marked enhancement of AGS susceptibility which occurs during the period of rapid amine decline rather than at the time of maximal NE depletion after treatment with reserpine or tetrabenazine. In my opinion, however, it is at this period of maximal depletion that reserpine and tetrabenazine would be expected to produce maximal suppression of noradrenergic activity. [As already discussed, reserpine and Ro 4-1284 (a benzoquinolizine similar to tetrabenazine) produce marked enhancement of AGS in rats at times of severe NE depletion.]

Recent observations show that DBA/2J mice (susceptible to AGS) have lower brain catechol-O-methyl transferase activity (COMT, an enzyme that catalyzes the degradation of NE and DA) than do C57BL/6J mice (resistant to AGS).[160] I believe that these observations do not provide sufficient evidence to support the noradrenergic hypothesis of AGS susceptibility. However, Schlesinger et al.[160] suggest that lower COMT activity in AGS-susceptible animals represents a compensatory mechanism designed to elevate synaptic NE levels by reduced catabolism. They contend that DBA/2J mice would be even more seizure-prone if it were not for the reduced COMT levels. Although plausible, this speculation has not been verified by experimentation.

Recent evidence presented by Kellogg[161] indicates that DBA/2J mice synthesize L-DOPA in the brain at a higher rate than nonsusceptible C57BL/6J mice. On the basis of these observations, coupled with the fact that the DBA/2J mice have lower NE levels in the hindbrain (at 14, 21, and 28 days of age), Kellogg suggested that in DBA/2J mice the mechanisms for intracellular retention of NE are deficient. The amount of physiologically releasable NE would consequently be decreased because storage is essential for release. As pointed out by Kellogg, her interpretation is equivocal because the method used for determining L-DOPA synthesis rate does not actually determine synthesis rate for NE.

An interpretation of her data that comes more readily to mind is that an increase in NE synthesis rate coupled with a decreased NE level occurs because of the more rapid release of NE into the synaptic cleft. This more rapid release would lower the NE content of the nerve ending so that there would be less feedback inhibition on tyrosine hydroxylase and the synthesis rate would increase as a consequence. It is also possible that the augmented level of synthesis results from greater resistance of the tyrosine hydroxylase of DBA/2J mice to feedback inhibition by cytoplasmic NE.

Other important investigations that point in the same diffuse directions as those already described have been conducted in mice: Kellogg,[162] Kellogg and Dobkin,[163] Anlezark and Meldrum,[164] Alexander et al.,[159,165-167] Plotnikoff and Kastin,[168] Schlesinger et al.,[169,170] Lehmann et al.,[171-173] Boggan et al.,[174,175] and Schlesinger.[47,176] Because of space limitations, these studies are not detailed.

In comparison to the observations in mice the emerging data relating AGS susceptibility in rats to a noradrenergic deficit are straightforward. This may be an indication that the etiology of AGS susceptibility in mice is more complex than in rats.

With regard to dopaminergic transmission, results in mice also differ from those in rats. Although, as already pointed out, DA does not appear to modulate AGS in rats, evidence indicates that it may do so in mice; for example, Boggan and Seiden[174] have attributed the anticonvulsant effects of L-DOPA to its conversion of DA in the brain of mice. Furthermore, Kellogg[161] has found that apomorphine (a dopaminergic agonist) decreases the incidence of clonic–tonic convulsions and death in DBA/2J mice. Anlezark et al.[164,177,178] have shown that in DBA/2J mice the potencies of various dopamine receptor agonists (*N-n*-propylnorapomorphine, apomorphine, and some ergot alkaloids) to suppress AGS are similar to their potencies in behavioral tests of dopaminergic function. Finally, Shaywitz et al.[179] reported that the turnover rate of DA in DBA/2J mice progressively increases from 3 weeks of age (when 94% of the animals are susceptible to AGS) to 6 weeks (when only 30% are susceptible) and finally to 12 weeks (when none of the animals exhibits seizures). An additional experiment by Shaywitz et al.,[179] which contrasts with the observations of Kellogg[161] described above, revealed that NE turnover rate is low at 3 weeks of age and that the turnover rate increases between this time and 6 weeks of age and remained stable thereafter. Although the latter observation could be interpreted as militating against an AGS-attenuating role for NE, an alternative and compatible explanation would be that the reduction in AGS susceptibility is caused by an increase in dopaminergic and noradrenergic transmission between 3 and 6 weeks of age and that it is caused only by an increase in dopaminergic transmission thereafter.

5-Hydroxytryptamine (5-HT)

Jobe et al.[180] and Prakhe[127] have studied the effects of various drugs on brain 5-HT levels in rats and compared their findings with the effect of these same treatments on AGS intensity. Although some of the treatments also altered NE and DA Levels, it was possible to observe differences in the depletion of these two catecholamines and 5-HT. The results indicate that depletion of 5-HT itself enhances AGS, whereas an increase in the content of this monoamine above physiological levels diminishes the intensity of seizure. Observations that support this concept include the following:

1. *p*-Chlorophenylalanine (PCPA, an inhibitor of tryptophan hydroxylase) produces enhancement of AGS and markedly decreases brain 5-HT levels.[127,180]
2. Iproniazid (a monoamine oxidase inhibitor) administered before Ro 4-1284 significantly inhibits the enhancement of seizure intensity associated with Ro 4-1284 alone.[180] Pretreatment with iproniazid also attenuates the decrease in brain 5-HT levels normally associated with Ro 4-1284 seizure enhancement but does not inhibit the accompanying decrease in NE and DA levels.[180]
3. Pretreatment with PCPA completely prevents the antagonistic effect of iproniazid on Ro 4-1284-induced enhancement of AGS intensity and on the reduction of 5-HT levels.[180]
4. Intraperitoneally administered 5-hydroxytryptophan (5-HTP, the precursor to 5-HT) in animals pretreated with a monoamine oxidase inhibitor significantly decreases the intensity of seizure.[180]

5 Deseryl, a 5-HT receptor blocking agent, abolishes the anticonvulsant effect of 5-HTP.[127]

In a recent paper Jerlicz et al.[181] confirmed the observation that PCPA enhances the intensity of AGS in rats. They also showed, however, the lesions in the nucleus raphe medianus and nucleus raphe dorsalis produce no changes in seizure intensity. These observations suggest that although some 5-hydroxytryptaminergic neurons may be involved in determining AGS intensity in the rat those that develop in the nucleus raphe medianus and nucleus raphe dorsalis do not function in this way.

A role for 5-HT in AGS intensity in rats is further emphasized by the work of Laird et al.[182] These investigators have found that ρ-chloromethamphetamine, a selective depletor of brain 5-HT content, causes marked enhancement of AGS intensity. Because this AGS enhancement occurred at a time when the cerebral hemispheres and midbrain showed greater depletion of 5-HT than the other regions of the brain, Laird et al.[182] suggested that these two parts of the brain are important sites for the seizure-modulating effect of 5-HT.

In contrast to these observations made in *rats* several investigators have reported that PCPA produces a distinct inhibition of AGS intensity in mice[159,165–167,183] and that this effect is accompanied by a marked reduction in the levels of brain 5-HT and 5-hydroxyindoleacetic acid (the major catabolite of 5-HT). Furthermore, drugs that have been reported to block 5-HT receptors also suppress AGS in mice.[183]

The effects of PCPA and 5-HT receptor blocking agents militate against the concept that 5-hydroxytryptaminergic neurons function as attenuators of AGS susceptibility and intensity in mice. However, the following findings support this hypothesis:

1 5-HTP suppresses AGS in various strains of susceptible mice.[183,184]
2 An inverse circadian correlation exists between changes in levels of brain 5-HT and intensities of AGS.[47,176]
3 6-Methoxy-1,2,3,4-tetrahydro-β-carboline increases brain 5-HT and suppresses AGS in mice.[185]
4 AGS susceptible mice have abnormally low brain 5-HT levels.[22,162]

An additional finding that DBA/2J mice also have faster rates of 5-HT production and disappearance[162] at the time of AGS susceptibility might be interpreted as arguing against an attenuating role of 5-HT in AGS. As Kellogg[162] suggests, however, the postsynaptic 5-HT receptors may be functionally immature at the age of AGS susceptibility and do not sufficiently regulate 5-HT synthesis. If this were true, a deficit in 5-hydroxytryptaminergic activity might exist despite a higher level of 5-HT in the synaptic cleft.

Other Neurotransmitters

γ-AMINOBUTYRIC ACID (GABA)

The nonmonoaminergic determinants of AGS intensity and susceptibility in rats are largely unknown. Benson and Salzberg[186] have reported that the convulsant drug thiosemicarbazide, which produces a decrease in brain GABA levels, also causes an increase in the incidence of AGS in rats. Although these observations are interesting, they should be interpreted with some degree of caution. Because thiosemicarbazide is a convulsant drug, it might cause the appearance of seizure activity in animals subjected to sound by mechanisms related to its convulsant action, whether or not the seizures have anything to do with genetically determined AGS susceptibility.

Duplisse[58] completed a series of experiments that, according to his interpretation, provides evidence that a defect in the GABA inhibitory system of the inferior colliculus in the rat is responsible for susceptibility to AGS. According to his concept, during sound stimulation inadequate containment of impulses within the inferior colliculus (due to a relative lack of GABA-ergic activity) results in the spread of discharges to other parts of the CNS. In my opinion, however, Duplisse's data more readily support the concept that repeated sound stimulation of genetically susceptible rats results in an abnormally high level of GABA-ergic transmission within the inferior colliculus which contains impulses in the auditory pathway so that seizure discharges can no longer be projected to other parts of the brain. In addition, recent observations by Laird and Huxtable[187] suggest that a GABA-ergic deficit does not exist in the brain of genetically susceptible rats.

Studies in *mice* do point toward a role of GABA-ergic neurons in AGS.[188–194] γ-Acetylenic GABA and γ-vinyl GABA, irreversible inhibitors of GABA transaminase, cause sustained elevations of brain GABA levels that correlate closely with decreases in AGS intensity and susceptibility.[188,189] Also, sodium valproate (a clinically effective antiepileptic drug) and ethanolamine-*o*-sulfate (a GABA-transaminase inhibitor) have suppressed AGS in mice in a manner that correlates with their capacity to increase brain GABA levels.[190,191]

TAURINE

Although taurine has not been firmly established as a neurotransmitter in CNS,[195] several studies indicate that this substance may play a role in AGS. Laird and Huxtable[187] have reported that ICV taurine and GABA produce dose-dependent anticonvulsant effects against AGS in rats, with taurine being the most potent. In a subsequent report Laird and Huxtable[43] showed that ICV taurine causes an anticonvulsant effect against electrically induced seizure only in AGS susceptible rats. These investigators have suggested that taurine may exert its anticonvulsant effect by one or the other of two mechanisms.[43,73] First, it may be taken up into neurons and/or glia cells and subsequently released to exert an inhibitory action. Second, it may exert an indirect effect by modifying metabolism of GABA. In this regard taurine given to mice (rendered "epileptic" by cobalt) causes an increase in cortical glutamic acid decarboxylase activity and a reduction in that of GABA aminotransferase.[196] Both effects would be expected to increase the GABA content of the synaptic cleft. More recent work by Huxtable and Laird,[197] however, has revealed that brain regions in genetically susceptible AGS rats have no lower taurine, GABA, glutamate, glutamine, or glycine levels than the brain regions of AGS-resistant rats. Also, the ratios of the concentrations of these amino acids in AGS rats were not different than those in resistant rats. On the basis of all of their results these investigators have concluded that no generalized theory of epilepsy based on disturbances in amino-acid regulation is possible at the present time.

ACETYLCHOLINE (ACH)

The role of Ach in AGS has received little attention and is not adequately understood. Kellogg[198] has reported that the muscarinic agonist oxotremorine protects against AGS in mice and that the centrally acting muscarinic blocking agent scopolamine prevents the protection provided by oxotremorine.

Observations of Jobe (unpublished) have shown that in rats the AGS itself has pronounced effects on whole-brain Ach levels. Young rats sacrificed in liquid nitrogen during the first running phase of AGS showed a nonsignificant decrease in Ach content. During the pause that occurs between the first and second running phases Ach levels appeared to be normal, whereas during the second running episode and tonic or clonic convulsion they were significantly reduced.

10.4.3 The Role of Central Nervous System Neurotransmitters in Audiogenic Seizure Priming

Two developmental and/or neuronal mechanisms appear to be operative in priming in mice.[199-204] One is responsible for the relatively slow onset susceptibility that occurs in most mice in response to acoustic priming or external ear plugging. The other is partly responsible for the rapid onset of susceptibility seen in C57BL/6J mice specifically in response to acoustic priming. The first mechanism involves a partial hearing loss that ultimately results in disuse supersensitivity in the brainstem auditory system. The second mechanism appears to involve a transient fall in brain GABA content described by Sze[199] as well as a dependency on corticosteroids[205] and brain protein synthesis.[201] GABA, however, has not been demonstrated to participate in the priming process in its role as a neurotransmitter. Maxson et al.[202] suggest that it may be involved in some metabolic process.

A role for other neurotransmitters in priming mechanisms in mice is also possible but it is not well documented. Boggan et al.[175] have observed that 5-HTP or L-DOPA (precursors to 5-HT and NE, respectively) or reserpine (a monoamine depleting agent) do not alter the onset of AGS susceptibility in primed C57BL/6J mice. In contrast, Kellogg[206] has observed that pharmacologic activation of noradrenergic transmission blocks appearance of susceptibility in mice exposed to the priming stimulus. Observations by Cooper et al.[207] suggest that a reduction in GABA in the brain stem of the rat may be involved in the development of audiogenic seizure susceptibility during the ethanol withdrawal syndrome.

The roles of the neurotransmitters in acoustic priming in rats have not been studied because these animals do not appear to become susceptible to AGS in response to a single acoustic stimulus[93] (also Jobe and Brown, unpublished observations). As already mentioned, however, Brown et al.[102c] have shown that multiple exposures of rat pups to the acoustic stimulus cause AGS susceptibility. Jobe and Brown (unpublished observations) are presently designing studies to determine whether CNS neurotransmitters are etiologically important in acoustically induced, developmentally dependent AGS susceptibility in rats.

10.4.4 The Role of Energy Reserves in Audiogenic Seizures

Evidence indicates that energy sources in the nervous system may play a role in priming induced or genetically determined AGS susceptibility in mice; for example, kanamycin may prime mice to AGS susceptibility by reducing the amount of glucose available to the cochlear hair cells. With regard to mechanism, Garcia-Quiroga et al.[208] have observed that alloxan-induced hyperglycemia clearly protects rats against kanamycin-induced ototoxicity as revealed by electrocochleographic and histologic examinations. According to the concept of these investigators, the ototoxicity of kanamycin may occur because the antibiotic reduces the amount of glucose available and that the hair cells are "less able to carry out repairs along with their normal functions and might die from lack of repair."

In addition, the possibility of a developmental abnormality in immediately available energy reserves in the *brains* of genetically susceptible mice and primed mice has been described by Schreiber.[209,210] According to his concept, AGS susceptible mice have such a low level of reserves that "coherent nervous activity" cannot be maintained during acoustic stimulation and seizures occur as a consequence. Whether this proposed developmental energy defect preferentially affects one or more neurotransmitter systems in CNS has not been determined.

10.4.5 Summary

The biological basis of AGS susceptibility and the regulatory mechanisms of AGS intensity have not been fully elucidated in the various species of AGS-susceptible animals or in the different types of AGS susceptibility observed in strains of the same species. At the present time, however, it could be concluded that there is more than one biological substrate. A cochlear abnormality characterized by hair-cell damage appears to be an important contributing factor, but this factor alone is insufficient to cause susceptibility unless it coexists with an abnormality in the CNS. Evidence indicates that this abnormality may be a deficit in one or more inhibitory neurotransmitter systems of the CNS. Findings are relatively consistent in supporting the concept that a deficiency in noradrenergic and/or 5-hydroxytryptaminergic transmission in rats may contribute to the severity and regulation of susceptibility. Similar deficits may also underlie AGS in mice, but interpretations of the supporting evidence are in some instances equivocal. Other neurotransmitter systems that may participate in AGS in the rat and mouse are GABA-ergic and cholinergic. Although dopaminergic systems may play a role in AGS in mice, they do not do so in rats. The role of endogenous taurine in AGS remains relatively obscure.

10.5 MEDICAL AND BIOLOGICAL SIGNIFICANCE OF STUDIES OF AUDIOGENIC SEIZURES

Audiogenic-seizure-susceptible rats and mice are of interest to neurobiologists partly because of a need to develop models by which a better understanding can be obtained for the genetic bases of behavior and of neurological diseases such as epilepsy. Because AGS susceptibility in rats and mice is a genetically determined trait, the key to correcting the underlying metabolic abnormalities may be discovered by the administration of specific chemical agents. By the development of these concepts a rational rather than a symptomatic approach to treatment may be obtained for human CNS disorders with similar neurochemical deficits. Preventive interventions may also be possible.

One application of these studies can be found in the parallelism between the multifaceted studies of genetically determined AGS in animals and human disorders of behavior. Although Fuller and Collins[21] specifically reject any implication that AGS is a model of schizophrenia or any other psychiatric disorder, they believe that the significance of AGS studies lies in the development of reasoning processes applicable to human disorders.

This same homology may exist between AGS and human epilepsy because considerable evidence indicates that these human disorders have genetic determinants (see review by Metrakos and Metrakos[211]). Although this is sufficient reason to study AGS in animals, the possibility that AGS *is* a model of human epilepsy should also be considered. In my opinion genetically determined AGS is more intimately associated with human epilepsy than seizures induced by electricity or drugs. As pointed out by Maxson and Cowan,[118] it may be particularly relevant to the brainstem component of grand mal seizures.

Furthermore, in one type of human epilepsy, seizures are triggered by sound stimulation. Overt similarities that exist in the AGS of animals and man include (1) seizures are induced by an exaggeration of stimuli present in the environment, (2) in some humans and animals, sound stimulation produces clonic convulsions, and (3) in other people or animals sound stimulation produces generalized tonic convulsions.

Audiogenic seizures in rats and mice also resemble other forms of human epilepsy such as those characterized by clonic or tonic–clonic seizure patterns but which are not caused by an acoustic stimulus. Audiogenic seizures in animals appear to be especially comparable to "cursive" epilepsy, a disorder characterized by extreme fear followed by frantic running, tonic–clonic convulsion, and postictal depression.[212]

Although clonic or tonic AGS in animals does not superficially resemble other human epileptic disorders like those characterized by cortical focal, psychomotor, atonic, petit mal, and akinetic seizures, they may have more in common than is initially suspected. Indeed, the similarity of AGS in animals to cursive and other clonic and tonic–clonic forms of epilepsy may imply a similarity to the forms that are not characterized by generalized clonic or tonic convulsions. This concept is supported by the findings of Metrakos and Metrakos[211] which indicate that the diverse types of human epilepsies (including those with and without clonic and tonic convulsions) may have more in common than divisions at the clinical seizure level would imply. Their review not only supports the concept that idiopathic epilepsy is determined by genetic factors but that "acquired" epilepsy is also genetically determined. They conclude that a genetically determined breakdown of normal negative feedback control results in the formation of an oscillatory mechanism capable of activation from a variety of points in the CNS and that this loss of inhibition is the common basis for at least three divergent forms of epilepsy; namely, centrencephalic, febrile, and focal. In patients who lack this genetically determined deficit an input of similar intensity would not initiate proxysmal activity and a seizure would not ensue.

In view of these considerations the similarity between AGS and the diverse forms of human epilepsy is more impressive than would otherwise be envisioned. Not only is AGS susceptibility genetically determined but sound-induced seizures appear to result from activation of an oscillator system which is abnormally sensitive to input from various sources in the brain.[27,213,214] As would be expected, if AGS animals have a genetically determined breakdown of inhibitory control that gives rise to a generalized seizure proneness, these animals also have lower electroshock, pentylenetetrazol, and bicuculline seizure thresholds than non-AGS animals.[43,58,215]

THUS AGS-SUSCEPTIBLE ANIMALS MAY PROVIDE RELEVANT MODELS FOR STUDIES OF HUMAN PREDISPOSITION TO SEIZURES. IN CONTRAST, OTHER MODELS BASED ON

INDUCED CONVULSIONS IN NORMAL ANIMALS WITH NO APPARENT GENETICALLY DETERMINED PREDISPOSITION TO SEIZURES MAY PROVIDE LITTLE OR NO INFORMATION REGARDING THE BIOLOGICAL BASIS OF PATHOLOGICALLY HIGH LEVELS OF SEIZURE SUSCEPTIBILITY.

Other models may clarify the appearance of seizures in humans without this predisposition. With regard to those models that have no predispositions to seizure the possibility that a focus could have such great intensity that it would produce seizures in a nongenetically predisposed human cannot be denied. It is also clear that seizures can occur in normal human subjects if they are exposed to sufficiently high doses of convulsant drugs or adequate currents of electricity. It must be emphasized, however, that genetically prone individuals would develop seizure activity in response to foci much too weak to precipitate seizures in normal subjects.

Neuropharmacological observations also support the concept that AGS in rats is a relevant model for studies of human epilepsy; for example, drugs such as phenytoin, phenobarbital, and clonazepam, which are clinically useful in the treatment of several forms of human epilepsy, are effective anticonvulsants against AGS in rats.[216] In addition, the neurochemical basis of AGS in rats and mice may be similar to that of human epilepsy. Shaywitz and coworkers[217] reported that epileptic children have significantly lower levels of metabolites of 5-HT and DA in the cerebrospinal fluid than nonepileptic children. Furthermore, Miras-Portugal et al.[218] have found that plasma DA-β-hydroxylase, the enzyme responsible for converting DA to NE, is significantly lower in epileptic patients than in control subjects. These findings suggest the possibility that a decrement in the functional state of one or more of the various monoaminergic pathways may be etiologically important in human epilepsy and in AGS in animals.

The importance of central monoaminergic activity in human epilepsy is further supported by observations that amphetamine, a drug that augments noradrenergic and dopaminergic activity in the CNS, is of some benefit in the treatment of certain forms of human epilepsy.[219] Phenytoin (a drug of choice in the treatment of grand mal seizures) inhibits the high-affinity uptake of NE into synaptosomes when used in concentrations that are well within the pharmacologic anticonvulsant range in human blood and brain.[220]

As research in this field progresses the primary neurotransmitter abnormalities may be elucidated. There may be one or more underlying deficits that are common to all forms of epilepsy. Alternatively, some kinds of seizures may develop from only *one* type of neurotransmitter deficit.

A practical application of the AGS model could be in the screening of antiepileptic drugs. Some investigators have commented that the effects of an ideal anticonvulsant drug should be confined to the abnormal neurons of a focus to prevent their excessive discharges. Unfortunately all neurons outside a focus may not be normal and, for that matter, not all epileptic patients have a seizure focus. Because a genetically determined inhibitory deficit may underlie human epilepsy, it is important to develop animal models that mimic this deficit accurately. If an animal model that lacks this deficit were used to screen for new antiepileptic drugs, the probable consequence would be to detect those agents that alter the functioning of normal neurons. As a result the side-effects associated with the use of these drugs might be pronounced. By using animals with the inhibitory deficit, however, it would be possible to detect treatments that specifically correct the deficit without altering the activities of normal neurons. Antiepileptic drugs detected by use of this type of model would therefore be expected to "normalize" the functioning of the defective neurons without directly inhibiting or exciting other components of the CNS.

ACKNOWLEDGMENTS

The excellent secretarial assistance of Ms. Susie Fessler, the typing of Ms. Kerry Turner, and the proofreading done by Ms. Susan Bairnsfather are sincerely appreciated. The past and present research support of the Pharmaceutical Manufacturers Association and the Veterans Administration (MRIS 525-76-9162-01 and MRIS 525-76-9162-02) is gratefully acknowledged as well.

REFERENCES

1. H. H. Donaldson, *The Rat: Data and Reference Tables*, 2nd ed., Wistar Institute, Philadelphia, 1924, p. 134.
2. F. W. Finger, *Psychol. Bull.*, **44,** 201 (1974).
3. N. R. F. Maier and N. M. Glaser, *Experimentally Produced Neurotic Behavior in the Rat*, Film. Bethlehem, A. Ford, 600 ft, 16 mm., 1938, in film library of the University of Arizona.
4. C. T. Morgan and J. D. Morgan, *J. Comp. Psychol.*, **27,** 505 (1939).
5. C. T. Morgan, *J. Genet. Psychol.*, **23,** 227 (1940).
6. E. T. Auer and K. U. Smith, *J. Comp. Psychol.*, **30,** 255 (1940).
7. M. M. Parker, *Psychol. Bull.*, **38,** 579 (1941).
8. R. A. Patton and H. W. Karn, *J. Comp. Psychol.*, **31,** 43 (1941).
9. F. W. Finger, *Am. J. Psychol.*, **55,** 68 (1942).
10. G. Humphrey, *J. Comp. Psychol.*, **33,** 315 (1942).
11. H. L. Sisk, *J. Psychol.*, **14,** 85 (1942).
12. T. J. Snee, C. F. Terrence, and M. E. Crowley, *J. Psychol.*, **13,** 233 (1942).
13. E. J. Stainbrook, *J. Psychol.*, **13,** 337 (1942).
14. J. Shohl, *J. Comp. Psychol.*, **37,** 243 (1944).
15. O. L. Lacey, *J. Comp. Psychol.*, **38,** 257 (1945).
16. C. T. Morgan and H. Waldman, *J. Comp. Psychol.*, **31** (1941).

17. G. Humphrey, *Bull. Can. Psychol. Assoc.*, **1,** 39 (1941).
18. K. U. Smith, *J. Comp. Psychol.*, **32,** 311 (1941).
19. I. A. Mirsky, S. Elgart, and C. D. Aring, *J. Comp. Psychol.*, **35,** 249 (1943).
20. W. J. Griffiths, Jr., *J. Comp. Psychol.*, **34,** 263 (1942).
21. J. L. Fuller and R. L. Collins, *Sem. Psychiat.*, **2,** 75 (1970).
22. K. Schlesinger, W. Boggan, and D. X. Freedman, *Life Sci.*, **4,** 2345 (1965).
23. P. C. Jobe, A. L. Picchioni, and L. Chin, *J. Pharmacol. Exp. Ther.*, **184,** 1 (1973).
24. J. L. Fuller, C. Easler, and M. E. Smith, *Genetics*, **35,** 622 (1950).
25. H. Frings and M. Frings, *Behaviour*, **5,** 305 (1953).
26. R. L. Collins, in D. P. Purpura, J. K. Penry, D. B. Tower, D. M. Woodbury, and R. D. Walter, Eds., *Experimental Models of Epilepsy*, Raven, New York, 1972, pp. 347–372.
27. E. A. Swinyard, in *Psychophysiologie, Neuropharmacologie et Biochimie de la Crise Audiogene*, Editions du Centre National de la Recherche Scientifique, Paris, 1963, pp. 405–421.
28. A. Lehmann and R. G. Busnel, in R. G. Busnel, Ed., *Acoustic Behavior of Animals*, Elsevier, New York, 1963, pp. 244–274.
29. E. M. Vicari, *Anat. Rec.*, **97,** 407 (1947).
30. G. Nellhaus, *Am. J. Physiol.*, **193,** 567 (1958).
31. G. Nellhaus, in *Psychophysiologie, Neuropharmacologie et Biochimie de la Crise Audiogene*, Editions du Centre National de la Recherche Scientifique, Paris, 1963, pp. 131–144.
32. J. J. Antonitis and J. P. Scott, *Genetics and Behavior*, Film. Psychol. Cinema Reg., 16 mm., 1953, in film library of the Pennsylvania State College, No. PCR-108K.
33. J. J. Antonitis, D. D. Crary, P. B. Sawin, and C. Cohen, *J. Hered.*, **45,** 278 (1954).
34. H. Parry, *Lancet*, **1,** 32 (1948).
35. R. A. Patton, *J. Comp. Physiol. Psychol.*, **40,** 283 (1947).
36. M. Critchley, *Brain*, **60,** 13 (1937).
37. M. Joynt and L. Green, *J. Am. Med. Assoc.*, **179,** 501 (1962).
38. D. C. Poskanzer, A. E. Brown, and H. Miller, *Brain*, **85,** 77 (1962).
39. F. M. Forster, in B. L. Welch and A. S. Welch, Eds., *Physiological Effects of Noise*, Plenum, New York, 1970, pp. 151–158.
40. J. L. Lush, *J. Hered.*, **21,** 242 (1930).
41. P. Bard, in C. Murchison, Ed., *A Handbook of General Experimental Psychology*, Clark University Press, Worcester, MA, 1934, pp. 264–311.
42. B. E. Ginsburg, *Proc. Assoc. Res. Nerv. Dis.*, **33,** 39 (1954).
43. H. E. Laird and R. J. Huxtable, in A. Barbeau and R. J. Huxtable, Eds., *Taurine and Neurological Disorders*, Raven, New York, 1978, pp. 339–357.
44. C. S. Hall, *J. Hered.*, **38,** 3 (1947).
45. P. C. Jobe, Relationship of Brain Amine Metabolism to Audiogenic Seizure in the Rat. Ph.D. dissertation, the University of Arizona, 1970, pp. 3–4.
46. C. W. N. Wilson, in *Psychophysiologie, Neuropharmacologie et Biochimie de la Crise Audiogene*, Editions du Centre National de la Recherche Scientifique, Paris, 1963, pp. 51–65.
47. R. A. Schreiber and K. Schlesinger, *Physiol. Behav.*, **8,** 699 (1972).
48. K. R. Henry and R. E. Bowman, in B. L. Welch and A. S. Welch, Eds., *Physiological Effects of Noise*, Plenum, New York, 1970, pp. 185–201.
49. G. J. Alexander and R. B. Alexander, *Life Sci.*, **19,** 987 (1976).

50. L. V. Krushninsky, L. N. Molodkina, D. A. Fless, L. P. Dobrokhotova, A. P. Steshenko, A. F. Semiokhina, Z. A. Zorina, and L. G. Romanova, in B. L. Welch and A. S. Welch, Eds., *Physiological Effects of Noise*, Plenum, New York, 1970, pp. 159–183.
51. J. R. Daube, *J. Nerv. Ment. Dis.*, **141,** 524 (1966).
52. W. Bevan, *Psychol. Bull.*, **52,** 473 (1955).
53. C. T. Morgan and R. Galambos, *Am. J. Psychol.*, **55,** 555 (1942).
54. J. F. Willott, K. R. Henry, and F. George, *Exp. Neurol.*, **46,** 542 (1975).
55. J. C. Saunders and K. A. Hirsch, *J. Comp. Physiol. Psychol.*, **90,** 212 (1976).
56. G. J. Alexander and R. Gray, *Fed. Proc.*, **29,** 779 (1970).
57. R. A. Schreiber, *Behav. Genet.*, **8,** 341 (1978).
58. B. Duplisse, Mechanism of Susceptibility of Rats to Audiogenic Seizure. Ph.D. Dissertation, University of Arizona, 1976, pp. 25–45.
59. C. Morgan and J. Gould, *Psychol. Rec.*, **4,** 258 (1941).
60. C. H. Norris, T. H. Cawthon, and R. C. Carroll, *Neuropharmacology*, **16,** 375 (1977).
61. J. C. Saunders, G. R. Bock, C.-S. Chen, and G. R. Gates, *Exp. Neurol.*, **36,** 426 (1972).
62. K. R. Henry, K. A. Thompson, and R. E. Bowman, *Exp. Neurol.*, **31,** 402 (1971).
63. F. M. Forster, P. Hansotia, C. Cleeland, and A. Ludwig, *Neurology*, **19,** 325 (1969).
64. W. D. Hohenboken and G. Nellhaus, *J. Hered.*, **61,** 107 (1970).
65. B. R. Alford and R. J. Ruben, *Ann. Otol. Rhinol. Laryngol.*, **72,** 237 (1963).
66. D. O. Mikaelian and R. J. Ruben, *Arch. Otolaryngol.*, **80,** 418 (1964).
67. D. O. Mikaelian and R. J. Ruben, *Acta Oto Laryngol.*, **59,** 451 (1965).
68. K. Kikuchi and P. Hilding, *Acta Oto Laryngol.*, **60,** 207 (1965).
69. H. Davis, *Physiol. Rev.*, **37,** 1 (1957).
70. P. Dallos and M. A. Cheatham, *J. Acoust. Soc. Am.*, **60,** 510 (1976).
71. E. M. Vicari, *J. Psychol.*, **32,** 79 (1951).
72. G. R. Gates and C.-S. Chen, *Exp. Neurol.*, **47,** 360 (1975).
73. R. Huxtable and H. Laird, *Can. J. Sci. Neurol.*, **5,** 215 (1978).
74. D. E. Crowley and M.-C. Hepp-Reymond, *J. Comp. Physiol. Psychol.*, **62,** 427 (1966).
75. I. Foss and G. Flottorp, *Acta Oto Laryngol.*, **77,** 202 (1974).
76. D. L. Jewett and M. N. Romano, *Brain Res.*, **36,** 101 (1972).
77. D. E. Crowley, V. L. Schramm, R. E. Swain, and S. N. Swanson, *Laryngoscope*, **83,** 264 (1973).
78. J. Darrouzet, M.-M. Niaussat, and A. Guilhaume, *Rev. Laryngol.*, **11–12,** 813 (1967).
79. M. Portmann, J. Darrouzet, and M.-M. Niaussat, *Audiology*, **10,** 298 (1971).
80. M.-M. Niaussat, *C. R. Soc. Biol.*, **161,** 529 (1967).
81. M.-M. Niaussat, *C. R. Soc. Biol.*, **163,** 2503 (1969).
82. H. Spoendlin, *Audiology*, **14,** 383 (1975).
83. M.-M. Niaussat, *C. R. Soc. Biol.*, **162,** 21 (1968).
84. D. W. Glenn, R. D. Brown, and P. C. Jobe, *Fed. Proc.*, **38,** 754 (1979).
85. K. Ralls, *Anim. Behav.*, **15,** 123 (1967).
86. P. C. Jobe, J. W. Dailey, and R. D. Brown, *Neurosci. Abstr.*, **3,** 141 (1977).
87. K. R. Henry, *Science*, **158,** 938 (1967).
88. W. B. Iturrian and G. B. Fink, *Fed. Proc.*, **26,** 737 (1967).
89. J. L. Fuller and R. L. Collins, *Dev. Psychobiol.*, **1,** 185 (1968).
90. W. O. Boggan, D. X. Freedman, R. A. Lovell, and K. Schlesinger, *Psychopharmacologia*, **20,** 48 (1971).

91. B. S. Deckard, J. M. Tepper, and K. Schlesinger, *Behav. Genet.*, **6,** 375 (1976).
92. C.-S. Chen and J. L. Fuller, *Behav. Genet.*, **5,** 91 (1975).
93. C.-S. Chen and G. R. Gates, *Medikon*, **4,** 19 (1975).
94. J. C. Saunders, *Laryngoscope*, **84,** 750 (1974).
95. R. A. Schreiber and L. M. Graham, *Develop. Psychobiol.*, **9,** 57 (1976).
96. R. A. Schreiber, *Develop. Psychobiol.*, **10,** 77 (1977).
97. R. A. Schreiber, *Exp. Neurol.*, **56,** 518 (1977).
98. C.-S. Chen, *J. Comp. Physiol. Psychol.*, **84,** 586 (1973).
99. C.-S. Chen, G. R. Gates, and G. R. Bock, *Exp. Neurol.*, **39,** 277 (1973).
100. K. R. Henry, *Science*, **176,** 689 (1972).
101. W. B. Iturrian and H. D. Johnson, *Experientia*, **27,** 1193 (1971).
102a. F. W. Finger, *J. Comp. Psychol.*, **35,** 227 (1943).
102b. P. C. Jobe, R. D. Brown, J. W. Dailey, T. B. Ray, T. W. Woods, M. E. Mims, and S. Bairnsfather, Society for *Neurosci. Abstr.* **6,** 824 (1980).
102c. R. D. Brown, P. C. Jobe, S. Bairnsfather, M. E. Mims, and T. W. Woods, Society for *Neurosci. Abstr.*, **6,** 825 (1980).
103. E. J. Farris and E. H. Yeakel, *J. Comp. Psychol.*, **34,** 75 (1942).
104. K. R. Henry and M. Saleh, *J. Comp. Physiol. Psychol.*, **84,** 885 (1973).
105. K. R. Henry, *J. Comp. Physiol. Psychol.*, **79,** 77 (1972).
106. J. C. Saunders, G. R. Bock, R. James, and C.-S. Chen, *Exp. Neurol.*, **37,** 388 (1972).
107. J. F. Willott and K. R. Henry, *J. Comp. Physiol. Psychol.*, **86,** 1 (1974).
108. G. R. Gates, C.-S. Chen, and G. R. Bock, *Exp. Neurol.*, **38,** 488 (1973).
109. J. Tonndorf and S. M. Khanna, *Ann. Otol Rhin. Laryngol.*, **79,** 743 (1970).
110. M. D. McGinn, J. F. Willott, and K. R. Henry, *Nature New Biol.*, **244,** 255 (1973).
111. M.-M. Niaussat, *Experentia*, **33,** 473 (1977).
112. G. Freund and D. W. Walker, *Psychopharmacologia*, **22,** 45 (1971).
113. B. E. Hunter, C. A. Boast, D. W. Walker, and S. F. Zornetzer, *Pharmacol. Biochem. Behav.*, **1,** 719 (1973).
114. W. M. Bourn and R. G. Buice, *Res. Comm. Psychol. Psychiat. Behav.*, **1,** 653 (1976).
115. R. G. Buice and W. M. Bourn, *Res. Comm. Chem. Path. Pharmacol.*, **19,** 75 (1978).
116. N.-S. Chu, K. C. Squires, and A. Starr, *Arch. Neurol.*, **35,** 596 (1978).
117. G. R. Gates and C.-S. Chen, *Nature*, **249,** 162 (1974).
118. S. C. Maxson and J. S. Cowan, *Physiol. Behav.*, **16,** 623 (1976).
119. D. W. Walker and S. F. Zornetzer, *Electroencephalog. Clin. Neurophysiol.*, **36,** 233 (1974).
120. K. R. Henry, M. Wallick, and M. Davis, *Physiol. Behav.*, **9,** 885 (1972).
121. E. Koenig, *J. Comp. Neurol.*, **108,** 383 (1957).
122. R. P. Kesner, *Exp. Neurol.*, **15,** 192 (1966).
123. C. L. Faingold, *Neuropharmacology*, **16,** 73 (1977).
124. C. L. Faingold and D. M. Caspary, *Neuropharmacology*, **16,** 143 (1977).
125. E. W. Maynert, T. J. Marczynski, and R. A. Browning, *Adv. Neurol.*, **13,** 79 (1975).
126. P. C. Jobe, A. L. Picchioni, and L. Chin, *Fed. Proc.*, **28,** 795 (1969).
127. I. B. Prakhe, *Bull. Eksp. Biol. Med.*, **76**(9), 23–26 (1973).
128. A. Picchioni, L. Chin, D. Choisser, and C. Breitner, *Pharmacologist*, **5,** 238 (1963).
129. W. M. Bourn, L. Chin, and A. L. Picchioni, *J. Pharm. Pharmacol.*, **24,** 913 (1972).
130. W. M. Bourn, L. Chin, and A. L. Picchioni, *J. Pharm. Pharmacol.*, **30,** 800 (1978).

131. R. M. Kostrzewa and D. M. Jacobowitz, *Pharmacol. Rev.*, **26,** 199 (1974).
132. P. C. Jobe, A. L. Picchioni, and L. Chin, *J. Pharm. Pharmacol.*, **25,** 830 (1973).
133. H. Corrodi, K. Fuxe, T. Hokfelt, and M. Schou, *Psychopharmacologia*, **11,** 345 (1967).
134. P. C. Jobe, A. L. Picchioni, L. Chin, and P. F. Geiger, *Fed. Proc.*, **35,** 270 (1976).
135. A. L. Picchioni, L. Chin, and C. Breitner, *Fed. Proc.*, **21,** 416 (1962).
136. H. G. Dengler, H. E. Spiegel, and E. O. Titus, *Nature*, **191,** 816 (1961).
137. G. Hertting, J. Axelrod, and L. G. Whitby, *J. Pharmacol. Exp. Ther.*, **134,** 146 (1961).
138. U. Trendelenburg, A. Muskus, W. W. Fleming, and B. G. Alonso de la Sierra, *J. Pharmacol. Exp. Ther.*, **138,** 170 (1962).
139. M. E. Rosenthale and J. R. Dipalma, *Arch. Int. Pharmacodyn. Ther.*, **146,** 529 (1963).
140. J. Glowinski and J. Axelrod, *Nature*, **204,** 1318 (1964).
141. R. A. Maxwell, *J. Pharmacol. Exp. Ther.*, **147,** 289 (1965).
142. W. C. Bowman, M. J. Rand, and G. B. West, *Textbook of Pharmacology*, Blackwell Scientific Publications, Oxford, 1968, pp. 734–775.
143. S. B. Ross, A. L. Renyi, and B. Burnfelter, *J. Pharm. Pharmacol.*, **20,** 283 (1968).
144. A. Carlsson, in U. S. Von Euler, S. Rosell, and B. Unnas, Eds., *Mechanisms of Release of Biogenic Amines*, Pergamon, New York, 1966, pp. 331–345.
145. F. Sulser, *Adv. Pharmacol.*, **6B,** 70 (1968).
146. R. A. Rutledge, W. E. Barrett, and A. J. Plummer, *Fed. Proc.*, **18,** 441 (1959).
147. A. Carlsson, H. Corrodi, K. Fuxe, and T. Holkfelt, *Eur. J. Pharmacol.*, **5,** 357 (1969).
148. S. Schanberg and N. J. Giarman, *Biochem. Pharmacol.*, **11,** 187 (1962).
149. A. Carlsson, M. Lindgvist, T. Magnusson, and B. Waldeck, *Science*, **127,** 471 (1958).
150. A. F. De Schaepdryver, Y. Piette, and A. L. Delaunois, *Arch. Int. Pharmacodyn. Ther.*, **140,** 358 (1962).
151. A. Carlsson, *Acta Neuroveg.*, **26,** 484 (1964).
152. K. Fuxe and U. Ungerstedt, *Life Sci.*, **5,** 1817 (1966).
153. K. Fuxe and U. Ungerstedt, *Histochemie*, **13,** 16 (1968).
154. J. Jones and D. J. Roberts, *Br. J. Pharmacol.*, **34,** 27 (1968).
155. A. Carlsson, *Handbuch. Exp. Pharmacol.*, **19,** 529, 1966.
156. R. D. Brown, P. C. Jobe, and J. W. Dailey, *Fed. Proc.*, **38**(3), 753 (1979).
157. W. M. Bourn, *Neurosci. Abstr.*, **1,** 710 (1975).
158. K. Schlesinger, W. Boggan, and D. X. Freedman, *Life Sci.*, **7,** 437 (1968).
159. G. J. Alexander and L. M. Kopeloff, *Psychopharmacol. Comm.*, **2,** 379 (1976).
160. K. Schlesinger, J. Harkins, B. S. Deckard, and G. Paden, *J. Neurobiol.*, **6,** 587 (1975).
161. C. Kellogg, *Brain Res.*, **106,** 87 (1976).
162. C. Kellogg, *J. Neurobiol.*, **2,** 209 (1971).
163. C. Kellogg and D. Dobkin, *Naunyn-Schmiedeberg's Arch. Pharmacol.*, **293,** 145 (1976).
164. G. M. Anlezark and B. S. Meldrum, *Br. J. Pharmacol.*, **53,** 419 (1975).
165. G. J. Alexander and L. M. Kopeloff, *Res. Comm. Chem. Path. Pharmacol.*, **14,** 437 (1976).
166. G. J. Alexander and L. M. Kopeloff, *Neuropharmacology*, **16,** 405 (1977).
167. G. J. Alexander, L. M. Kopeloff, and R. B. Alexander, *Life Sci.*, **10,** 877 (1971).
168. N. P. Plotnikoff and A. J. Kastin, *Life Sci.*, **18,** 1217 (1976).
169. K. Schlesinger, K. L. Stravens, and W. O. Boggan, *Psychopharmacologia*, **15,** 226 (1969).
170. K. Schlesinger, W. O. Boggan, and D. X. Freedman, *Life Sci.*, **9,** 721 (1970).

171. A. Lehmann, *Life Sci.*, **6,** 1423 (1967).

172. A. G. Lehmann, in B. L. Welch and A. S. Welch, Eds., *Physiological Effects of Noise*, Plenum, New York, 1970, pp. 227–257.

173. A. G. Lehmann, *Life Sci.*, **20,** 2047 (1977).

174. W. O. Boggan and L. S. Seiden, *Physiol. Behav.*, **6,** 215 (1971).

175. W. O. Boggan, D. X. Freedman, R. A. Lovell, and K. Schlesinger, *Psychopharmacologia*, **20,** 48 (1971).

176. R. A. Schreiber and K. Schlesinger, *Physiol. Behav.*, **6,** 635 (1971).

177. G. M. Anlezark, R. W. Horton, and B. S. Meldrum, *Adv. Biochem. Psychopharmacol.*, **19,** 383 (1978).

178. G. Anlezark, C. Pycock, and B. Meldrum, *Eur. J. Pharmacol.*, **37,** 295 (1976).

179. B. A. Shaywitz, R. D. Yager, and J. W. Gordon, *Dev. Psychobiol.*, **11,** 243 (1978).

180. P. C. Jobe, A. L. Picchioni, and L. Chin, *Life Sci.*, **13,** 1 (1973).

181. M. Jerlicz, W. Kostowski, A. Bidzinski, and M. Hauptmann, *Pol. J. Pharmacol. Pharm.*, **30,** 63 (1978).

182. H. E. Laird, L. Chin, and A. L. Picchioni, *Proc. West. Pharmacol. Soc.*, **17,** 46 (1974).

183. W. Kostowski, A. Bidzinski, M. Hauptmann, J. E. Malinowski, M. Jerlicz, and J. Dymecki, *Pol. J. Pharmacol. Phar.*, **30,** 41 (1978).

184. W. O. Boggan and L. S. Seiden, *Physiol. Behav.*, **10,** 9 (1973).

185. N. S. Buckholtz, *Pharmacol. Biochem. Behav.*, **3,** 65 (1975).

186. E. E. Benson and H. C. Salzberg, *Psychol. Rep.*, **19,** 525 (1966).

187. H. E. Laird and R. Huxtable, in Ryan Huxtable and Andre Barbeau, Eds., *Taurine*, Raven, New York, 1976, pp. 267–274.

188. P. J. Schecter, Y. Tranier, M. J. Jung, and P. Bohlen, *Eur. J. Pharmacol.*, **45,** 319 (1977).

189. P. J. Schecter, Y. Tranier, M. J. Jung, and A. Sjoerdsma, *J. Pharmacol. Exp. Ther.*, **201,** 606 (1977).

190. R. W. Horton, G. M. Anlezark, C. B. Sawaya, and B. S. Meldrum, *Eur. J. Pharmachol.*, **41,** 387 (1977).

191. S. Simler, L. Ciesielski, M. Maitre, H. Randrianarisoa, and P. Mandel, *Biochem. Pharmacol.*, **22,** 1701 (1973).

192. R. Tapia, H. Pasantes-Morales, E. Taborda, and M. P. De La Mora, *J. Neurobiol.*, **6,** 159 (1975).

193. G. Anlezark, J. Collins, and B. Meldrum. *Neurosci. Lett.*, **7,** 337 (1977).

194. J. Yamashita and Y. Hirata, *Neurosci. Lett.*, **8,** 89 (1978).

195. J. R. Cooper, F. E. Bloom, and R. H. Roth, *The Biochemical Basis of Neuropharmacology*, Oxford University Press, New York, 1978, pp. 225–256.

196. N. Van Gelder, *Brain Res.*, **47,** 157 (1972).

197. R. J. Huxtable and H. E. Laird, *Neurosci. Lett.*, **10,** 341 (1978).

198. C. Kellogg, in E. Giacobini, A. Vernadakis, and G. Filogamo, Eds., *Maturation of Neurotransmission*, Karger, Basel, 1978, pp. 217–225.

199. P. Y. Sze, in B. L. Welch and A. S. Welch, Eds., *Physiological Effects of Noise*, Plenum, New York, 1970, pp. 259–269.

200. S. Siporin and J. L. Fuller, *Pharmacol. Biochem. Behav.*, **4,** 269 (1976).

201. S. C. Maxson, A. C. Towle, and P. Y. Sze, *Behav. Biol.*, **18,** 111 (1976).

202. S. C. Maxson, A. G. Towle, and P. Y. Sze, *Psychopharmacology*, **53,** 217 (1977).

203. S. C. Maxson, J. S. Cowen, and P. Y. Sze, *Pharmacol. Biochem. Behav.*, **7,** 221 (1977).

204. S. C. Maxson, *Exp. Neurol.*, **62,** 482 (1978).

205. P. Y. Sze, and S. C. Maxson, *Psychopharmacologia*, **45,** 79 (1975).
206. C. Kellogg, *Neurosci. Abstr.*, **1,** 793 (1975).
207. B. R. Cooper, K. Viik, R. M. Ferris, and H. L. White, *J. Pharmacol. Exp. Ther.*, **209,** 396 (1979).
208. J. Garcia-Quiroga, C. H. Norris, L. Glade, C. M. Bryant, M. Tachibana, and P. S. Guth, *Res. Comm. Chem. Path. Pharmacol.*, **22,** 535 (1978).
209. R. A. Schreiber, *Res. Comm. Psychol. Psychiat. Behav.*, **3,** 27 (1978).
210. R. A. Schreiber, *Pharmacol. Biochem. Behav.*, **8,** 619 (1978).
211. K. Metrakos and J. D. Metrakos, in O. Magnus and A. M. Lorentzdehass, Eds., *Handbook of Clinical Neurology*, Vol. 15, American Elsevier, New York, 1974, pp. 429–439.
212. H. Geist, *The Etiology of Idiopathic Epilepsy*, Exposition, New York, 1962.
213. J. Bures, in *Psychophysiologie, Neuropharmacologie et Biochimie de la Crise Audiogene*, Editions du Centre National de la Recherche Scientifique, Paris, 1963, pp. 165–177.
214. W. B. Iturrian and H. D. Johnson, *Pharmacology*, **5,** 65 (1971).
215. H. Laird, P. Consroe and A. Straussner, *Pharmacologist*, **18,** 136 (1976).
216. P. Consroe and A. Wolkin, *J. Pharmacol. Exp. Ther.*, **201,** 26 (1977).
217. B. A. Shaywitz, D. J. Cohen, and M. B. Bowers, *Neurology*, **25,** 72 (1975).
218. M. T. Miras-Portugal, D. Aunis, P. Mandel, J. M. Warter, G. Coquillat, and D. Kurtz, *Psychopharmacologia*, **41,** 75 (1975).
219. S. Livingston and L. Pauli, *J. Am. Med. Assoc.*, **233,** 278 (1975).
220. J. Weinberger, W. J. Nicklas, and S. Berl, Neurology, **26,** 162 (1976).

CHAPTER 11

Vestibular Pharmacology

CHARLES H. NORRIS, Ph.D.

Associate Professor
Department of Otolaryngology
Tulane University Medical School
New Orleans, Louisiana

CONTENTS

11.1 INTRODUCTION

It would be inappropriate to discuss the cochlea without also directing some attention to the vestibular apparatus. Although the central nervous system activity that results from stimulation of the auditory and vestibular receptors is different, these cells share many common traits at the level of the inner ear. The receptor cells of both systems are mechanoreceptors and have many similar physiologic and anatomical features. This is also true of the afferent and efferent nerves that subserve the cochlear and vestibular receptor cells. The two systems of mechanoreceptors share common fluid spaces and many chemical agents that affect cells in one system have similar effects on the cells in the other; for example, aminoglycoside antibiotics are toxic to both systems.

More clinical drugs have been developed for use in the vestibular than in the auditory system, however. The apparent reason is that it is often useful to suppress activity in the vestibular system but seldom desirable to do so in the auditory system. The similarity, yet clinical dichotomy, between the two systems is exemplified by the use of streptomycin. In the past some clinicians have used this drug to destroy the peripheral vestibular apparatus while retaining useful cochlear function.

In addition to peripherally acting drugs, many vestibular drugs have sites of action at various locations in the central nervous system, beginning with the vestibular nuclei. Thus drugs affecting the vestibular system can be divided into two main classes: those reputed to have their major effects on the vestibular portions of the inner ear and others acting on areas more central than the primary vestibular afferent nerves. No clear separation exists between these two classes because drugs like alcohol appear to have actions in both places.

11.2 ANATOMY

In the central nervous system the vestibular system is one part of a triumvirate that makes up the body's overall arrangement for maintaining equilibrium. The other members are the visual and proprioceptive systems. Information developed by the sensors in each of these subsystems is sent to the brain stem and cerebellum where it is coordinated, processed, and passed on to other parts of the central nervous system.

11.2.1 Vestibular Nuclei

Primary vestibular neurons originating from sensory areas in the inner ear synapse centrally in the vestibular nuclei of the brainstem. These nuclei are located just below the floor of the IVth ventricle in the medulla. There are four principal vestibular nuclei: *inferior, lateral, medial,* and *superior*.

The inferior vestibular nucleus begins caudally in the medulla, medial to the accessory cuneate nucleus and extends rostrally, medial to the inferior cerebellar peduncle, to a point near the brainstem entrance of the vestibular nerve. The lateral vestibular nucleus is located laterally in the ventricular floor near the entrance of the vestibular nerve and extends rostrally to the level of the abducens nucleus. The medial vestibular nucleus occupies the floor of the IVth ventricle medial to the inferior and lateral vestibular nuclei. Its rostral and caudal boundaries are indistinct. Rostrally, it fuses dorsolaterally with the superior vestibular nucleus and becomes small at the level of the abducens nucleus. The superior vestibular nucleus lies dorsal and mostly rostral to the lateral vestibular nucleus in the angle formed by the floor and lateral wall of the IVth ventricle. The superior cerebellar peduncle forms the dorsolateral border of the nucleus throughout most of its rostrocaudal extent. The mesencephalic and principal sensory nuclei of the trigeminal nerve are adjacent to the nucleus medially and ventrally respectively in its rostral two-thirds. The rostral pole of the superior vestibular nucleus is also indistinct.

In addition to the four nuclei described above, there are several smaller accessory nuclei, one of which is diffusely spread between the fibers of the vestibular nerve as it enters the brainstem (interstitial nucleus of the vestibular nerve).

Primary vestibular fibers from the periphery project on to all four principal vestibular nuclei and the interstitial nucleus. The *inferior* vestibular nucleus receives input from all areas of the peripheral sensory epithelium and sends its output to the cerebellum and other brainstem nuclei. The function of this primary pathway seems to be to facilitate the control of body movements and to allow a smooth interrelationship of various body parts. The primary fibers to the *lateral* vestibular nucleus originate mostly in the utricular macula and the output of this nucleus is fed mainly to the vestibulo-spinal tract for the control of body musculature. The *medial* vestibular nucleus receives most of its primary input from the cristae of the semicircular canals and sends its output to the occulomotor nuclei and to the cervical area of the spinal cord via the medial longitudinal fasciculus. This provides information for eye and neck control for the position of the head when it is moved in relation to the body. The *superior* vestibular nucleus receives its primary input from the cristae of the three semicircular canals and sends its output mainly to the occulomotor, trochlear, and abducens nuclei via the medial longitudinal fasciculus. The information on this pathway is used for control of eye movements when the head or head and body are in motion. Clinically, the activity of this pathway is used to measure the functioning of the peripheral vestibular sense organs quantitatively.

The previously described primary vestibular pathways are not the only connections to the vestibular nuclei. All receive important inputs from a number of other areas of the CNS, such as the cerebellum and the pontine paramedian reticular formation. Important secondary fibers also lead from the vestibular nuclei to the cerebellum, reticular formation, and other cranial nerve nuclei. The vestibular system, however, is primarily a sensory system designed to convert changes in head position, spatial acceleration and deceleration, gravitational effects, and vibration into neural impulses for central processing and the foregoing are the primary pathways by which this is accomplished.

11.2.2 Sensory Areas of Vestibular Apparatus

The sensory areas of the vestibular system are the cristae of the three semicircular canals and the maculae of the utricle and saccule. The three cristae respond to angular acceleration and the utricular macula responds to gravitational forces and horizontal accelerations; the function of the saccular macula is still unproved but it appears to respond to vibrations and vertical accelerations. These sensory areas are innervated by the primary vestibular neurons, which are grouped into two bundles that constitute the superior and inferior vestibular nerves. The primary vestibular neurons are bipolar and the cell bodies are located in Scarpa's superior and inferior vestibular ganglia. The superior vestibular nerve innervates the cristae of the horizontal and superior semicircular canals, the ultricular macula, and part of the saccula macula. The inferior vestibular nerve innervates the rest of the saccular macula and the crista of the posterior semicircular canal.

11.2.3 Vestibular Hair Cells

The cristae and the maculae contain receptor cells that function to convert mechanical environmental stimuli to electrical (or chemical) changes which, in turn, are used to stimulate the primary afferent fibers of the vestibular nerve. There are two different types of sensory cell which act as the receptor units in the epithelium of the cristae and maculae. Type I has a rounded, flask shape with a narrow neck that leads to an expanded peripheral end. The bottom of the hair cell is surrounded by the nerve chalice which is the origin of the afferent dendrite that runs toward the vestibular ganglia (Scarpa's ganglia). In proximity to the nerve chalice (presumably in synaptic contact with it) are a number of other vesicle-containing nerve endings that carry efferent feed-back impulses from the central nervous system. Type II differs slightly from Type I. Its shape is cylindrical and it is often longer. It possesses no nerve chalice but only small afferent, boutonlike endings and some efferent nerve-fiber endings on the basal part of the cell.

About 50 or more hair processes project from the polar or upper end of both types of hair cell. One of the hair processes on each cell is called a *kinocilium;* and others are *stereocilia*. The kinocilium is always located toward an edge of the hair cell and is thicker and longer than the stereocilia.

The kinocilia are arranged spatially with relation to the stereocilia and are found on the same side of the hair tufts in all cristae. The kinocilia always lie on the utricular side of the cells in the horizontal canal and face away from the utricle in the superior and posterior canals. The arrangement of the kinocilia in the maculae is quite different. In most of the hair cells, the kinocilia lie along the side that faces the central midline of the utricular macula; in the saccular macula the kinocilia face away from the midline. This meridianlike arrangement permits spatial orientation in a full 360° arc. The orientation of the kinocilia is important because mechanical deformation of the stereocilia toward the side of the sensory cell containing the kinocilia is excitatory. Movement away from the kinocilium is inhibitory and hyperpolarizes the cell. The otolithic membrane, which covers the cilia of both maculae, consists of gelatinous masses of tissue with fine channels for the passage of the sensory cilia. On the surface of the otolithic membrane are pure white crystals of calcium carbonate (aragonite concretions) known as *otoliths* or *otoconia*. Gravitational and linear acceleration forces acting on the otoconia cause the cilia to bend, which in turn excites or inhibits the sensory cells, depending on the direction of the forces.

The hair processes of the sensory cells of the cristae ampullaris of the semicircular canals are also covered with a gelatinous mass of protein material known as the cupula which contains many small channels running from the base to the apex through which the processes travel. Even though it is capable of deformation from side to side, the cupula forms an effective seal for the lumen of the ampulla of the semicircular canal. This seal is so effective that it prevents leakage of endolymph from one side of the cupula to the other. After movement the cupula returns to its original position by virtue of its intrinsic mechanical elasticity. Movement of the cupula causes bending of the cilia on the surface of the sensory cells, which again excites or inhibits, depending on the direction of the mechanical acceleration forces acting on the cupula.

11.3 PHYSIOLOGY

Polarization and orientation of the sensory cells give rise to the following observations, known as Ewald's laws:

1. A horizontal semicircular canal is maximally stimulated by a movement of endolymph toward the utricle (ampullopetal flow); a vertical semicircular canal is maximally stimulated by a movement of endolymph away from the utricle (ampullofugal flow).
2. When a semicircular canal is stimulated it tends to elicit nystagmus in its own plane.
3. When a semicircular canal is maximally stimulated it elicits a nystagmus that has its quick phase to the ipsilateral side of the head.

Nystagmus is a repetitive, sawtoothlike oscillation of the eyes, to and fro, in the horizontal or vertical plane. The steepest slope of the sawtooth (fastest movement of the eyes) is known as the quick phase of the nystagmus. Clinically horizontal nystagmus is induced, quantitatively measured, and used to detect vestibular system disorders.

When the head is accelerated in a rotary fashion in the horizontal plane the fluid in the horizontal semicircular canals (endolymph) pushes the horizontal canal cupula on one side of the head toward the utricle and the horizontal canal cupula on the other side of the head away from the utricle. Thus the sensory cells in one ear become excited as those in the other ear are inhibited. A resting firing rate in the vestibular neurons rapidly increases when the sensory cells are excited and decreases when the sensory cells are inhibited. Therefore during angular acceleration there is disparity between the firing rates in the afferent vestibular neurons that develop in each ear. This disparity is stimulatory to the vestibular reflexes and observation of these reflexes indicates whether the vestibular system is functioning in a normal fashion.

There are four important vestibular reflexes among which only the vestibulo-occular reflex can be recorded and quantitated with present-day instrumentation: (1) the vestibulo-ocular reflex (cranial nerves III, IV, and VI), (2) the vestibulo-vegetative reflex (cranial nerve X), (3) the vestibulo-spinal reflex, and (4) the vestibulo-cerebellar reflex. Activity in the other reflexes (nausea, vomiting, ataxia, etc.), however, is also an important clinical observation that helps the modern otologist diagnose conditions in the vestibular system.

The vestibulo-occular reflex arc consists of the primary afferent vestibular neurons that discharge into the ipsilateral superior and medial vestibular nuclei, the secondary vestibular neurons that connect the vestibular nuclei to the occulomotor nuclei (III, IV, and VI), and the motor neurons from the occulomotor nuclei to the extraoccular muscles. Motor neurons in cranial nerve III (occulomotor) supply the inferior oblique muscle and the superior, internal, and inferior rectus muscles. Motor neurons in cranial nerve IV (trochlear) supply the superior oblique muscle and in cranial nerve nerve VI they supply the lateral rectus (abducens) muscle.

When excitatory stimuli in the ipsilateral horizontal semicircular canal cause increased firing in the ipsilateral VIIIth nerve, the occulomotor muscles move the eyes slowly to the contralateral side. Two sources of fast return commands are available to return the eyes quickly to their starting position. One source is activity in the reticular activating system (mainly the paramedian pontine reticular formation) which is transmitted to the accessory occulomotor nucleus and then to the main occulomotor nuclei. The second source is visual fixation transmitted from the retina via the superior colliculus to the main occulomotor nuclei. If both "fast return" channels are working and the peripheral vestibular labyrinth is stimulated, the eyes remain relatively stationary. If, however, one of the fast return channels is blocked (i.e., the eyes are closed, thus removing visual clues), nystagmoid eye movement results with slow rotation contralaterally and fast return rotation ipsilaterally. If both fast return channels are blocked (i.e., eyes closed in conjunction with a brainstem lesion), the eyes move to the contralateral side and stay there.

Controlled head and body angular rotary stimulations are used to test vestibular function and the effects of drugs thereon. Such stimuli are physiologic but unfortunately they test both labyrinths simultaneously. It is diagnostically more useful to test each labyrinth individually. This can be accomplished with a thermal stimulus rather than a mechanical stimulus. The head is positioned such that the horizontal semicircular canals are placed in a vertical plane; the external auditory meatus is then irrigated with warm stimuli (water or air) or cool stimuli (water or air). Warm stimuli will cause the endolymph to push the cupula toward the utricle, thus eliciting a nystagmus with an ipsilateral fast phase. Cool stimuli will cause a nystagmus with a contralateral fast phase. Thus with four stimulations (two temperatures in each ear) it is possible to differentiate between abnormalities in the right and left labyrinths.

Although nystagmoid movements of the eyes always appear to be involved with that part of the vestibulo-occular reflex arc between the vestibular nuclei and the occulomotor muscles, it is possible to generate nystagmus without involving the primary vestibular neurons. Nystagmus can be elicited optokinetically by looking at a rotating cylinder with vertical stripes (railroad nystagmus). In addition, nystagmus can be elicited by electrical stimulation or lesions placed in various areas of the CNS; for example, medullary nystagmogenic areas (vestibular nuclei, medial longitudinal fasciculus, and reticular formation), mesencephalic nystagmogenic areas (superior colliculus and upper areas of the reticular formation), diencephalic nystagmogenic areas (lateral geniculate nuclei and optic tracts), and finally cortical nystagmogenic areas (Brodal's area 18).

Thus it can be difficult to evaluate some drug studies that use recorded nystagmus and report an influence on the vestibular areas of the inner ear; that is, in some studies it is not clear that the nystagmus under influence of the drug is nystagmus which uses activity from the primary vestibular neurons. Nystagmus generated in nonperipheral vestibular areas can be differentiated from peripheral vestibular nystagmus by use of the bithermal caloric test. If warm stimulation in one ear produces results equal to those from cool stimulation in the contralateral ear and this is also true when cool stimulation in one ear equals warm stimulation in the contralateral ear, then it is unlikely that the problem under study is the result of some activity in the peripheral labyrinth.

A much more detailed description of the anatomy and physiology of the peripheral vestibular areas can be found in the review by Kornhuber[1] and the central vestibular system is well described by Brodal and Pompeiano[2] and Truex and Carpenter.[3] Precht[4] nicely integrates activity in the peripheral vestibular system with that of the central vestibular system.

11.4 PHARMACOLOGY

11.4.1 Peripherally Acting Drugs

Drugs reputed to have direct action on the vestibular portions of the inner ear include osmotic agents, diuretics, vasodilators, vestibulotoxic antibiotics, and a miscellaneous group that includes such substances as lithium, alcohol, and heavy water.

Vestibulotoxic Agents

AMINOGLYCOSIDE ANTIBIOTICS

Streptomycin was probably the first drug with a site of action that could definitely be attributed to the vestibular areas of the inner ear.[5–7] The ototoxicity of the aminoglycoside antibiotics is well known and has been reviewed extensively (see Chapter 7). Streptomycin's vestibular toxicity was first reported when it became widely used as an antituberculosis agent. When streptomycin is infused in the carotid artery of a cat whose basilar artery has been altered such that the blood supply to the ear is almost entirely from the carotid there is unilateral vestibular ablation with preservation of cochlear function.[8] In the cat streptomycin vestibulotoxicity results in a decrease in the slow-phase velocity of nystagmus induced by caloric stimulation.[9] The effect is much more easily discerned in the ampullar cristae than in the maculae.[10] The intratympanic administration of streptomycin causes sensory-cell destruction (in order of vulnerability) in the central area of the cristae and the striola (midline) of the utricular macula; the saccular macula is extremely resistant.[11]

In addition, streptomycin preferentially affects Type I cells, but in the guinea pig the Type II cells located in the central region of the cristae are more vulnerable than the Type I cells in the periphery.[12] It is also interesting to note that, furosemide, another ototoxic agent and a potent saluretic agent, has been suggested for use in the management of streptomycin-induced vestibular damage. The possible mechanisms underlying this treatment include a local site of action in the vestibular system, alterations in the electrolyte-fluid balance, and a "flushing out" of streptomycin from the blood and vestibular system.[13–14]

In the squirrel monkey gentamicin has been reported as having a higher liability in the vestibular system with hair-cell loss in the crista and macula, as shown by light microscopy; electron micrographs delineate the higher vulnerability of Type I cells.[10] This effect is dose-dependent, with longer exposure that involves sensory cell loss in the utricle and cristae ampullaris and no loss of supporting cells. The evidence has been duplicated in guinea pigs which were given the drug for 30 days at a level of 250 mg/kg/day.[15] In the same species, also, doses of 100 mg/kg/day I.M. for 13 days or local application of 0.2 ml of a 0.3% solution of gentamicin have produced subcellular changes which include clumping of the chromatin and mitochondrial alterations. Merging of the sensory hairs is followed by destruction of a "stabilizing factor" in the cell membrane which results in the final deterioration of the hair cell with its contents streaming into the endolymph.[16] In man vestibular damage from gentamicin and other aminoglycoside antibiotics can occur from systemic or topical application. Burn patients treated with topical gentamicin have exhibited both cochlear and vestibular damage.[17] Some individuals demonstrate an idiosyncrasy in that one ear may be more susceptible to the drugs than the other, with the result that unilateral rather than bilateral vestibular damage occurs.*[18] When aminoglycoside antibiotics are used it is important to note the condition of the kidneys. Concomitant renal failure will exacerbate the vestibular damage and compound it with peripheral neuropathy.[17]

Minocycline, a semisynthetic tetracycline that attacks sulfonamide-resistant meningococci, has also been reported to be vestibulotoxic.[19,20] The moderate-to-severe vestibular symptoms that appeared in a group of hospital personnel after as little as 200 mg were reversible.[21] It has also been reported, however, that minocycline may lack ototoxicity in guinea pigs,[22] but this difference could be due to species specificity or to its reversible nature.

Viomycin sulfate in squirrel monkeys follows the characteristic destruction pattern in the vestibular system seen with streptomycin. Either systemic or topical administration of viomycin will cause vestibular damage.[23] In contrast, spectinomycin, another similar antibiotic, has shown little ototoxicity, possibly because it lacks an amino sugar moeity; instead it is a fused tricyclic molecule, an aminocyclitol.[24]

LOOP DIURETICS

Ethacrynic acid and furosemide are known to have auditory toxicity, but vestibular toxicity has been reported only for ethacrynic acid.[25] The greater vulnerability of the vestibular system to ethacrynic acid may be due to a number of situations: (1) the system itself is more sensitive to the drug, (2) the method of assessing damage to the vestibular system (electronystagmography) is more sensitive to ethacrynic acid-induced damage, and (3) there is a distinctly different mechanism of action in the destruction of sensory cells in the vestibular apparatus compared with the cochlea.[26] By using the cat as an experimental animal ethacrynic acid was specified as affecting the vestibulo-ocular reflex rather than the optokinetic reflex, as tested by its effect on nystagmus induced by caloric stimulation and optokinetic methods, respectively.[26] The effect of ethacrynic acid has been reported capable of potentiating the vestibulotoxic effect of streptomycin

*The presence of a unilateral otitis media may explain this phenomenon; see Chapter 7 for further details.

because pretreatment with the diuretic followed by increasing dosages of streptomycin delayed recovery from the depression of slow-phase-velocity nystagmus in response to caloric stimulation in a dose-dependent manner.[9]

Osmotic Agents, Diuretics, and Vasodilators

Over the years these drugs have been popular in the treatment of Meniere's disease[27] which is characterized by fluctuant low-frequency hearing loss, vertigo, tinnitus, and a sense of fullness in the ear.[28] The pathological changes that accompany this disease include distension of the endolymphatic system, vacuolization of its epithelium, and degeneration of the sensory epithelium.[29,30] The pathological picture suggests that a disturbance of the balance between the osmotically active components of the endolymphatic space and those of its environment may be a part of the etiology of the disease. It also suggests that the endolymphatic space may be swollen because of an overproduction of endolymph, defective absorption of endolymph, or a combination of these factors[31] (see also Chapter 4). It is not surprising, therefore, that many clinical treatments for Meniere's disease assume one or more of these etiologies and use drugs that are known to affect vascular tissues or to change tissue osmolarity. One of the earliest clinical studies that related variations in body fluids and electrolytes to Meniere's disease was that of Dederding.[32] This study was extended by Furstenberg et al.,[33] who advocated a combination of low sodium diets with diuretics as therapy. Hydrochlorthiazide has been used successfully in the "fluctuating stage" of the disease.[34,35] Although diuretics such as ammonium chloride, hydrochlorothiazide, and chlorthalidone may have beneficial effects in the reduction of the endolymphatic space,[33,36–37] one must be careful in the choice of diuretics because some of them, such as ethacrynic acid and furosemide, have been reported to be ototoxic.[38–40]

Possible "dehydration" of the endolymphatic space by an osmotic agent is the basis of the glycerol test.[41] Klockhoff and his coworkers[42–44] have shown that serum osmolarity increases after ingestion of glycerol and a reduction in inner-ear and cerebrospinal fluid pressure occurs. These findings have also been reported by Juhn et al.[45] and both Juhn's group[46] and that of Angelborg[31] have supported the osmolarity theory of glycerol's action by demonstrating similar results with urea. Also lending support to the osmotic hypothesis is another clinical report that diaphoresis provides transient relief for patients in the early stages of Meniere's disease.[47]

The idea that diuretics, such as the ammonium chloride used by Furstenberg et al.,[33] acidify tissues and the importance of the maintenance of endolymphatic ionic balance (high potassium, low sodium)[48] have lead some investigators to question the role of acid/base balance in Meniere's disease. Calestine et al.[49] found that acidifying drugs were beneficial in relieving Meniere's patients who had proved alkalosis. The number of patients in this category in their study was small, however, and in others, in which the acidifying drugs had benefit, there was no strong evidence of metabolic alkalosis. In fact, four of the patients who achieved relief were in acidosis at the start of the study. It appears that such results are merely supportive of the diuretic results of Furstenberg and others.[33] Also negative to the acidifying theory are the reports of Hasegewa[50] and, later, Elia[51] that injection of a 7% solution of sodium bicarbonate can relieve acute attacks of the disease. The proposed mechanism of action of this drug is the reversal of a presumed microcapillary angioneurosis caused by intense constriction of arterioles. Sodium bicarbonate neutralizes acid metabolites and produces CO_2 and water. These conditions would lead to vasodilation, improved blood flow, and reabsorption of the edematous fluid in the endolymphatic space.

Vasodilators are used by many clinicians who treat Meniere's disease and one in particular, betahistine hydrochloride, is the subject of a number of reports.[52-55] This drug has a structure and mechanism of action similar to that of histamine[56]; that is, it increases capillary permeability and capillary blood flow.[57] Improvement of local capillary blood flow by betahistine or histamine would therefore theoretically improve the exchange between the endolymphatic and vascular spaces and reduce the amount of excess fluid in the endolymphatic space. Double blind studies like those by Bertrand[56] and Segers and Boedts[54] apparently support this idea; but as Hommes[52] points out Meniere's disease is one of *natural* remissions and exacerbations that make evaluation of any treatment modality difficult.

Other vasodilators used to treat hydrops of the peripheral vestibular endolymphatic system include naftidrofuryl,[58] ergot alkaloids and papaverine,[59] ethyl apovincaminate,[60] niacin,[61] intravenous procaine, nicotinic acid,[62-63] cyclandelate,[64] and carbon dioxide.[63,65] Evidence of improvement in the function of the local microvascular supply to the inner ear is either sparse or nonexistent for many of these drugs. It should also be pointed out that accumulation of local tissue metabolites in areas of compromised blood flow is by itself a powerful, localized, physiological, vasodilator stimulus.[66] Therefore the use of drugs to increase the localized vasodilation in the face of compromised blood flow may be of questionable value. It is also possible that it is not the vasodilator effects of some of these drugs that provide therapeutic benefits; for example, nicotinic acid is a powerful peripheral vasodilator but it has little effect in CNS[63]; it also has a strong lipolytic effect and the accumulation of excess lipids has been implicated as the possible etiology in some forms of Meniere's disease.

Lithium

Lithium carbonate has also been tested for therapeutic use in Meniere's disease. Lutz[67] reported the success of this treatment for one patient who had a 14-year history. In 1974 Thomsen et al.[68] reported improvement in 70% of the 21 patients in their study (0.7 to 1.3 mmole/liter of serum lithium).

Thomsen et al.,[68] however, later concluded from a double-blind crossover study that lithium carbonate was not effective. The problem with agreeing with their conclusion is that the sample size for the study was rather small ($N = 10$) and each of the patients had been on $LiCO_3$ therapy for the 18 months immediately preceding the initiation of the experiment. The mechanism of lithium's effect evades precise definition, but it is believed that it affects electrolyte balance. Glenn and Reading[69] suggest that lithium can correct imbalances in the distribution of Na^+ and K^+ across the cellular membranes and that lithium is especially useful in regulating high or low intracellular Na^+ concentrations. Much more basic and clinical research will be required, however, before lithium's usefulness can be determined.

Heavy Water, Alcohol, and General CNS Depressants

Because alcohol appears to be such a general and continuous depressant of the central nervous system, it is not surprising that it has influenced vestibular pathways.[70] These vestibular effects have been known for a long time.[71-72]

Positional alcoholic nystagmus (PAN) quantitatively recorded by means of electronystagmography was first described by Aschan and his coworkers in 1955.[73] Aschan[74] described two phases for PAN. PAN I occurs 20 to 40 min after ingestion of an amount of alcohol sufficient to produce a blood alcohol level of 0.3 to 0.6%. It is characterized by the appearance of nystagmus when the head is placed in a lateral position. The direction of the fast phase of the nystagmus correlates with the side of the head that is down (side of head on the pillow if the subject is in a supine position). Pan II begins approximately 4 hr postalcohol ingestion and is also characterized by the appearance of horizontal nystagmus when the head is in a lateral position. The direction of the nystagmus in PAN II is exactly opposite that in PAN I. This sensitivity to head position seen with nystagmus produced by alcohol ingestion suggests that alcohol affects not only the central vestibular pathways but also may have a direct affect on the vestibular sensory cells of the inner ear. Lending support to this thesis is the observation[75-77] that PAN cannot be induced in animals or humans in which the peripheral organs have been destroyed bilaterally, nor can it be induced during periods of weightlessness.[78] Osterveld[77] proposed that the otoliths are responsible for PAN because he could eliminate PAN in rabbits if he cut both utricular nerves. It is not clear, however, from his paper how he severed surgically just the utricular part of the vestibular nerve but spared the innervation of the semicircular canals. In addition, he did not test specifically for semicircular canal function to show that it was still intact after surgery. Other investigators[79-80] propose that the semicircular canals are responsible for the effects of alcohol because discrete lesions in individual canals apparently can also eliminate PAN. Bearing on the question which of the vestibular end organs are responsible for PAN is the interesting finding made by Money and

Miles[81] that ingestion of heavy water also produces positional nystagmus with two phases. However, the direction of the positional nystagmus produced by heavy water is the opposite of that produced by alcohol. It was therefore suggested that differential absorption of heavy water or alcohol between the cupula and endolymph causes the cupula to rise or fall in its endolymph environment rather than to assume its normal floating position. Thus immediately after the ingestion of heavy water positioning the head laterally will cause the horizontal canal cupula, now heavier than endolymph, to be displaced downward and horizontal nystagmus will be elicited. In a normal animal the cupula would float and no nystagmus could be induced by this positioning. It is further hypothesized that after alcohol ingestion the cupula is lighter than endolymph and similar head positioning conditions will cause the cupula to be displaced upward to produce a nystagmus with the direction reversed from that seen after heavy-water ingestion. Greven et al.[82] measured the time for diffusion of tritiated water from blood into endolymph in pigeons and found that equilibrium occurred within 45 min. This may cast some doubt on the theory of Money and Miles[81] but there is enough variability in the data and in the species used to explain the time discrepancies between the two sets of experiments.

The effects of alcohol on the central vestibular pathways become apparent when the vestibular apparatus is dynamically stimulated by rotation or calorization rather than by static head positioning. Schroeder[83] points out that some researchers have found that alcohol enhances dynamic vestibular responses,[84-86] whereas others have found an inhibitory effect for alcohol.[87-89] In a series of papers Schroeder and his colleagues[83,90-92] showed that alcohol suppresses vestibular responses when the eyes are closed but enhances them when the eyes are open. Thus, as far as the vestibular system is concerned, the primary effect of alcohol appears to be a blockade of the visual system's normal ability to suppress nystagmus, vertigo, and nausea. This is consistent with the view that alcohol is a general CNS depressant and that a disinhibition[93] causes its apparent excitatory responses.

Alcohol and barbiturates and other anesthetic agents have a direct depressant effect on the reticular formation[94] and in sufficient doses produce sleep, unconsciousness, and the deeper stages of anesthesia.[70,93] Under these conditions the quick component of induced nystagmus is blocked and therefore rotation or calorization cannot be successfully used to stimulate the vestibular system. Also, under these conditions the eyes are closed and visual fixation on a target is impossible. If the level of consciousness is raised to the point at which visual fixation is possible but the reticular formation is still depressed, opening the eyes will restore the quick component of eye movement and increase occulomotor neuron activity and a brisk nystagmus can be elicited by rotary or caloric stimulation. The latter phenomenon can be seen best if the depressed subject is aroused[95] by another external stimulus, such as a loud noise, or induction of minor pain (pinch or squeeze). The anesthetic combination of fantanyl and droperidol has also been used to suppress vestibular function[96-97] clinically and experimentally, as has intravenous lidocaine. Again these drugs appear to produce their vestibular system influences via the reticular formation. Because many of the anesthetics influence vestibular activity in this manner, the selection of an appropriate animal anesthetic for vestibular research becomes a problem. Fluur and Siegborn[98] have suggested the use of ketamine for these experiments. Although there are no specific experiments for a study of ketamine's pharmacology in the reticular formation, it does appear to be without vestibular suppressant effect.[98]

11.4.2 Drugs Presumed to Act on Central Portions of the Vestibulotoxic System

Antihistamines, CNS depressants, tranquilizers, antiemetics, and autonomic drugs are agents that have important clinical effects on the vestibular system, but it is unlikely that these substances act directly on the peripheral vestibular apparatus. In fact, most evidence now points to the paramedian pontine reticular formation and higher CNS structures as the sites of action for many of the popular vestibular suppressant drugs.

Autonomic Drugs and Motion Sickness

The compounds with the longest history of usefulness in treating motion sickness are atropine and scopolamine, which were first used empirically. Their subsequent, continued use was probably on the basis of their anticholinergic effects in the GI tract. However, because they both also have central effects and because synthetic analogs that have no similar central effects are not effective aginst motion sickness,[99] it now appears that it is the central actions of atropine and scopolamine that are responsible for their influence on the vestibular system. Early evidence in this regard was provided by Himwich et al.,[100] who injected the anticholinesterase diisopropylfluorophosphate into the carotid arteries of animals and found that they would circle in a direction opposite to the side of injection. Simultaneously, the animals displayed abnormal EEG changes. These effects could be at least partly blocked by a variety of drugs with anticholinergic activity. Additional evidence is provided by the fact that physostigmine, another anticholinesterase, has the ability to induce occulomotor activity that can be abolished by bilateral surgical ablation of the vestibular nuclei.[101] It has also been shown that certain field potentials in the lateral vestibular nucleus can be dramatically enhanced by physostigmine and that this effect can be reduced by scopolamine.[102] Furthermore, iontophoretically applied acetylcholine, methacholine, and carbamylcholine can excite cells in the medial and lateral vestibular nuclei.[103] Physostigmine will enhance this excitation but atropine will block it.

Although it is possible that these cholinergic effects may be partly mediated in the peripheral vestibular system (e.g., Ross[104] has found acetylcholinesterase in Scarpa's ganglion), it is more likely that they can be attributed to actions of reticular neurons on the vestibular nuclei and to direct action of the cholinergic and anticholinergic drugs on the vestibular nuclei.[102] In this regard Shute and Lewis[105-106] have described pathways that apparently are cholinergic and that develop, at least in part, from the reticular formation and project into the vestibular nuclei. There is some evidence that these pathways enhance activity in the vestibulo-occular reflex system and perhaps in other vestibular reflex systems as well.[99]

Another reticulo-vestibular connection of interest is apparently monoaminergic.[101,107-109] This pathway can be stimulated by amphetamine[109] and has an inhibitory influence on activity provoked by electrical stimulation of the VIIIth nerve. Thus it appears that the reticular formation has an excitatory-cholinergic and an inhibitory-monoaminergic influence on the vestibular system and this gives some basis to the use of scopolamine and amphetamine as vestibular suppressant medications. Direct electrophysiological support for this thesis is provided by Yules et al.[110] who have, by means of electrical stimulation, mapped the specific mesencephalic reticular formation areas that inhibit and excite vestibular activity. Amphetamine was first combined with scopolamine in antimotion-sickness preparations to counteract the sedative effects of scopolamine.[99] It has since been shown that amphetamine has some vestibular suppressant effects of its own that are synergistic to those of scopolamine.[111-113] Based on this evidence, Wood and Graybiel[112] have proposed that most of the effective antimotion sickness drugs have a cholinolytic component, an alpha-sympathomimetic component, or both. It is true that many antihistamines, antiemetics, tranquilizers, and CNS depressants have one or both of these components in their total spectrum of activity, but it is also true that many of these drugs have an additive effect when combined with scopolamine or amphetamine.[114-116] If these other drugs have an additive effect when combined with a maximally effective dose of scopolamine *and* a maximally effective dose of amphetamine, then a third mechanism of action would definitely be implied.

Antihistamines

For the last 25 years antihistamines have gained ever increasing popularity for the prevention of vertigo. Now they may be considered the drug class of choice for blocking vestibular-induced symptoms. Many antihistamines have some anticholinergic activity and some of them also enhance sympathetic activity by blocking the reuptake mechanisms in monoaminergic nerve terminals.[57] In fact, it appears that the antihistamines that are most effective for treating motion sickness are those with the strongest anticholinergic- and/or monoaminergic-enhancing components.[117-118] However, antihistamines have a variety of effects that can also influence the vestibular system; for example, one of the prominent side effects of many of these drugs is drowsiness, which results from a depression of reticular formation activity.[57] This may or may not be related to anticholinergic activity. Also, some antihistamines are vasodilators[119] and may have direct actions on the peripheral vestibular vascular system. Another possible explanation for the action of antihistamines is that they have local anestheticlike activity and can depress activity in many forms of excitable tissue, including neurons.

Antiemetics

A number of antiemetic medications like metoclopromide,[120-122] sulpiride,[123-124] diphenidol,[125-127] and trimethobenzamide[128-130] have been used to ameliorate vestibular system disturbance. It is not clear, however, that these drugs act directly on the vestibular system. It is more likely that they have an indirect, perhaps reflexive, action because most are known to block apomorphine-induced emesis, which implies a direct action of the chemoreceptive trigger zone in the area postrema.

11.4.3 Piracetam

A relatively new drug with possible vestibular activity is piracetam,[131] which has been termed a nootrophic drug (Noos is greek for intelligence) because it seems to have selective action to restore function to failing neurons of the cerebral cortex.[132] It is unlikely that piracetam has direct action on the peripheral vestibular apparatus, although definitive experiments have not yet been reported.

11.5 SUMMARY

Thus drugs with pharmacological effects on the vestibular system include osmotic agents, vasodilators, antibiotics, antiemetics, antihistamines, alcohol, tranquilizers, CNS depressants, anticholinergics, sympathomimetics, and a miscellaneous group that includes lithium, heavy water, and piracetam, a relatively new drug. Among these drugs, osmotic agents, vasodilators, aminoglycoside antibiotics, alcohol, lithium and heavy water very likely exhibit their effects because of direct action on the inner ear, whereas the effects of the rest of the drugs are more likely due to central nervous system activity.

ACKNOWLEDGMENTS

I wish to acknowledge the assistance of Dr. Kathrine L. Parrish who read the manuscript and made useful additions. Thanks also are due to Ms. Audria Brook whose assistance in the library research was invaluable.

REFERENCES

1. H. H. Kornhuber, Ed., *Handbook of Sensory Physiology*, Vol. 6/1, Springer, Berlin, 1974.
2. A. Brodal and O. Pompeiano, Eds., *Progress in Brain Research*, Vol. 37, Elsevier, Amsterdam, 1972.
3. R. C. Truex and M. S. Carpenter, *Human Neuroanatomy*, 6th ed., Williams and Wilkins, Baltimore, 1969.
4. W. Precht, *Neuronal Operations in the Vestibular System*, Springer, Berlin, 1978.
5. R. D. Brown and A. M. Feldman, *Ann. Rev. Pharmacol. Toxicol.*, **18,** 233 (1978).
6. J. E. Hawkins, *Handbook of Sensory Physiology*, Vol. 5/3, Springer, Berlin, 1976, pp. 707–748.
7. J. E. Hawkins and R. E. Preston, *The Vestibular System*, Academic, New York, 1975, pp. 321–349.
8. D. N. F. Fairbanks, H. Shimizu, and D. Warfield, *Arch. Otolaryngol.*, **93,** 590 (1971).
9. R. H. Mathog and M. J. Capps, *Ann. Otol.*, **86,** 158 (1977).
10. M. Igarashi, *Audiology*, **12,** 337 (1973).
11. H. H. Lindeman, *Acta Oto Laryngol.*, **67,** 177 (1969).
12. K. Watanuki and A. M. Z. Gottesberge, *Acta Oto Laryngol.*, **72,** 59 (1971).
13. S. D. Purohit, G. S. Shauma, and B. S. Bomb, *J. Assoc. Phys. Ind.*, **24,** 99 (1976).
14. S. D. Purohit, B. S. Bomb, and G. S. Shauma, *Indian J. Chest Dis. Allied Sci.*, **18,** 111 (1976).
15. K. Watanuki, H. F. Stupp, and A. M. Gottesberge, *Laryngoscope*, **82,** 363 (1972).
16. J. Wersall, P. G. Lundquist, and B. Bjarkroth, *J. Infect. Dis.*, **119,** 410 (1969).
17. V. S. Dayal, E. L. Smith, and W. G. McCain, *Arch. Otolaryngol.*, **100,** 338 (1974).
18. R. M. Meyers, *Arch. Otolaryngol.*, **92,** 160 (1970).
19. Center for Disease Control, *Morbid. Mortal. Week Rep.*, **24,** 9 (1975).
20. D. N. Williams, L. W. Laughlin, and Y. H. Lee, *Lancet*, **2,** 744 (1974).
21. J. J. Jacobson and B. Daniel, *Antimicrob. Agents Chemother.*, **8,** 453 (1975).
22. V. Kepenis, N. Yuda, G. Gordon, H. F. Diermeier, and B. M. Sparano, *Toxicol. Appl. Pharmacol.*, **34,** 327 (1975).
23. T. Kanda and M. Igarashi, *Acta Oto Laryngol.*, **68,** 177 (1969).
24. E. Novak, J. E. Gray, and R. J. Pfeifer, *J. Infect. Dis.*, **130,** 50 (1974).
25. R. M. Levinson, M. J. Capps, and R. H. Mathog, *Ann. Otol.*, **83,** 223 (1974).
26. R. H. Mathog, *Laryngoscope*, **87,** 1791 (1977).
27. P. Meniere, *Gaz. Med. Paris*, **16,** 597 (1861).
28. J. Shea, *J. Miss. St. Med. Assoc.*, **6,** 411 (1965).
29. H. F. Schuknecht, *Pathology of the Ear*, Harvard University Press, Cambridge, MA, 1974.
30. C. S. Hallpike and H. Cairns, *Proc. Roy. Soc. Med.*, **31,** 1317 (1938).
31. C. Angelvorg, I. Klockhoff, and J. Stahle, *Scand. Audiol.*, **6,** 143 (1977).
32. D. Dederding, *Acta Oto Laryngol.*, **16,** 404 (1931).
33. A. C. Furstenberg, F. H. Lashmet, and F. Lathrop, *Ann. Otol. Rhinol. Laryngol.*, **43,** 1035 (1934).
34. I. Klockhoff and U. Lindblom, *Acta Oto Laryngol.*, **63,** 347 (1967).
35. I. Norell and J. Stahle, *Acta Oto Laryngol.*, **54,** 447 (1961).
36. I. Klockhoff and U. Lindblom, *Acta Oto Laryngol.*, **63,** 349 (1967).

37. I. Klockhoff, U. Lindblom, and J. Stahle, *Arch. Otolaryngol.*, **100**, 262 (1974).
38. R. D. Brown, *Toxicol. Appl. Pharmacol.*, **31**, 270 (1975).
39. R. H. Mathog and W. J. Klein, *N. Engl. J. Med.*, **280**, 1223 (1969).
40. R. M. Levinson, M. J. Capps, and R. H. Mathog, *Ann. Otol.*, **88**, 223 (1974).
41. I. Klockhoff and U. Lindblom, *Acta Oto Laryngol.*, **61**, 459 (1966).
42. J. Stahle, I. Klockhoff, and C. Angelborg, Proceedings Barany Society, 1st Extraordinary Meetings, **227** (1978).
43. C. Angelborg, I. Klockhoff, and J. Stahle, *Acta Oto Laryngol.*, **76**, 450 (1973).
44. C. Angelborg and B. Agerup, *Acta Oto Laryngol.*, **79**, 81 (1975).
45. S. K. Juhn, S. Prado, and J. Pearce, *Arch Otolaryngol.*, **102**, 683 (1976).
46. J. N. Youngs and S. K. Juhn, *Pract. Otorhinolaryngol.*, **34**, 140 (1972).
47. L. E. Herman, M. H. Stroud, W. F. Carver, and I. Arenberg, *Arch. Otolaryngol.*, **103**, 700 (1977).
48. C. A. Smith, O. H. Lowry, and H. L. Wei, *Laryngoscope*, **64**, 141 (1954).
49. D. Celestino, N. Cerulli, G. Iannetti, and G. Sagliaschi, *J. Laryngol. Otol.*, **90**, 263 (1976).
50. Takatoshi Hasegawa, *Acta Oto Laryngol. Suppl.*, **192**, 113 (1963).
51. Joseph C. Elia, *Rocky Mountain Med. J.*, **56**, 33 (1959).
52. O. R. Hammes, *Acta Oto Laryngol. Suppl.*, **305**, 70 (1970).
53. Robert A. Bertrand, *Laryngoscope*, **81**, 889 (1971).
54. J. M. Segers and D. Boedts, *Acta Oto. Rhino. Laryngol. Belg.*, **29**, 5 (1975).
55. T. J. Wilmot and G. N. Menon, *J. Laryngol. Otol.*, **90**, 833 (1976).
56. R. A. Bertrand, *Acta Oto Laryngol. Suppl.*, **305**, 48 (1970).
57. W. W. Douglas, in L. S. Goodman and A. Gilman, Eds., *The Pharmacological Basis of Therapeutics*, 5th ed., Macmillan, New York, 1975, p. 592.
58. W. P. R. Gibson, R. T. Ramsden, and D. A. Moffat, *J. Laryngol. Otol.*, **91**, 679 (1977).
59. Herbert J. Rosen, *J. Am. Geriatrics Soc.*, **23**, 169 (1975).
60. O. Ribari, B. Zelen, and B. Kollar, *Arzneim. Forsch.*, **26**, 1977 (1976).
61. Fred T. Shaia, *Va. Med. Mon.*, **102**, 1054 (1975).
62. Fred T. Shaia, *Laryngoscope*, **86**, 389 (1976).
63. W. Rubin, *Arch. Otolaryngol.*, **97**, 135 (1973).
64. E. Markey Pullen and John R. Surber, *Curr. Ther. Res.*, **4**, 317 (1962).
65. W. Shea and A. E. Kitabichi, *Arch. Otolaryngol.*, **97**, 118 (1973).
66. P. Bard, in V. B. Mantcastle, Ed., *Medical Physiology*, Vol. 1, Mosby, 1968, p. 174.
67. E. G. Lutz, *J. Med. Soc. N.J.*, **71**, 502 (1974).
68. J. Thomsen, P. Bech, A. Geisler, M. B. Jorgensen, O. J. Rafaelsen, K. Terkildsen, J. Udsen, and K. Zilstorff, *Acta Oto Laryngol.*, **78**, 59 (1974).
69. A. M. Glenn and H. W. Reading, *Lancet*, **2**, 1239 (1973).
70. J. M. Ritchie, in L. S. Goodman and A. Gilman, Eds., *The Pharmacological Basis of Therapeutics*, 5th ed., Macmillan, New York, 1975, p. 137.
71. R. Barany, *Mschr Ohrenheilk*, **45**, 959 (1911).
72. J. Rothfield, *Mschr Ohrenheilk*, **47**, 1392 (1913).
73. G. Aschan, M. Bergstedt, L. Goldberg, and L. Laurell, *Tr. Swed. Otol. Soc.* (December 1955), and *Quart. J. Stud. Alcohol*, **17**, 381 (1956).
74. G. Aschan, *Acta Oto Laryngol. Suppl.*, **140**, 69 (1958).
75. A. R. Fregly and A. Graybeil, *Acta Oto Laryngol.*, **65**, 469 (1968).

76. K. E. Money, W. H. Johnson, and B. M. Carlett, *Am. J. Physiol.*, **208,** 1065 (1965).
77. W. J. Oosterveld, *Acta Oto Laryngol.*, **75,** 252 (1973).
78. W. J. Oosterveld, *Aerospace Med.*, **40,** 382 (1970).
79. K. E. Money, W. A. Johnson, and B. M. Carlett, *Am. J. Physiol.*, **208,** 1065 (1965).
80. J. I. Suzuki, *Prog. Brain Res.*, **37,** 507 (1972).
81. K. E. Money and W. S. Myles, *Nature*, **247,** 404 (1974).
82. A. J. Greven, W. J. Oosterveld, and G. Samson, *Adv. Oto. Rhino. Laryngol.*, **22,** 152 (1977).
83. D. J. Schroeder, *Aerospace Med.*, **42,** 959 (1971).
84. R. Mantz, *Dtsch. Z. Gesamte Gerichtl Med.*, **32,** 301 (1940).
85. B. Taschen, *Dtsch. Z. Gesamte Gerichtl Med.*, **44,** 436 (1956).
86. D. Ingle, *Behav. Biol.*, **9,** 479 (1973).
87. B. Forster, *Dtsch. Z. Gesamte Gerichtl Med.*, **47,** 282 (1958).
88. Z. Bochenek and F. C. Ornerod, *J. Laryngol. Otol.*, **76,** 39 (1962).
89. Y. Mizoi, T. Ishido, and N. Ohga, *J. Forensic Med.*, **12,** 19 (1965).
90. D. J. Schroeder, *Ann. Otol.*, **81,** 218 (1972).
91. W. E. Collins, D. J. Schroeder, and R. J. Hill, *Adv. Oto. Rhino. Laryngol.*, **19,** 295 (1973).
92. F. E. Guedry, R. D. Gilson, D. J. Schroeder, and W. E. Collins, *Aviation Space and Environmental Med.*, **46,** 1008 (August 1975).
93. A. Berthot, L. Young, and F. Oliveras, *Acta Oto Laryngol.*, **84,** 317 (1977).
94. D. T. Haciska, *Acta Oto Laryngol.*, **75,** 477 (1973).
95. R. Eckmiller and M. Mackeben, *Pfluegers Arch.*, **363,** 33 (1976).
96. E. G. Dowdy, N. Gaksen, G. E. Arnold, W. T. Moore, and L. W. Fabian, *Arch. Otolaryngol.*, **89,** 482 (1969).
97. J. Kanzaki, M. Igurashi, H. Migata, and W. K. Wright, *Keio J. Med.*, **22,** 77 (1973).
98. E. Fluur and J. A. Siegborn, *Exp. Neurol.*, **413,** 594 (1974).
99. H. I. Chinn and P. K. Smith, *Pharm. Rev.*, **7,** 33 (1955).
100. H. E. Himwich, A. Morillo, and W. G. Steiner, *J. Neuropsychiat. Suppl.*, **3**(1), 15 (1962).
101. P. C. Magherini, O. Pompeiano, and U. Thoden, *Arch. Ital. Biol.*, **110,** 235 (1972).
102. I. Matsuoka and E. F. Domino, *Neuropharmacology*, **14,** 201 (1975).
103. E. B. Kirsten and J. N. Sharma, *Neuropharmacology*, **15,** 743 (1976).
104. M. D. Ross, *J. Comp. Neurol.*, **135,** 453 (1969).
105. C. C. D. Shute and P. R. Lewis, *Nature*, **199,** 1160 (1963).
106. C. C. D. Shute and P. R. Lewis, *Nature*, **205,** 242 (1965).
107. E. B. Kirsten and J. N. Sharma, *Brain Res.*, **112,** 77 (1976).
108. A. Dahlstrom and K. Fuye, *Acta Physiol. Scand. Suppl.*, **64,** 247 (1965).
109. E. B. Kirsten, E. P. Schoener, and S. C. Wang, *J. Pharm. Exp. Ther.*, **191**(3), 377 (1974).
110. R. B. Yules, C. Q. Krebs, and F. P. Gault, *Exp. Neuro.*, **16,** 349 (1966).
111. A. Graybiel, C. D. Wood, J. Knepton, J. P. Hoche, and G. F. Perkins, *Aviation Space and Environmental Med.*, **46**(9), 1107 (1975).
112. C. D. Wood and A. Graybiel, *Aerospace Med.*, **43**(3), 249 (1972).
113. C. D. Wood, A. Graybiel, and R. McDonough, *Aerospace Med.*, **37,** 187 (1966).
114. D. J. Schroeder and W. E. Collins, *Ergonomics*, **17,** 613 (1974).
115. H. Sugano and H. Tominaga, *Symposium International de Posturographie Paris*, **23–26,** 63–67 (1975).

116. A. Graybiel and J. Knepton, *Aviation Space and Environmental Medicine*, **48,** 867 (1977).
117. J. R. Leonard and R. A. Lawrence, *Eye, Ear, Nose, Throat Mon.*, **50,** 391 (1971).
118. *Medical Letter on Drugs and Therapeutics*, **16,** 47 (1974).
119. S. Cobb, L. W. Coen, S. L. Gitomer, and R. Iles, *Eye, Ear, Nose, Throat Mon.*, **55,** 24 (1976).
120. L. Justin-Basancon, C. Laville, and M. Thominet, *C.R. Acad. Sc. Paris*, **258,** 4384 (1964).
121. G. N. McMurray, *Postgraduate Medical Journal Suppl.*, **38,** 38 (1973).
122. J. J. Brand and W. L. M. Pert, *Pharmacol. Rev.*, **18,** 895 (1966).
123. G. A. Molinari and M. Cenzi, *Current Ther. Res.*, **16,** 812 (1974).
124. L. Justin-Besancon, M. Thominet, C. Laville, and J. Margarit, *C.R. Acad. Sc. Paris*, **265,** 1253 (1967).
125. A. C. Smoot, *Delaware Med. J.*, **37,** 234 (1965).
126. T. Futaki, M. Kitahara, and M. Morimoto, *Acta Oto Laryngol. Suppl.*, **330,** 122 (1975).
127. C. A. Leonard, *J. Pharm. Exp. Ther.*, **154,** 339 (1966).
128. J. Elia, *Medical Times*, **93,** 597 (1965).
129. F. H. Stern, *J. Am. Geriat. Soc.*, **11,** 884 (1963).
130. F. Schwartz, *Eye, Ear, Nose, Throat Mon.*, **42,** 50 (1963).
131. A. J. Stegink, *Arzneim. Forsch.*, **22,** 977 (1972).
132. H. Hakkarainen and L. Hakamies, *Eur. Neurol.*, **17,** 50 (1978).

CHAPTER 12

Clinical Application of Auditory Electrophysiology

CHARLES I. BERLIN, Ph.D.

Professor of Otorhinolaryngology and Physiology and
Director of the Kresge Hearing Research
Laboratory of the South
Louisiana State University Medical Center
New Orleans, Louisiana

JOHN N. GARDI, Ph.D.

University of California
Department of Otorhinolaryngology
Coleman Memorial Laboratory,
San Francisco

CONTENTS

12.1 BACKGROUND

12.1.1 Introduction

For many years behavioral methods, borrowed from psychology and acoustics, have been used to describe the type, severity, and treatability of hearing losses. In the last two decades attempts have been made to supplant a patient's behavioral response primarily by the specialized use of the electroencephalogram (EEG).

Many techniques have been tried, but for purposes of brevity four unique response configurations are described in this chapter:

1 Auditory brainstem response (ABR).
2 Middle latency response (MLR).
3 Frequency-following response (FFR).
4 Binaural interaction component-auditory brainstem response (BIC-ABR).

All four techniques have signal averaging paradigms that allow the investigator to extract small-amplitude, time-locked synchronous discharges out of the larger amplitude, on-going EEG. These simultaneous and/or synchronous firings of many neurons from diverse sources throughout the central auditory nervous system constitute the complex response configurations.

After the four responses of interest are outlined the recent pertinent auditory-evoked response literature is summarized. One section is devoted to a theoretical and technical consideration of evoked-response measurement. In a final section examples of results from patients, drawn from our files and the reports of other investigators, are discussed.

12.1.2 General Overview

The Auditory Brainstem Response (ABR)

The ABR (called the BSER or brainstem-evoked response in Chapter 2) represents the synchronous discharge of onset-sensitive neurons to brief rise-time tone pips or clicks; the resultant compound action potentials appear as a six-wave complex, all of which occur in humans within the first 12 msec after stimulation, depending on the intensity of stimulation and the age of the subject (Figure 12.1). At 75 to 80 dB above threshold (i.e., 75 to 80 dB sensation level or SL) the first wave is positive with respect to the reference electrode and has a latency of roughly 1.5 msec. It is followed by positive deflections that occur at approximately 1-msec intervals (2.5, 3.5, 4.5, 5.5, 6.5, and 7.5 msec).

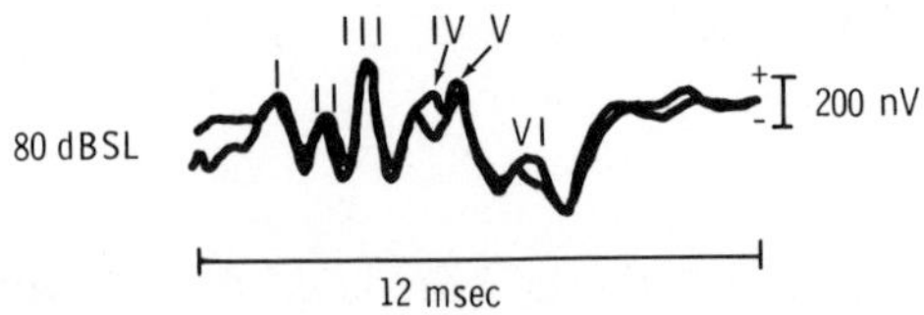

Figure 12.1 Two superimposed auditory brainstem responses to 1024 repetitions of a 10/sec 75 dB SL (i.e., 75 dB above threshold) click (100-μsec square wave). Subject, P.B., a 17-year-old normal-hearing female, was also the source of the other normal sample potentials in this chapter. The positive waves are labeled with successive Roman numerals. Records displayed as duplicates for crosschecking purposes.

The Middle Latency Response (MLR)

The MLR has its earliest reliably recorded waveform (the negative N_a) about 14 to 18 msec after stimulus onset (Figure 12.2). Following this wave, a series of larger-amplitude, lower frequency waveforms is typically recorded (the positive P_a, with a latency of 28 to 32 msec, N_b, 45 to 50 msec, and P_b, 60 to 70 msec). These responses can be elicited equally well by click or brief-duration (5- to 10-msec) tone.

The Frequency-Following Response (FFR)

The FFR differs from the first two types in that it is a continuous or sustained response that roughly reproduces the frequency of the tonal stimulus. The FFR is most dependably recorded in human subjects at low frequencies (200 to 1000 Hz) when a tone burst of moderate duration and slow rise/fall time is used (15- to 20-msec duration, 5-msec rise/fall time). The FFR, like the ABR, also originates in auditory nuclei and tracts in the brainstem and therefore has a short latency similar to the latency of the second and/or third wave(s) of the ABR. When the FFR is elicited by low-intensity tonal stimuli it has the advantage of being low-frequency specific (i.e., it is mediated by localized, low-frequency regions along the basilar membrane), in contrast to the high-frequency bias of the ABR.

The Binaural Interaction Component (BIC)

The BIC-ABR is a derived potential and is defined as the numerical difference between the sum of the two ABR responses obtained when each ear is

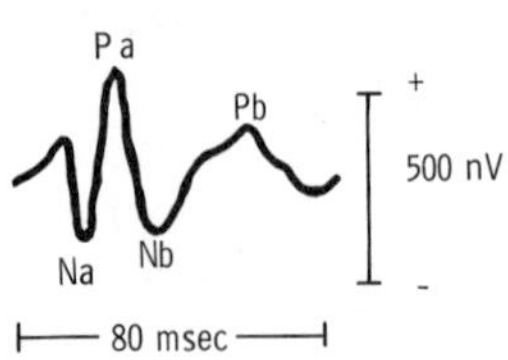

Figure 12.2 MLR to 60 dB SL click. P on wave name indicates positivity with respect to the reference electrode; *N* indicates negativity.

stimulated *individually* and the response obtained when both ears are stimulated *simultaneously*. The primary advantage of studying a derived response is that the technique offers a means of studying two-ear interactions in the auditory information-processing machinery. The technique has already been applied to longer latency periods (MLRs) so that in the future BICs may be classified according to the latency of the primary components of interest.[1]

12.1.3 Historical Perspective

Recording of the EEG in conjunction with the presentation of auditory signals has been used for many years in an attempt to define hearing sensitivity physiologically in uncooperative patients. It was not until 1958, however, that researchers focused on early time epochs (less than 50 msec) after acoustic stimulation.[2] Although Lowell et al.[3] corroborated the findings of Geisler and his colleagues,[2] an erroneous claim by Bickford et al.[4] that the middle latency components were completely myogenic rather than neurogenic in origin brought about a four-year hiatus in research in the middle latency response area. Goldstein and Rodman[5] reasserted the importance of studying middle latency components by describing a polyphasic waveform that could be recorded in the first 50 msec after acoustic stimulation.

Jewett, during his midsixties postdoctoral fellowship at Yale, investigated higher frequency-evoked activity that could be recorded in the first 10 msec after stimulus onset. He published an abstract[6] in 1969 and his first paper[7] on the ABR (at that time referred to as auditory far-field potentials) in 1970. Subsequent to Jewett's publication it was noted by other researchers in the field that Sohmer and Feinmesser[8] had, in fact, also recorded ABR waveforms, although they had not precisely defined them as components derived from central auditory neurons; they believed erroneously that they had obtained recordings of multiple firings of the N_1 and N_2 response arising from the cochlea.

Three years after Jewett's initial observations Moushegian et al.[9] showed that scalp-recorded, auditory-evoked activity could be obtained with low-frequency, tone-burst stimuli rather than click stimuli. These responses were referred to as FFRs from work done by Worden and Marsh,[10] who used near-field recording electrodes placed in the vicinity of auditory nuclei in the brainstem. Therefore by the early 1970s research was being conducted on three separate types of auditory-evoked response, the MLR, the ABR to click stimuli, and the FFR or auditory-evoked potential to a sustained or continuous low-frequency tone (FFR). It was not until 1978 that Huang and Buchwald[11] described the possibility of using the ABR to investigate binaural interaction in the auditory system. They presented data from cats that showed small differences in ABRs obtained under binaural stimulation conditions, as opposed to summed monaural recording conditions; true binaural interaction differences in the ABR have also been shown in humans[1,12] and guinea pigs.[12]

12.2 REVIEW OF THE LITERATURE

12.2.1 Auditory Brainstem Response (ABR)

Stimulus Variables

As click stimulus intensity is increased, ABR amplitude increases and response latency (of individual peaks and valleys) decreases (Figure 12.3).[7,13,14] As repetition rate of the stimulus is increased from low values below 10 stimuli/sec to high values around 80 to 90 stimuli/sec the ABR waveforms appear to be less distinct and exhibit longer latencies (Figure 12.4).[13,15,16] Figure 12.4 shows that at low-stimulus repetition rates the human ABR is multipeaked, with a pronounced IV–V complex and clear earlier waves I, II, and III. As the repetition rate is increased this distinctive pattern is lost; waves I, II, and III are diminished, although a prominent IV–V complex remains.

Tone pips also have been used successfully to generate frequency-selective ABR recordings.[17-19] The use of high-frequency, low-intensity tone pips produces clear ABRs that appear to be derived from narrow regions along the basilar membrane. With modified response-filtering techniques 500-Hz tone pips have also been used to investigate lower frequency regions along the basilar membrane. Stimulus rise/fall time is a critical factor, however, in generating clear ABR waveforms.[17] Fast or instantaneous rise times are required to obtain synchronous firing of many individual neurons in the VIII nerve. Acoustic clicks, therefore, are ideal stimuli for ABR recording, for they have nearly instantaneous rise times. Tone-pip stimuli with narrow

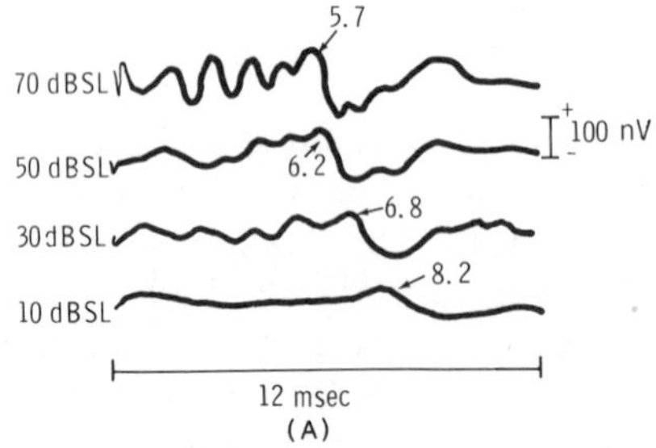

Figure 12.3A The effect of intensity on the ABR. Note how the only remaining wave at low intensities is analogous to wave V. This synchronous response at low intensities is most often used as an index of auditory sensitivity. Numbers at arrows indicate latencies of wave V in milliseconds.

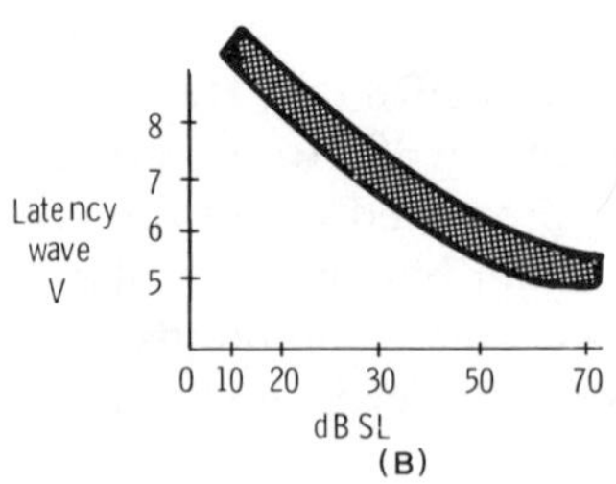

Figure 12.3B Latency-intensity function of the ABR. Latency is, of course, given in milliseconds.

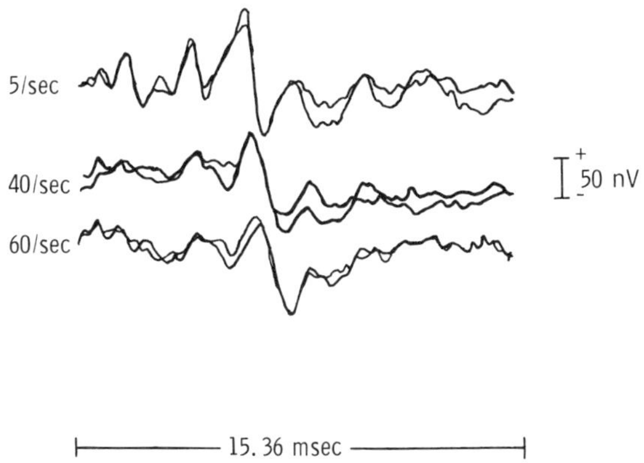

Figure 12.4 The effect of increasing stimulus repetition rate on the ABR. Duplicate traces were obtained at each repetition rate.

spectra are less effective because they must have prescribed rise/fall times. In general, a two- to three-period rise/fall time is the maximum that can be tolerated without losing response synchrony from 500 Hz and above. This limitation is reflected in the frequency components of these signals. Stimuli with faster rise times produce uncontrolled spread of energy across the spectrum and as a result evoke ABRs with inappropriately short latencies and exaggerated amplitudes. Caution must be used when interpreting ABR recordings obtained with tone-pip stimuli. When knowledge of the spectrum of the acoustic signal is lacking, limitations must be placed on conclusions of a patient's sensitivity for specific frequencies. Duration of tone pips is not a crucial parameter in ABR recording, although one study has been directed toward this question.[20]

Additional Factors Affecting the Auditory Brainstem Response (ABR)

The active electrode is placed on the vertex, or forehead, with a reference electrode on the earlobe or mastoid (ipsilateral to the stimulated ear). The ground electrode is usually positioned on the contralateral earlobe or mastoid. Placing the active electrode at the hairline reduces the apparent size of wave V and enlarges the apparent size of wave III. A reference at the neck is also useful.[21]

Drugs and/or variations in "attention state" do not significantly affect the latency and/or amplitude values obtained from ABR waveforms.[22,23] Age effects, however, are quite pronounced. In general, only waves I, III, and V are commonly observed in term babies at birth.[14,24] As the infant matures latency values decrease and the smaller amplitude waves (II, IV, and VI) begin to appear. Amplitude measures, however, unlike latency measures, do not systematically vary as a function of age.

Premature infants show longer wave V latencies and somewhat longer central conduction times than term infants.[25]

The interaction between drugs and response parameters of the ABR has also been studied to a limited extent. In general the application of sedatives and/or anesthetic agents has little or no effect on response properties.[26]

Clinical Overview

Subjects with various types of hearing disorder have been tested in an attempt to validate the use of ABR testing in audiological and/or otological diagnosis.[27-32] When ABRs are collected at a variety of stimulus-intensity levels the diagnostician can construct a latency-intensity (L–I) curve. An example of these data is shown in Figure 12.3B. Typically, latency to wave V is plotted against stimulus intensity to create an asymptotic function (the L–I curve). Patients suffering from conductive hearing loss show similarly shaped curves, except that their curves fall parallel but to the right of the curves collected from patients with normal hearing. The L–I curve of hearing-impaired patients with sensorineural losses appears to be composed of a mixture of two curves obtained from a conductively impaired patient for low-stimulus intensities and a normal-hearing patient at moderate-to-high stimulus levels. It must be recalled, however, that the ABR maximally reflects activity generated only along mid- to high-frequency regions (2 to 6 kHz) of the basilar membrane, and therefore hearing losses primarily affecting frequency regions outside this area may not be reflected in the ABR procedure.

Neurological disorders, especially demyelinating diseases and brainstem tumors, reveal themselves in their disruption of ABR synchrony.[33-35] Dyssynchrony reflects itself as an apparent increase in latency to individual peaks in the ABR, often with concomitant distortion of the typical ABR waveform shape. Based on the presence or absence of definable peaks in the waveform and an understanding of the primary anatomic origin of these individual peaks (see Chapter 2), the clinician can often approximate the location and size of the lesion.

Uses

There are many new applications of the ABR in a variety of medical disciplines; for example, the ABR has been tested as a feedback, or monitoring, agent in the selection of hearing aids.[36] The use of ABR as a physiologic measurement tool may increase the precision with which hearing aids are prescribed and developed.

The ABR technique has been used to monitor the success of cochlear implants in patients who have been implanted with electrical stimulators.[37] In such cases ABR can determine whether discrete channels of current are still flowing normally and/or whether simultaneous stimulation of multiple channels will produce complexlike stimuli that excite neurons along large portions of the cochlear partition.

Many psychophysical, adaptation, fatigue, and masking studies have also been completed with ABR.[15,38,39] In addition, it is possible to use the ABR to monitor drug administration of ototoxic agents needed in particularly severe cases of general systemic infection; ABR has also been used to monitor safe drug levels for hearing when nornal renal clearance is impaired. Likewise, in the future, the ABR may be used as a monitor for ototoxic drug effects in patients difficult to test.

Finally, the ABR separates comatose patients likely to recover normal brain function from comatose patients who exhibit extensive neurophysiological damage and are unlikely to recover function.[40]

12.2.2 Frequency-Following Response (FFR)

Stimulus Parameters

The FFR is recorded with low frequencies, continuous or pulsed tone-burst stimulation, or pulsed noise bursts of rapid repetition rate. Recording conditions (electrode positions, etc.) are essentially the same as those required for recording the ABR response. Filter settings for optimal FFR recording, like those used in recording the ABR, are 100 to 3000 Hz. The number of stimulus trials necessary to record an FFR in humans is about 2000. Changes in FFR interstimulus intervals have not been thoroughly investigated. Stillman et al.,[41] however, showed that the FFR waveform is essentially unchanged as the repetition rate increases from 5 to 25 stimuli/sec. Suter et al.[42] have demonstrated that FFRs can also be obtained with rapidly presented clicks at rates of 100 to 500 stimuli/sec.

Tone bursts of 500 Hz have been used by most investigators to elicit the FFR, although Moushegian et al.[9] recorded FFRs at frequencies up to 2000 Hz and Glaser et al.,[43] to frequencies as low as 70 Hz. In general lower frequency stimuli produce FFR waveforms of greater amplitude.

Changes in FFR amplitude or latency due to variations in signal duration or rise/fall time have not been systematically investigated. The duration of tone bursts selected by investigators have ranged from the shortest value of 2 1/2 msec[21] to the longest value of 20 msec.[44] Other durations between these two extremes, as well as various rise times (1 to 5 msec), have been used. Continuous-tone stimulation has also been applied.[43]

The amplitude of the FFR varies as a function of stimulus intensity. Glaser et al.[43] and Marsh et al.[44] have shown that as stimulus intensity increases FFR amplitude increases as well. Although binaural presentation of stimuli increases FFR amplitude, no study has been published to quantify precisely the increase in amplitude due to binaural stimulation. As expected, latency to the first peak in the FFR decreases as stimulus intensity increases, but it is not clear why this should be so. Three theories have been postulated to explain this result (all of which could coexist). First, as stimulus intensity is increased, the spread of excitation basalward along the basilar membrane recruits additional high-frequency neurons, which, because of their position, are recruited earlier than the primary lower frequency contributing neurons. Second, as stimulus intensity is increased cochlear and neuronal generation sites contribute to the scalp-recorded FFR. A cochlear contribution (cochlear microphonic) would, of necessity, reduce the latency to the first peak in the FFR. Third, at higher stimulus levels the level of the few cycles contained in the rising envelope of the signal is also increasing. At these levels, therefore, the first few cycles begin to evoke FFR activity. This activity, of course, precedes the major sustained FFR activity and results in a reduction in the measured latency to the first response peak.

FFR threshold varies widely from 20[41,45] to 50 dB SL. Most investigators agree, however, that an easily identifiable response can be recorded about 40 dB SL.

Subject Parameters

Subject parameters have been less critically studied because of the results of analogous studies carried out on ABR. The effect of attention, sleep, and drug-induced sleep has not been systematically explored in FFR. Various investigators have observed that these parameters do not produce changes in the FFR waveform.[43,45,46] In addition, it has been shown that the shape of the FFR waveform is stable over long periods.[45]

Hearing-impaired adults have been investigated with FFR by Stillman et al.[41] and Daly et al.[47]; both groups of investigators used low-frequency tone bursts (500 Hz). Subjects with profound hearing loss were tested by the first group. Stimulus presentation to the impaired ear failed to elicit FFRs recorded with the reference electrode at both ears. Stimulus presentation to the unimpaired ear produced normal FFRs on either side. In the report by Stillman and his colleagues a 500-Hz, 5-msec duration tone burst was used to elicit FFRs from subjects in four different patient groups: normal, hearing-impaired, and deaf-blind subjects and others who exhibited learning disorders and mild speech-discrimination deficits. The results from normal-hearing adults showed that FFRs could be elicited at a level of 10 to 30 dB SL. Results from hearing-impaired and deaf-blind subjects showed elevated FFR thresholds that corresponded to the subjects' behavioral thresholds. FFR waveforms obtained from some of the subjects that exhibited learning disorders did not show the characteristic frequency-following peaks, although a slow-wave positive plateau was seen.

The FFR has also been described in neonatal populations.[48] Results from this study suggest that the FFR in neonates is mature at birth, although there are slight differences in the amplitude and latency values obtained from neonatal populations.

For the audiological assessment of low-frequency sensitivity in infants and difficult-to-test adults the FFR holds great promise. It has been shown, in both animal and human studies,[49-51] that the FFR at low-stimulus intensities is generated by restricted regions along the cochlear partition. This technique can therefore be used to augment the ABR by providing low-frequency threshold information. It is perhaps even more important that a macroscopic, physiological view of the dynamic processes in neural encoding of sound may be possible. A masked FFR audiogram or tuning curve can be derived[51,52] with gap, pure-tone masking or high-pass, noise-masking techniques. At high stimulus-intensity levels the derived tuning curve (in a normal-hearing subject) would be broad or almost flat across the masker-frequency range, but for patients with high-frequency, sensorineural hearing loss the loss of high-frequency regions along their cochleae should ensure a less broadly tuned or more V-shaped tuning curve.

The application of the FFR to neurological disorders has not been thoroughly investigated. It is assumed that patients exhibiting demyelinating disease will show various abnormalities in their ability to follow high frequencies. Patients who have discrete, lower brainstem lesions (specifically in areas around and including the cochlear nuclei and superior olivary complex) should also be amenable to FFR analysis based on the anatomical origin of the FFR.[53]

Uses

The FFR, like the ABR, is used in audiological assessment of difficult-to-test patients to aid in the selection of hearing aids; it may be used in monitoring the capacities of patients implanted with cochlear prostheses and may help to bridge and gap between human psychophysical and physiological studies in animals.[54,55] Complex analyses, such as FFR gap-masking studies,[52] may lead to an understanding of how "frequency" is coded as "pitch" in the nervous system.

12.2.3 MIddle Latency Response (MLR)

Stimulus Parameters

Goldstein and Rodman[5] and Mendel and his colleagues[56-60] described recordings of the MLR. Stimulus parameters are similar in many ways to the two previously defined categories of response measures; for example, as stimulus intensity is increased response amplitude increases and response latency decreases. One advantage in the use of MLR is that it is easily obtainable with both click and tone-burst stimuli. This has enabled investigators to test frequency-specific regions all along the cochlear partition, something that has not been demonstrated with any other technique, although in combination the FFR and ABR could test similar ranges of the auditory sensitivity. Again, stimulus rise/fall time is an important parameter.

Faster rise times lead to greater spectral spread and, as a result, greater synchrony of firing among fibers of the auditory nerve. This may lead to MLRs that have earlier latencies and greater amplitudes than obtained with tone bursts. Electrode positions, again, are similar to those used for the FFR and ABR. Repetition rates above approximately 8/sec greatly decrease the amplitude of the MLR.[56] This finding suggests that MLRs are originating in higher centers in the nervous system because they are more susceptible to adaptation and fatigue effects.

The MLR's have peak-to-peak amplitudes of about .05 to 2.0 μV. These amplitudes are, in general, an order-of-magnitude greater than ABR amplitudes; therefore the number of sweeps needed to visualize the response is reduced to 500. Typically, maximal MLR activity is seen with bandpass-filter settings of 25 to 175 Hz.[5]

Subject Parameters

Like the early responses, MLRs also show remarkable stability during changes in subject alertness. Although the effects of attention have not been thoroughly explored, Mendel and Goldstein[56] found no significant differences in the response properties of MLR caused by changes in test conditions (i.e., eyes closed in the dark, eyes open in lighted room or reading). Picton and Hillyard[23] found no MLR amplitude differences as a function of attention state. MLRs also show long-term stability when tested at 3-hr intervals over a 24-hr sleepless period[57] and/or during overnight sleep.[58]

MLRs also appear to be unaffected by light sedation.[59,61] True anesthesia, however, may depress the amplitude of the MLRs. Recent evidence obtained from animals[62a] has shown that MLRs recorded from pentobarbital-anesthetized cats are profoundly attenuated; in fact, no information beyond about 15 msec is typically observed under deep anesthesia. The use of a lighter anesthetic agent, such as urethane and/or ketamine, allows a full complement of cat MLR waveforms to be recorded.

In general, infant MLR amplitude was somewhat smaller than adult MLR amplitude tested under similar circumstances.[60] It is interesting that latency values tended to be *shorter* for infants than adults. (Usually, longer latency values would be expected for an immature organism because of incomplete myelinization.) In the Mendel et al. study[60] threshold determinations were successfully obtained in 27 of 28 infants who ranged in age from 1 month to 2 years.

Uses

The primary use of the MLR has been in the audiological assessment of infants and uncooperative adults. No additional audiologic information is necessarily gained by the use of MLRs that a combination of ABR and FFR techniques would not yield, but because the MLR originates, at least, in part from rostrally located structures (perhaps including auditory cortex) information can be gleaned about the *level* of auditory processing available to the patient. This information may be especially useful to neurologists and other clinicians interested in auditory-perceptual problems.

12.2.4 Binaural Interaction Component (BIC)

The Response

The ordinary brainstem response is a representation of the synchronous discharge of *onset-sensitive* single units in the auditory system. There are, of course, many different types of unit in the auditory nervous system, some sensitive to offset of the stimuli, others to rising- or falling-frequency configurations. The BIC–ABR measures the activity of those units that discharge only on *simultaneous* stimulation from both auditory input paths. These units are "coincidence detectors" and respond only when impinged on from both sides by neural representations of clicks or tone bursts that have similar spectra and similar intensities, and coincide in their onsets within a few hundred microseconds.[12]

Figure 12.5 shows an example of such a recording. Here the right ear is stimulated first, the left ear is stimulated second, and last a binaural recording is obtained from the subject. At this point the responses from the right and left ears are added together and the sum is subtracted from the response generated by binaural stimulation. The acquired "difference potential" is a representation of the activity of those units that have been activated by binaural stimulation.

Stimulus and Subject Parameters

Because the BIC is a derived ABR, all the comments concerning the effects of stimuli appropriate to the ABR are applicable here. However, the electrode-recording configuration for the BIC is radically different from the

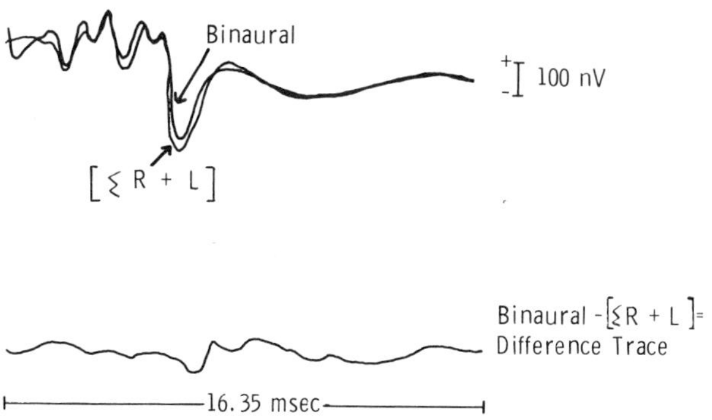

Figure 12.5 The BIC–ABR. Tracings show a "difference trace" at the bottom of the figure which represent the subtraction of the sum of the right and left ear responses from the responses obtained binaurally.

configuration used in simple ABR recording. It is imperative that the recording montage not favor one ear over the other (otherwise binaurally evoked ABRs will be recorded with a particular ear bias). As a result, linked references (with a forehead ground), or a single midline reference on the neck (with a forehead ground), are necessary to avoid biased records. The active or hot electrode (as before) remains on the vertex. In a recently completed study, using two preamplifiers and simultaneously recording from both sides of the head during monaural and binaural stimulation, we found what may be a *brainstem asymmetry in favor of one side in humans,* which is not seen in animals.[62b]

Uses

The BIC has only recently been investigated in detail. Dobie and Berlin[12] have characterized the BIC in guinea pigs as a function of stimulus intensity and differences in intra-aural time and intensity. Also, the BIC has been studied in humans.[1,12,63] It is likely to be useful in diagnosing subtle lesions of the central auditory pathway. Preliminary findings in animals suggest that normal BIC waveforms are not observed in mice reared in auditory deprivation. The application of this technique to populations of infants and/or children with chronic otitis media may reveal that children with these medical histories do not develop normal monaural or binaural central auditory pathways.[64] Other recent findings (Berlin, unpublished observations) suggest that children diagnosed as autistic may not exhibit normal BIC waveforms.

12.3 THEORETICAL AND TECHNICAL CONSIDERATIONS

The ABR, as well as the other responses described here, is often less than 1 μV in peak-to-peak amplitude. Common-mode-rejection recordings and response averaging are almost always necessary to extract such a small signal from high-amplitude background noise.

Common-mode rejection is used to extract a desired signal from background noise by placing the "hot" and "reference" electrodes across the source of the potential desired. As the potential moves toward the hot electrode, it hopefully is moving *away from* the reference electrode. This configuration gives the desired potential a positive algebraic sign with respect to the hot electrode and a negative algebraic sign with respect to the reference electrode. The contents of these two electrodes are *subtracted* from one another in the differential preamplifier. Thus, although externally generated electrical activity such as 60-Hz noise, radio stations, EMG, and any other electrical signals *common* to both electrodes are subtracted in the preamplifier, the *target* electrical activity is enhanced because of its differential sign with respect to the two electrodes. It is imperative, therefore, that the electrodes be attached to the skin with similar impedance, an impedance that is as *low* as possible. In this way the rejection of any electrical activity common to both electrodes is uniform and effective; uneven electrode impedance leads to uneven rejection of electrical activity to both electrodes and leads to uneven enhancement of the target potential. Some commercial manufacturers have large tolerances of acceptable electrode impedance mismatch, whereas others are not so generous. Impedance of the electrodes in human subjects should be below 10,000 Ω and, if possible, below 5000 Ω, although some preamps function well at higher levels of impedance.

The digital computer use, of course, also enhances the extraction of the time-locked target waveforms. It is axiomatic that the clicks and tone bursts are selected to generate a maximum amount of temporal synchrony of discharge in the auditory nervous system. By triggering the computer in time registration with the stimulus to the ear, synchronous neural discharges are summed linearly in the computer. However, random discharges, or discharges unrelated either to the stimulus or the computer trigger, generate electrical activity that is added into the overall waveform as the *square root* of the number of times the stimulus is presented. This effectively enhances the signal-to-noise ratio as a function of the number of sweeps. Thus, if only one "sweep" were taken, the signal-to-noise ratio would be $1/\sqrt{1}$ and no enhancement or special detectability of the target waveform would be possible. After 100 sweeps signal-to-noise ratio would improve by 10 to 1, and by 2000 sweeps the ratio would be roughly 45 to 1, or $2000/\sqrt{2000}$.

For clinical purposes between 1000 and 2000 sweeps are sufficient to reveal a normal response to high-intensity stimulation, and, if collected parsimoniously, recordings are best displayed as duplicates and "crosschecks" of one another to assess the validity of the latency and peak assessments.

The filter-band pass and stimulus selection for all four potentials were outlined earlier. If stimuli *other* than pure tones are used (a condition that is virtually always necessary in these types of recording), one must remain alert to an unusual set of constraints: typically, in auditory research as the stimulus intensity of the signal *drops* no concern need be given to the spectral content of the stimulus other than to note that its harmonic purity to the subject is relatively constant. When clicks or other transients are used the high-intensity spectrum is clearly different than the low-intensity spectrum that reaches the subject's ear. The lower the intensity of the transient reaching the subject's ear, the more likely the examiner is to be assessing very narrow ranges of spectral sensitivity. As the intensity drops the spectrum of the signal to which the subject is being asked to respond also narrows (Figure 12.6). Thus, if a very synchronous response to a faint click of 100-μsec duration into a TDH/39 earphone is obtained, the conclusion is quite justified that the subject has adequate peripheral and probably lower brainstem auditory sensitivity in a narrow range from about 2500 to 4000 Hz. Because it is physiologically impossible to have a perfectly normal island of hearing in the presence of absolutely *no* auditory sensitivity on either side of that island, the assumption of adequate hearing for speech and language is

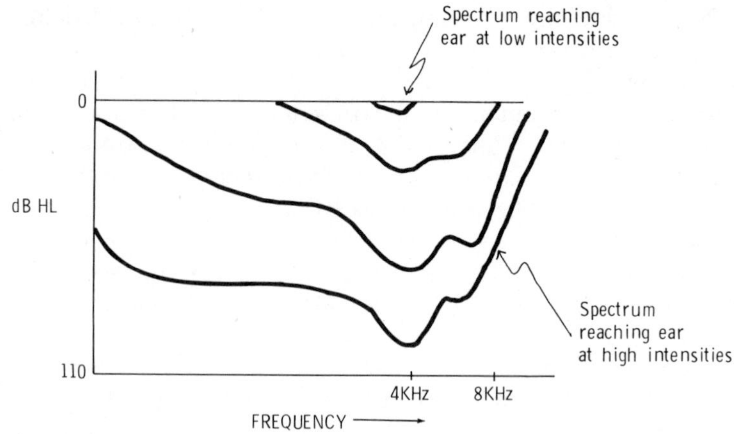

Figure 12.6 Schematization of changes in spectrum of a click as intensity is reduced. Spectral levels are plotted as if they were in a common audiogram format (dB HL = dB hearing level = dB ISO; see Chapter 2 for explanation).

often justified. There are rare but important occasions when that conclusion may be incorrect.[65]

12.4 SAMPLE PATIENTS

Patients from our files and others who show the application and utility of the potentials discussed in this chapter are discussed.

Patient 1 was a 3-year, 2-month-old, right-handed female with slow speech development. She was alternately diagnosed as "mentally retarded," "autistic," and finally "hard-of-hearing" by a number of well-respected clinics throughout the country. We saw her in three sessions and, including impedance audiometry and clinical observations, we were able to complete an ABR to click stimuli, to pure tones at 1000 and 2000 Hz, and a FFR to a 250-Hz stimulus. Figure 12.7 outlines each of the responses obtained from this patient. It was our conclusion, subsequently confirmed by voluntary audiometry, that this child had normal peripheral hearing sensitivity. One might ask why all these data were collected on such a subject if the ABR to a broad-band click was normal. At the time of referral there was a possibility—in fact, a strong likelihood, in the mother's mind—that this child was clearly not "deaf" but had considerable residual hearing. The question then was how close could we approximate an audiogram with her and could we pick up any mild-to-moderate sensorineural losses that would be contributing to her auditory imperception? In summary, then, we have an example of auditory electrophysiology being used to resolve a conflict in a young child in whom definitive auditory diagnosis had not heretofore been possible.

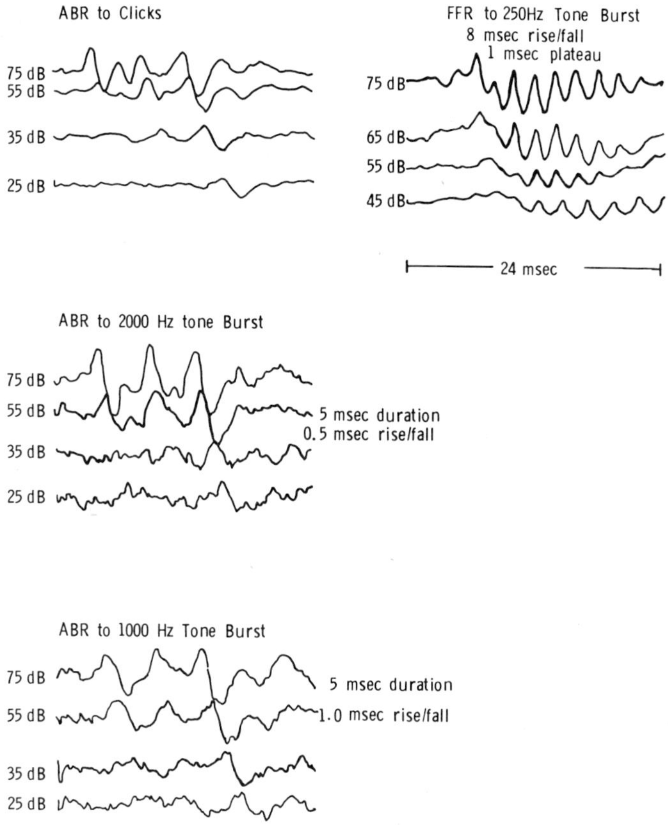

Figure 12.7 Summary of ABR responses to clicks, 1000- and 2000-Hz tone pips, and an FFR to a 250-Hz tone burst in a child later shown to have normal hearing. dB are dB HL.

Patient 2 was a 4-week-old baby whose mother suspected deafness because of the child's inattentiveness to loud sounds. Despite assuagement from her pediatrician that "the child would outgrow the problem," she sought electrophysiological assessment and the child was brought in for ABR studies. Figure 12.8 shows the absence of response synchrony from this patient's ears; immediately below those tracings is a set of tracings run from the mother's scalp, done to confirm the functioning of the equipment and to show the mother what normal responses should look like. The child had no residual bone conduction to ABR nor responses to any other potentials recorded, and it was our belief that she was severely hearing-impaired. Subsequent audiological assessment 1 1/2 years later confirmed this diagnostic picture, and we have here an example of a child properly diagnosed as being severely hearing-impaired by age 2 months. The early management led to excellent speech and language development.

Patient 3 was brought to us at age 2 weeks by an adoption agency. His mother was deaf and his father's hearing status was unknown. Before the

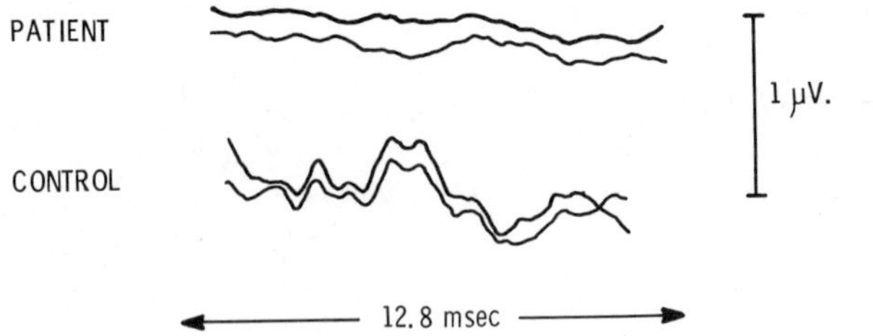

Figure 12.8 Top two traces from a child ultimately shown to be deaf. Bottom two traces are from the child's mother; the mother's data were taken at the time of the child's test to confirm that all systems were working properly.

adoption was made final both the social agency and potential adoptive parents wanted to know whether they were dealing with a child with impaired hearing. Figure 12.9 shows a perfectly normal response for a child of this age and the family adopted the child with the knowledge that at least at the time of adoption the auditory system was functioning normally. Subsequent audiological studies as this child matured confirmed the original diagnosis of normal hearing.

Patient 4 was a normal-hearing adult who complained of lightheadedness and a numbness on one side of his face. His audiological assessment was unremarkable, but a number of objective tests, including ABR, were markedly suspicious. Figure 12.10 shows that despite the normal latency of the first wave in both ears, which implied normal synchrony of the VIII nerve after cochlear stimulation on both sides, a gross dyssynchrony and slowing of central-conduction time was observed in the patient's left ear. This unusually prolonged latency is a common finding in patients with neoplastic processes in and around the VIII nerve and is an example from our files of the kind of patient reports obtained by Coats and Martin[28] and Selters and Brackmann.[66]

Patient 5 is a 23-year-old male who was worked up and studied by David Pillsbury of the North Carolina Baptist Hospital (this case is described with

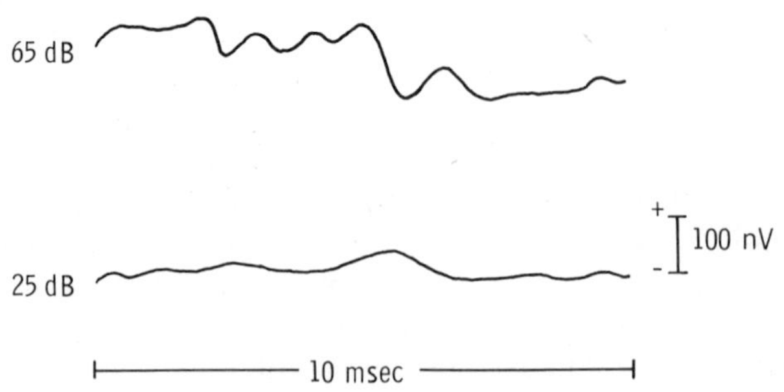

Figure 12.9 ABR from a 2-week-old adoptive child. Latencies and central conduction times in children this age are usually longer than in adults. dB are dB HL.

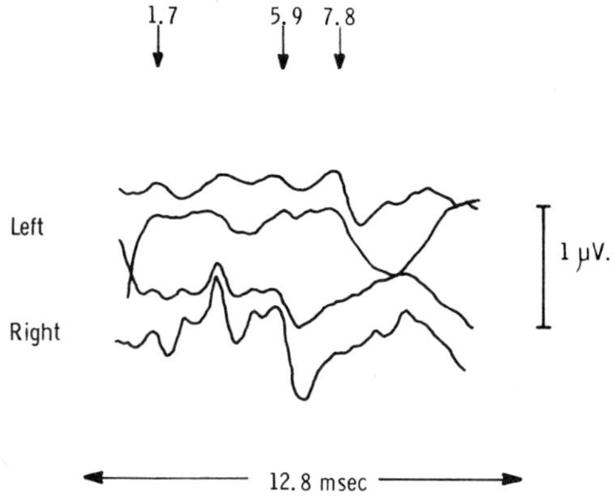

Figure 12.10 ABR in a patient with an acoustic tumor. Duplicate tracings shown for each ear. Numbers above arrows indicate latencies (in milliseconds) for Waves I and V. Wave V from affected ear was 7.8 milliseconds.

his permission and cooperation). The patient had normal pure-tone audiograms, normal auditory discrimination, but complaints of dysarthric-like speech, limb weakness, and facial numbness lasting for about six months. Impedance audiometry (measurement of middle-ear mechanics) showed normal middle-ear function but auditory reflexes were present only by ipsilateral stimulation and not by contralateral stimulation. This unusual condition implicates the crossed fibers from the IV ventricle of the dorsal brain stem. Figure 12.11 shows normal waves I and II but an abnormal morphology of wave III and absent later components. The final diagnosis was pontine glioblastoma. The electrophysiological tests were involved in the location of the lesion and could then be used to monitor the efficacy of radiation therapy.

In summary, electrophysiological results can be obtained on patients to aid audiologists and otolaryngologists in the diagnosis of hearing loss, location of lesions in the auditory system, early detection and diagnosis of neurological impairment, and monitoring for ototoxicity. Safe drug levels can thereby be established when aminoglycosides are used to treat severe systemic infection and/or when severe renal impairment exists in patients given aminoglycosides.

These procedures can also be used as gross physiological indicators of

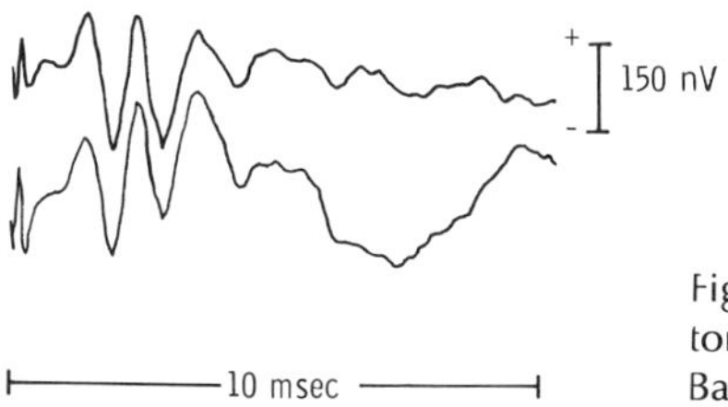

Figure 12.11 ABR in a patient with a pontine glioblastoma (courtesy of David Pillsbury, North Carolina Baptist Hospitals, Winston-Salem, NC).

auditory sensitivity in animals and are recommended to our colleagues in auditory research as powerful indices of peripheral auditory synchrony.

ACKNOWLEDGMENTS

We thank Patti Berlin, Gae Decker, Fred Drake, Michelle Paige, David Pillsbury, and Nancie Roark for their contributions. This work was supported in part by the National Institutes of Health, USPHS Grants No. NS-11647 (Clinical Research Center), NS-07058 (National Research Service Award), and NS-06094 (National Research Service Award). Laboratory facilities were provided, in part, by The Kresge Foundation.

REFERENCES

1. R. A. Dobie and S. Norton, *Electroencephalogr. Clin. Neurophysiol.*, **49,** 303–313 (1980).
2. L. D. Geisler, L. S. Frishkopf, and W. A. Rosenblith, *Science*, **128,** 1210–1211 (1958).
3. E. L. Lowell, C. T. Williams, R. M. Ballinger, and D. P. Alvig, *J. Speech Hear. Res.*, **4,** 105–112 (1961).
4. R. G. Bickford, J. L. Jacobsen, D. Cody, and E. H. Lambert, *Trans. Am. Neurol. Assoc.*, **89,** 56–58 (1964).
5. R. Goldstein and L. Rodman, *J. Speech Hear. Res.*, **12,** 697–705 (1967).
6. D. Jewett, *Physiologist*, **12,** 262 (1969).
7. D. Jewett, *Electroencephalogr. Clin. Neurophysiol.*, **28,** 609–618 (1970).
8. H. Sohmer and M. Feinmesser, *Ann. Otol. Rhinol. Laryngol.*, **76,** 427–435 (1967).
9. G. Moushegian, A. L. Rupert, and R. D. Stillman, *Electroencephalogr. Clin. Neurophysiol.*, **35,** 665–667 (1973).
10. F. G. Worden and J. T. Marsh, *Electroencephalogr. Clin. Neurophysiol.*, **25,** 42–52 (1968).
11. C. M. Huang and J. S. Buchwald, *Electroencephalogr. Clin. Neurophysiol.*, **44,** 177–186 (1978).
12. R. A. Dobie and C. I. Berlin, *Arch. Otolaryngol.*, **105,** 391–398 (1979).
13. D. Jewett and J. Williston, *Brain*, **94,** 681–696 (1971).
14. K. Hecox and R. Galambos, *Arch. Otolaryngol.*, **99,** 30–33 (1974).
15. M. Don, A. R. Allen, and A. Starr, *Ann. Otol. Rhinol. Laryngol.*, **86,** 186–195 (1977).
16. M. L. Scott and S. W. Harkins, *Int. J. Neurosci.*, **8,** 147–152 (1978).
17. K. Kodera, H. Yamane, O. Yamada, and J.-I. Suzuki, *Scand. Audiol.*, **6,** 205–210 (1977a).
18. K. Kodera, H. Yamane, O. Yamada, and J.-I. Suzuki, *Audiology*, **16,** 469–479 (1977b).
19. T. Suzuki and K. Noriuchi, *Scand. Audiol.*, **6,** 123–126 (1977).
20. K. Hecox, N. Squires, and R. Galambos, *J. Acoust. Soc. Am.*, **60,** 1187–1192 (1976).
21. K. Terkildsen, P. Osterhammel, and F. Huist 'n veld, *Scand. Audiol.*, **4,** 167 (1975).
22. M. Amadeo and C. Shagass, *Psychophysiology*, **10,** 244–250 (1973).
23. T. Picton and S. A. Hillyard, *Electroencephalogr. Clin. Neurophysiol.*, **36,** 191–200 (1974).
24. A. Salamy and C. McKean, *Electroencephalogr. Clin. Neurophysiol.*, **40,** 418–426 (1976).

25. J. J. Stockard, J. E. Stockard, and F. W. Sharbrough, *Am. J. EEG Tech.*, **18,** 177–189 (1978).

26. J. J. Stockard, V. S. Rossiter, T. A. Jones, and F. W. Sharbrough, *Electroencephalogr. Clin. Neurophysiol.*, **43,** 550–551 (1977).

27. A. Møller and B. Blegvad, *Scand. Audiol.*, **5,** 115–127 (1976).

28. A. C. Coats and J. L. Martin, *Arch. Otolaryngol.*, **103,** 605–622 (1977).

29. J. Jerger and L. Mauldin, *Arch. Otolaryngol.*, **104,** 456–461 (1978).

30. M. J. Rowe, *Electroencephalogr. Clin. Neurophysiol.*, **44,** 459–470 (1978).

31. K. H. Chiappa, K. J. Gladstone, and R. R. Young, *Arch. Neurol.*, **36,** 81–87 (1979).

32. M. E. Glasscock, C. G. Jackson, A. F. Josef, J. R. E. Dickins, and R. J. Wiet, *Laryngoscope*, **89,** 1021–1034 (1979).

33. A. Starr and J. Achor, *Arch. Neurol.*, **32,** 761–768 (1975).

34. K. Robinson and P. Rudge, *Brain*, **100,** 19–40 (1977).

35. J. J. Stockard, J. E. Stockard, and F. W. Sharbrough, *Mayo Clin. Proc.*, **52,** 761–769 (1977).

36. B. Mokotoff, C. Schulman-Galambos, and R. Galambos, *Arch. Otolaryngol.*, **103,** 38–43 (1977).

37. M. M. Merzenich, M. White, M. C. Vivion, and P. Leak-Jones, *Acta Oto Laryngol.*, **87,** 196–203 (1979).

38. M. Don and J. J. Eggermont, *J. Acoust. Soc. Am.*, **63,** 1084–1092 (1978).

39. M. Don, J. J. Eggermont, and D. E. Brackmann, *Ann. Otol. Rhinol. Laryngol.*, **88**(S57), 1–20 (1979).

40. A. Starr and A. E. Hamilton, *Electroencephalogr. Clin. Neurophysiol.*, **41,** 595–608 (1976).

41. R. D. Stillman, G. Moushegian, and A. L. Rupert, *Audiology*, **15,** 10–22 (1976).

42. C. Suter, E. Glaser, A. Goldberg, and R. Dasheiff, *J. Acoust. Soc. Am. Suppl.*, **60,** 1, S16 (1976).

43. E. M. Glaser, G. M. Suter, R. Dasheiff, and A. Goldberg, *Electroencephalogr. Clin. Neurophysiol.*, **40,** 25–32 (1976).

44. J. T. Marsh, W. S. Brown, and J. C. Smith, *Electroencephalogr. Clin. Neurophysiol.*, **38,** 113–119 (1975).

45. H. Davis and S. K. Hirsh, *Audiology*, **15,** 181–195 (1976).

46. H. Davis, *Ann. Otol. Rhinol. Laryngol.*, **85**(S28), 1–96 (1976).

47. D. M. Daly, R. J. Roeser, and G. Moushegian, *Electroencephalogr. Clin. Neurophysiol.*, **40,** 132–142 (1976).

48. J. Gardi, A. Salamy, and T. Mendelson, *Audiology*, **18,** 494–506 (1979a).

49. O. Yamada, H. Yamane, and K. Kodera, *Electroencephalogr. Clin. Neurophysiol.*, **43,** 362–370 (1977).

50. S. C. Bledsoe, Jr. and G. Moushegian, *Electroencephalogr. Clin. Neurophysiol.*, **48,** 654–663 (1980).

51. J. Gardi and M. Merzenich, *J. Acoust. Soc. Am.*, **65,** 1491–1500 (1979).

52. J. N. Gardi, S. C. Bledsoe, Jr., and C. I. Berlin, FFP tone-on-tone masking studies in cats and guinea pigs, *Abstracts of the Second Midwinter Research Meeting of the Association for Research in Otolaryngology* (*ARO*), St. Petersburg Beach, Florida, January 22–24, 1979b, pp. 8–9.

53. J. Gardi, M. Merzenich, and C. McKean, *Audiology*, **18,** 353–380 (1979c).

54. J. C. Smith, J. T. Marsh, S. Greenberg, and W. S. Brown, *Science*, **201,** 639–641 (1978).

55. J. W. Hall, III, *Science*, **205,** 1297–1299 (1979).

56. M. I. Mendel and R. Goldstein, *J. Speech Hear. Res.*, **12,** 344–350 (1969a).

57. M. I. Mendel and R. Goldstein, *J. Speech Hear. Res.*, **12,** 351–361 (1969b).

58. M. I. Mendel and R. Goldstein, *J. Speech Hear. Res.*, **14,** 829–840 (1971).

59. M. I. Mendel and E. C. Hosick, *Rev. Laryngol. Otol. Rhinol.*, **96,** 178–184 (1975).

60. M. I. Mendel, C. D. Adkinson, and L. A. Harker, *Ann. Otol. Rhinol. Laryngol.*, **86,** 293–299 (1977).

61. G. L. Kupperman and M. I. Mendel, *Audiology*, **13,** 379–390 (1974).

62a. J. N. Gardi and S. C. Bledsoe, Jr., Preliminary observations on the origins of middle latency components of the auditory-evoked response in the cat, International Electric Response Audiometry Study Group, Santa Barbara Conference, August 1979.

62b. P. Lobaugh, D. Parker, A. R. D. Thornton, and C. I. Berlin. *J. Acous. Soc. Am.*, **68** (Suppl. 1), S20 (1980).

63. H. L. Hosford, B. C. Fullerton, and R. A. Levine, *J. Acoust. Soc. Am.*, **65**(S1), S86 (1979).

64. R. A. Dobie and C. I. Berlin, *Ann. Otol. Rhinol. Laryngol.*, **80**(5), Suppl. 60, Part 2, 48–53 (1979).

65. C. I. Berlin, K. F. Wexler, J. J. Jerger, H. H. Halperin, and S. Smith, *Otolaryngology*, **86,** ORL-111–ORL-116 (1978).

66. W. Selters and D. Brackmann, *Arch. Otolaryngol.*, **103,** 181–187 (1977).

INDEX